Glioblastoma, Part I: Surgical Management and Adjuncts

Editor

MICHAEL A. VOGELBAUM

NEUROSURGERY CLINICS OF NORTH AMERICA

www.neurosurgery.theclinics.com

Consulting Editors
DANIEL K. RESNICK
RUSSELL R. LONSER

January 2021 • Volume 32 • Number 1

ELSEVIER

1600 John F. Kennedy Boulevard • Suite 1800 • Philadelphia, Pennsylvania, 19103-2899

http://www.theclinics.com

NEUROSURGERY CLINICS OF NORTH AMERICA Volume 32, Number 1
January 2021 ISSN 1042-3680, ISBN-13: 978-0-323-79094-9

Editor: Stacy Eastman
Developmental Editor: Laura Fisher

Neurosurgery Clinics of North America (ISSN 1042-3680) is published quarterly by Elsevier Inc., 360 Park Avenue South, New York, NY 10010-1710. Months of issue are January, April, July, and October. Business and Editorial Offices: 1600 John F. Kennedy Blvd., Suite 1800, Philadelphia, PA 19103-2899. Customer Service Office: 11830 Westline Industrial Drive, St. Louis, MO 63146. Periodicals postage paid at New York, NY, and additional mailing offices. Subscription prices are $438.00 per year (US individuals), $1,013.00 per year (US institutions), $470.00 per year (Canadian individuals), $1,059.00 per year (Canadian institutions), $545.00 per year (international individuals), $1,059.00 per year (international institutions), $100.00 per year (US students), $255.00 per year (international students), and $100.00 per year (Canadian students). International air speed delivery is included in all *Clinics* subscription prices. All prices are subject to change without notice. **POSTMASTER:** Send address changes to *Neurosurgery Clinics of North America*, Elsevier Periodicals Customer Service, 11830 Westline Industrial Drive, St. Louis, MO 63146. **Customer Service: 1-800-654-2452 (US and Canada). From outside the US and Canada, call: 1-314-453-7041. Fax: 1-314-453-5170. E-mail: JournalsCustomerService-usa@elsevier.com (for print support) and journalsonlinesupport-usa@elsevier.com (for online support).**

Reprints. For copies of 100 or more, of articles in this publication, please contact the Commercial Reprints Department, Elsevier Inc., 360 Park Avenue South, New York, NY 10010-1710. Tel. 212-633-3874; Fax: 212-633-3820; E-mail: reprints@elsevier.com.

Neurosurgery Clinics of North America is covered in *MEDLINE/PubMed (Index Medicus), EMBASE/Excerpta Medica,* and *Current Contents/Clinical Medicine (CC/CM).*

Contributors

CONSULTING EDITORS

DANIEL K. RESNICK, MD, MS
Professor and Vice Chairman, Program
Director, Department of Neurosurgery,
University of Wisconsin-Madison School of
Medicine and Public Health, Madison,
Wisconsin, USA

RUSSELL R. LONSER, MD
Professor and Chair, Department of
Neurological Surgery, The Ohio State
University Wexner Medical Center, Columbus,
Ohio, USA

EDITOR

**MICHAEL A. VOGELBAUM, MD, PhD,
FAANS**
Program Leader of NeuroOncology, Chief of
Neurosurgery, Department of NeuroOncology,
H. Lee Moffitt Cancer Center and Research
Institute, Professor, University of South Tampa
Morsani School of Medicine, Tampa, Florida,
USA

AUTHORS

LORENZO BELLO, MD
Department of Oncology and Hemato-
Oncology, IRCCS Istituto Ortopedico Galeazzi,
U.O. Neurochirurgia Oncologica, Milan, Italy

ANGELA BOHNEN, MD
NeurosurgeryOne, Littleton, Colorado,
USA

ADOMAS BUNEVICIUS, MD, PhD
Department of Neurosurgery, University of
Virginia Health System, Charlottesville,
Virginia, USA

DANIEL P. CAHILL, MD, PhD
Associate Professor, Department of
Neurosurgery, Massachusetts General
Hospital, Harvard Medical School, Boston,
Massachusetts, USA

MANUELA CAROLI, MD
Unit of Neurosurgery, Fondazione IRCCS Ca'
Grande Ospedale Maggiore Policlinico, Milan,
Italy

ANTONELLA CASTELLANO, MD, PhD
Neuroradiology Unit and CERMAC, Vita-Salute
San Raffaele University, IRCCS San Raffaele
Scientific Institute, Milan, Italy

MARCO CONTI NIBALI, MD
Department of Oncology and Hemato-
Oncology, Unit of Neurosurgery, Fondazione
IRCCS Ca' Grande Ospedale Maggiore
Policlinico, Milan, Italy

GAETANO DE BIASE, MD
Department of Neurological Surgery, Mayo
Clinic, Jacksonville, Florida, USA

CHIBAWANYE ENE, MD PhD
Department of Neurosurgery, The Brain Tumor
Center, The University of Texas MD Anderson
Cancer Center, Houston, Texas, USA

DIOGO P. GARCIA, MD
Department of Neurological Surgery, Mayo
Clinic, Jacksonville, Florida, USA

LORENZO G. GAY, MD
Department of Oncology and Hemato-Oncology, IRCCS Istituto Ortopedico Galeazzi, U.O. Neurochirurgia Oncologica, Milan, Italy

ALEXANDRA J. GOLBY, MD
Department of Neurosurgery, Department of Radiology, Brigham and Women's Hospital, Harvard Medical School, Boston, Massachusetts, USA

MATTHEW M. GRABOWSKI, MD
Department of Neurosurgery, Rose Ella Burkhardt Brain Tumor and Neuro-Oncology Center, Cleveland Clinic, Cleveland, Ohio, USA

CONSTANTINOS HADJIPANAYIS, MD, PhD
Department of Neurosurgery, Icahn School of Medicine at Mount Sinai, Mount Sinai Health System, Department of Neurosurgery, Mount Sinai Beth Israel, New York, New York, USA

SARA HARTNETT, MD
Chief Resident, Department of Neurosurgery, USF Morsani School of Medicine, Tampa, Florida, USA

SHAWN L. HERVEY-JUMPER, MD
Department of Neurological Surgery, Helen Diller Family Comprehensive Cancer Center, University of California, San Francisco, San Francisco, California, USA

SEBASTIAN ILLE, MD
Department of Neurosurgery, Technical University of Munich, Germany, School of Medicine, Klinikum rechts der Isar, Munich, Germany

BRITTANY PARKER KERRIGAN, PhD
Department of Neurosurgery, The Brain Tumor Center, The University of Texas MD Anderson Cancer Center, Houston, Texas, USA

SANDRO M. KRIEG, MD, MBA
Department of Neurosurgery, Technical University of Munich, Germany, School of Medicine, Klinikum rechts der Isar, Munich, Germany

DEREK KROLL, DO
Fellow in Neurosurgical Oncology, Department of NeuroOncology, Moffitt Cancer Center, Tampa, Florida, USA

FREDERICK F. LANG, MD
Department of Neurosurgery, The Brain Tumor Center, The University of Texas MD Anderson Cancer Center, Houston, Texas, USA

ANTHONY T. LEE, MD PhD
Department of Neurological Surgery, Helen Diller Family Comprehensive Cancer Center, University of California, San Francisco, San Francisco, California, USA

EGESTA LOPCI, MD, PhD
Unit of Nuclear Medicine, Humanitas Clinical and Research Center - IRCCS, Rozzano, Milan, Italy

ALIREZA M. MOHAMMADI, MD
Associate Professor of Neurosurgery, Department of Neurological Surgery, Cleveland Clinic Lerner College of Medicine at CWRU, Rose Ella Burkhardt Brain Tumor and Neuro-Oncology Center, Cleveland Clinic, Cleveland, Ohio, USA

RAMIN A. MORSHED, MD
Department of Neurological Surgery, Helen Diller Family Comprehensive Cancer Center, University of California, San Francisco, San Francisco, California, USA

MARTINA MUSTROPH, MD, PhD
Department of Neurosurgery, Brigham and Women's Hospital, Harvard Medical School, Boston, Massachusetts, USA

MARCO CONTI NIBALI, MD
Department of Oncology and Hemato-Oncology, IRCCS Istituto Ortopedico Galeazzi, U.O. Neurochirurgia Oncologica, Milan, Italy

THOMAS NOH, MD
Department of Neurosurgery, Brigham and Women's Hospital, Boston, Massachusetts, USA; Hawaii Pacific Health, John A Burns School of Medicine, Honolulu, Hawaii, USA

BALINT OTVOS, MD, PhD
Department of Neurosurgery, Rose Ella Burkhardt Brain Tumor and Neuro-Oncology Center, Cleveland Clinic, Cleveland, Ohio, USA

ALFREDO QUIÑONES-HINOJOSA, MD
Department of Neurological Surgery, Mayo Clinic, Jacksonville, Florida, USA

MARCO RIVA, MD
Department of Medical Biotechnology and
Translational Medicine, Università degli Studi
di Milano, IRCCS Istituto Ortopedico Galeazzi,
U.O. Neurochirurgia Oncologica, Milan, Italy'
Grande Ospedale Maggiore Policlinico, Milan,
Italy

MARCO ROSSI, MD
Department of Oncology and Hemato-
Oncology, IRCCS Istituto Ortopedico Galeazzi,
U.O. Neurochirurgia Oncologica, Milan, Italy

ALEXANDER J. SCHUPPER, MD
Department of Neurosurgery, Icahn School of
Medicine at Mount Sinai, Mount Sinai Health
System, New York, New York, USA

TOMMASO SCIORTINO, MD
Department of Oncology and Hemato-
Oncology, IRCCS Istituto Ortopedico Galeazzi,
U.O. Neurochirurgia Oncologica, Milan, Italy

JASON P. SHEEHAN, MD, PhD
Department of Neurosurgery, University of
Virginia Health System, Charlottesville,
Virginia, USA

ADAM M. SONABEND, MD
Assistant Professor and Attending
Neurosurgeon, Department of Neurological
Surgery, Lou and Jean Malnati Brain Tumor
Institute, Robert H. Lurie Comprehensive
Cancer Center, Northwestern University,
Chicago, Illinois, USA

VISISH M. SRINIVASAN, MD
Department of Neurosurgery, The University of
Texas MD Anderson Cancer Center,
Department of Neurosurgery, Baylor College of
Medicine, Houston, Texas, USA

ROGER STUPP, MD
Paul C. Bucy Professor of Neurological
Surgery, Departments of Neurological Surgery,
Neurology, and Medicine, Division of
Hematology and Oncology, Lou and Jean
Malnati Brain Tumor Institute, Robert H. Lurie
Comprehensive Cancer Center, Northwestern
University, Chicago, Illinois, USA

**MICHAEL A. VOGELBAUM, MD, PhD,
FAANS**
Program Leader of NeuroOncology, Chief of
Neurosurgery, Department of NeuroOncology,
H. Lee Moffitt Cancer Center and Research
Institute, Professor, University of South Tampa
Morsani School of Medicine, Tampa, Florida,
USA

JEFFREY S. WEINBERG, MD, FAANS, FACS
Professor and Deputy Chair, Department of
Neurosurgery, The University of Texas MD
Anderson Cancer Center, Houston, Texas,
USA

JACOB S. YOUNG, MD
Department of Neurological Surgery, Helen
Diller Family Comprehensive Cancer Center,
University of California San Francisco, San
Francisco, California, USA

MARK W. YOUNGBLOOD, MD, PhD
Resident Physician, Department of
Neurological Surgery, Northwestern University,
Northwestern Medicine, Chicago, Illinois, USA

RASHEED ZAKARIA, PhD, FRCS
Fellow, Department of Neurosurgery, The
University of Texas MD Anderson Cancer
Center, Houston, Texas, USA

Contents

The clinical presentation of glioblastomas is varied, and definitive diagnosis requires
pathologic examination and study of the tissue. Management of glioblastomas includes surgery and adjuvant chemotherapy and radiotherapy, with surgery playing
an important role in the prognosis of these patients. Awake craniotomy plays a
crucial role in tumors in or adjacent to eloquent areas, allowing surgeons to maximize resection, while minimizing iatrogenic deficits. However, the prognosis remains
dismal. This article presents the perioperative management of patients with glioblastoma including tools and surgical adjuncts to maximize extent of resection and minimize poor outcomes.

Whenever possible, maximal safe resection is the first intervention for management
of glioblastoma. Resection offers tissue for diagnosis, decompression of the brain,
cytoreduction, and has been associated with prolonged survival in numerous retrospective studies. In this review, we provide a critical overview of the literature asso-
ciating glioblastoma resection with survival. We discuss techniques that enhance
extent of resection, and the role of clinical and surgeon-variables. At last, we analyze
the covariates and confounders that might influence the relationship between extent
of resection and survival for glioblastoma, as these might ultimately also influence
outcomes and other therapeutic interventions tested in trials.

The work of modern neurosurgical glioma practice combines securing accurate diagnoses, under the 2016 revised World Health Organization (WHO) Classification of
Tumors of the Central Nervous System, with an aggressive and safe surgical pursuit
of tumor removal. The evidence base that drives clinical decision-making has undergone a critical reevaluation with the incorporation of molecular classifiers into the updated WHO diagnoses including the 3 most common diffuse gliomas in adults:
glioblastoma IDH wild-type, astrocytoma IDH mutant, and oligodendroglioma IDH
mutant 1p/19q codeleted. The studies that form the foundation of modern practice,
and the areas for future inquiry are reviewed.

> Conventional magnetic resonance imaging (cMRI) has an established role as a crucial disease parameter in the multidisciplinary management of glioblastoma, guiding diagnosis, treatment planning, assessment, and follow-up. Yet, cMRI cannot provide adequate information regarding tissue heterogeneity and the infiltrative extent beyond the contrast enhancement. Advanced magnetic resonance imaging and PET and newer analytical methods are transforming images into data (radiomics) and providing noninvasive biomarkers of molecular features (radiogenomics), conveying enhanced information for improving decision making in surgery. This review analyzes the shift from image guidance to information guidance that is relevant for the surgical treatment of glioblastoma.

> This article discusses intraoperative imaging techniques used during high-grade glioma surgery. Gliomas can be difficult to differentiate from surrounding tissue during surgery. Intraoperative imaging helps to alleviate problems encountered during glioma surgery, such as brain shift and residual tumor. There are a variety of modalities available all of which aim to give the surgeon more information, address brain shift, identify residual tumor, and increase the extent of surgical resection. The article starts with a brief introduction followed by a review of the latest advances in intraoperative ultrasound, intraoperative MRI, and intraoperative computed tomography.

 Video content accompanies this article at http://www.neurosurgery.theclinics.com.

> Fluorescence-guided surgery provides surgeons with improved visualization of tumor tissue in the operating room to allow for maximal safe resection of brain tumors. Multiple fluorescent agents have been studied for fluorescence-guided surgery. Both nontargeted and targeted fluorescent agents are currently being used for glioblastoma multiforme visualization and resection. Fluorescence detection in the visible light or near infrared spectrum is possible. Visualization device advancements have permitted greater detection of fluorescence down to the cellular level, which may provide even greater ability for the neurosurgeon to resect tumors.

> Although intraoperative mapping of brain areas was shown to promote greater extent of resection and reduce functional deficits, this was shown only recently for some noninvasive techniques. Yet, proper surgical planning, indication, and patient consultation require reliable noninvasive techniques. Because functional magnetic resonance imaging, tractography, and neurophysiologic methods like navigated transcranial magnetic stimulation and magnetoencephalography allow identifying eloquent areas prior to resective surgery and tailor the surgical approach, this article provides an overview on the individual strengths and limitations of each modality.

Intraoperative functional mapping of tumor and peri-tumor tissue is a well-established technique for avoiding permanent neurologic deficits and maximizing extent of resection. Motor, language, and other cognitive domains may be assessed with intraoperative tasks. This article describes techniques used for motor and language mapping including awake mapping considerations in addition to less traditional intraoperative testing paradigms for cognition. It also discusses complications associated with mapping and insights into complication avoidance.

Although surgical resection of the solid tumor component of glioblastoma has been shown to provide a survival advantage, it will never be a curative procedure. Yet, systemically applied adjuvants (radiation therapy and chemotherapy) also are not curative and their options are limited by the inability of most agents to cross the blood–brain barrier. Direct delivery of adjuvant therapies during a surgical procedure potentially provides an approach to bypass the blood–brain barrier and effectively treat residual tumor cells. This article summarizes the approaches and therapeutics that have been evaluated to date, and challenges that remain to be overcome.

Despite significant improvement in understanding of molecular underpinnings driving glioblastoma, there is minimal improvement in overall survival of patients. This poor outcome is caused in part by traditional designs of early phase clinical trials, which focus on clinical assessments of drug toxicity and response. Window of opportunity trials overcome this shortcoming by assessing drug-induced on-target molecular alterations in post-treatment human tumor specimens. This article provides an overview of window of opportunity trials, including novel designs for incorporating biologic end points into early stage trials in context of brain tumors, and examples of successfully executed window of opportunity trials for glioblastoma.

The previous decade has seen an expansion in the use of laser interstitial thermal therapy (LITT) for a variety of pathologies. LITT has been used to treat both newly diagnosed and recurrent glioblastoma (GBM), especially in deep-seated, difficult-to-access lesions where open resection is otherwise infeasible or in patients who would not tolerate craniotomy. This review aims to describe the current state of the technology and operative technique, as well as summarize the outcomes data and future research regarding LITT as a treatment of GBM.

Glioblastoma (GBM) is infiltrative neoplasm with limited treatment options and poor overall survival. Stereotactic radiosurgery (SRS) allows spatially precise and conformal delivery of high doses of radiation. Salvage SRS for locally recurrent GBM was shown to improve patient survival and have more favorable safety profile than repeated surgical resection. Boost SRS after fractionated radiation therapy is sometimes attempted; however, Radiation Therapy Oncology Group 93–05 randomized clinical trial did not demonstrate benefits of upfront SRS that was administered before fractionated radiation. Administration of bevacizumab with SRS is associated with improved survival and can allow SRS dose escalation.

Reoperation for glioma is increasingly common but there is neither firm agreement on the indications nor unequivocally proven benefit from clinical trials. Patient and tumor factors should be considered when offering reoperation and a clear surgical goal set. Reoperation is challenging because of placement of previous incisions, wound devascularization by preceding radiotherapy and/or chemotherapy, chronic steroid use, the need for further adjuvant therapy, and adherent and defective dura. This article reviews indications, challenges, and recommendations for repeat surgery in the patient with glioma.

The management of glioblastoma in the elderly population represents a field of growing interest owing a longer life expectancy. In this age group, more than in the young adult, biological age is much more important than chronologic one. The date of birth should not exclude a priori access of treatments. Maximal safe resection is proved to be the first option when performance status and general health is good. Adjuvant therapy and decision about management of recurrence should be choose in a multidisciplinary group according to performance of the patients and O^6-methylguanine-DNA methyl-transferase methylation.

NEUROSURGERY CLINICS OF NORTH AMERICA

SERIES OF RELATED INTEREST

Neurologic Clinics
https://www.neurologic.theclinics.com/
Neuroimaging Clinics
https://www.neuroimaging.theclinics.com/

THE CLINICS ARE AVAILABLE ONLINE!
Access your subscription at:
www.theclinics.com

Preface

Surgical Management of Glioblastoma: More Than Just Diagnosis and Decompression

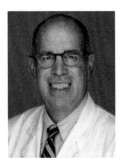

Michael A. Vogelbaum, MD, PhD, FAANS
Editor

Despite recent advances in our understanding of the biology of glioblastoma (GBM) and the completion of multiple, multiple clinical trials aimed at using this knowledge to evaluate the effectiveness of novel targeted therapies, immunotherapies, gene therapies, and locoregional therapies, GBM remains an unrelentingly fatal form of cancer. There is an understandable sense of nihilism and fatalism that drives the approach of many clinicians to consider GBM (and gliomas in general) to fall into the realm of general neurosurgical practice, with the goals of surgery limited to diagnosis and decompression followed by transfer of care to radiation and medical oncologists for all subsequent care. Yet, such an approach discounts developments over the past decade that have helped us understand how best to use specialized neurosurgical approaches to provide more than a diagnosis, but also to potentially provide survival benefit in the operating room (OR). Furthermore, there are ways that neurosurgeons can use the OR to advance our ability to care for GBM patients. We can explore the basis for failure of promising systemically administered agents, which may help to drive the design of agents that are more likely to achieve therapeutics concentrations in both contrast-enhancing and non-centrations in both contrast-enhancing and non-enhancing parts of GBM, and we can provide direct approaches to the central nervous system for the more effective delivery of adjuvant treatments.

This issue of *Neurosurgery Clinics of North America* focuses on how appropriately trained and equipped neurosurgical oncologists can derive the most benefit from their surgical intervention on patients with GBM. First, there is a focus on the tools that we currently have to maximize the extent of tumor resection while minimizing the neurologic morbidity associated with surgery (the so-called maximally safe resection). This is followed by a discussion of additional value that neurosurgical oncologists can provide in the OR, ranging from surgically delivered adjuvants to engaging in "window of opportunity" clinical trials that permit us to obtain tissue for laboratory analysis in the setting of a systemically applied treatment. Next, there are several articles that critically examine the use of other therapeutic technologies and the value that they may, or may not, bring to extending patient survival. Finally, we evaluate special circumstances in which a carefully considered plan of care, that may involve surgery, should be developed in coordination with a multidisciplinary neurooncology team.

Neurosurg Clin N Am 32 (2021) xiii–xiv
https://doi.org/10.1016/j.nec.2020.09.007
1042-3680/21/© 2020 Published by Elsevier Inc.

neurosurgery.theclinics.com

Surgical resection alone will never be the cure for GBM. It is hoped that readers will recognize that the specific skills and knowledge developed and put into practice by specialized neurosurgical oncologists can bring valuable survival benefit to patients, and that they also provide a path to overcoming the barriers to finding more effective cures for our patients. Specific ways in which we are evaluating novel therapeutic approaches will be covered in the second part (edited by Dr Linda Liau) of this 2-part series on Glioblastoma.

I would like to thank Drs Russ Lonser and Dan Resnick for inviting me to be Guest Editor of this issue of *Neurosurgery Clinics of North America*, my colleagues, who have contributed their valuable time and effort to bring you the benefits of their experience and knowledge, and Laura Fisher, who had the unenviable job of making sure that everything was completed on time!

Michael A. Vogelbaum, MD, PhD, FAANS
H. Lee Moffitt Cancer Center and Research Institute
12902 Magnolia Drive
Tampa, FL 33612, USA

University of South Florida Morsani School of Medicine
Tampa, FL 33612, USA

E-mail address:
michael.vogelbaum@moffitt.org

Perioperative Management of Patients with Glioblastoma

Gaetano De Biase, MD[a], Diogo P. Garcia, MD[a], Angela Bohnen, MD[b], Alfredo Quiñones-Hinojosa, MD[a],*

KEYWORDS

- Glioblastoma • Awake brain surgery • Temozolamide

KEY POINTS

- The aim of glioma surgery is to maximize the extent of the resection while minimizing the risk of neurologic deficit.
- Interindividual differences in function location exist. Awake brain mapping provides a personalized, safe approach to lesion resection.
- Neoadjuvant modalities for brain mapping include: positron emission tomography scan, DTI, and functional MRI.
- Multidisciplinary teams are crucial to produce a successful outcome both intraoperatively and post-operatively.

INTRODUCTION

The first credible report of intracranial surgery for an intracranial glioma appears to have been that of Bennet and Godlee in 1884,[1] with the patient succumbing to cerebral herniation and meningitis 4 weeks after surgery. For most of the first half of the twentieth century, because of the high rate of surgical morbidity and mortality, surgical resection of glioblastomas was still perceived as controversial, with Bender and Elizan in 1962 recommending the use of radiation exclusively for all malignant tumors of the brain.[2]

During the past decades, accumulating evidence has consistently demonstrated improvement in overall survival and progression-free survival after surgical treatment of intracranial gliomas. Multiple factors contribute to this advancement, including the introduction of standard adjuvant therapeutic protocols[3] and better understanding of tumor biology[4]; however, aggressive surgical resection has proven to be a main component of treatment success.

Early studies have shown that at least 98% removal of the gadolinium-enhanced portion of glioblastoma was associated with significant survival benefit; however, more recent volumetric studies from different institutions/groups have demonstrated that statistically significant prognostic advantage begins at a level of volumetric resection of 70% to 78% and steadily increases as it approaches 100%.[5–7] Chaichana[5] and colleagues were the first to show that not only the extent of resection is significantly associated with survival and recurrence benefits, but also

Funding: A. Quiñones-Hinojosa was supported by the Mayo Clinic Professorship and a Clinician Investigator award, and Florida State Department of Health Research Grant, and the Mayo Clinic Graduate School, as well as the National Institutes of Health (R43CA221490, R01CA200399, R01CA195503, and R01CA216855).
[a] Department of Neurological Surgery, Mayo Clinic, Jacksonville, FL, USA; [b] NeurosurgeryOne, Littleton, CO, USA
* Corresponding author. Brain Tumor Stem Cell Laboratory, Department of Neurologic Surgery, Mayo Clinic, Florida, 4500 San Pablo Road South, Jacksonville, FL 32224.
E-mail address: quinones@mayo.edu

Neurosurg Clin N Am 32 (2021) 1–8
https://doi.org/10.1016/j.nec.2020.09.005
1042-3680/21/

residual tumor volume, with a threshold of 5 cm³. Overall, these results emphasize the importance of maximal resection of the tumor. Aggressive surgery, however, may be associated with risk of neurologic deterioration, especially if the neoplasm is located within, or in close proximity to, eloquent structures.[8,9]

Because of the infiltrative nature of glioblastoma (GBM), it is not always possible to achieve gross total resection while preserving neurologic function. Obtaining maximal resection with the least amount of morbidity is thus considered the goal of surgery.

This article illustrates clinical, radiographic, and pathologic features of GBM, and delves into the perioperative medical and surgical management of patients with GBM.

DISCUSSION
Clinical Presentation of Patients with Glioblastomas

The clinical presentation of GBM is varied and depends on the function of the involved area of the brain, with focal signs such as hemiparesis, sensory loss, and visual field disturbances being common. Headaches are present in about half of patients newly diagnosed, usually assuming a nonspecific pattern,[10] and frequently being associated with mass effect, either directly or indirectly via the obstruction of the ventricular system. Cognitive and personality changes may occur and are frequently mistaken for psychiatric disorders or dementia, particularly in older patients. Gait imbalance and incontinence might be present in larger tumors with significant mass effect. Language difficulties might be mistaken for confusion or delirium.[11]

Age at diagnosis and Karnofsky Performance Status (KPS) are important and established prognostic factors in high-grade glioma patients.[12,13] Seizures occur in up to 40% of all newly diagnosed GBMs and are usually focal at onset.[14] Importantly, the role of antiseizure medication in patients without seizures is not clearly established in GBMs.

In the setting of a clinical suspicion of a brain tumor, brain MRI with and without contrast is the modality of choice for presumptive diagnosis, with computed tomography (CT) being reserved for patients unable to undergo MRI.[15] Multiple non-neoplastic syndromes are similar on neuroimaging, including abscess, subacute stroke, and multiple sclerosis, with the patient's history being crucial in the deliberation before surgery.[16] Additional testing, such as lumbar puncture or cerebral angiogram for diagnostic purposes, is rarely needed.[11]

Imaging Features of Patients with Glioblastomas

Imaging is a crucial component in the diagnosis, surgical planning, and follow-up of patients with GBMs. Multiple imaging modalities can be used in its characterization, although MRI plays a central role, allowing the integration of conventional anatomic images with physiologic and metabolic information obtained at the same examination.

On CT, the lesion is usually hypointense, when compared with adjacent brain tissue. On MRI, the lesions are usually hypointense on T1-weighted images, hyperintense on T2-weighted images and on proton density-weighted images.[17] T2-weighted fluid-attenuated inversion recovery (FLAIR) sequence shows the lesion with high intensity compared with normal gray and white matter (**Fig. 1**).[18–20]

The administration of intravenous contrast agents allows the study of regions where there is disruption of the blood-brain barrier, allowing the leakage of the contrast agent. On contrast-enhanced T1-weighted images, the lesions are heterogenous in appearance, with abnormal contrast enhancement being observed in most GBMs, presumably representing macroscopic tumor. Importantly, the aforementioned characteristics are not enough for a diagnosis, with some low-grade gliomas exhibiting contrast enhancement and some glioblastomas not showing any enhancement.[17]

Magnetic resonance spectroscopic imaging (MRISI) allows the characterization of the cellular metabolism. Using a clinical field strength of 1.5 T with echo times of 144 to 280 milliseconds, the major peaks observed in normal brain tissue correspond to choline-containing compounds (Cho), creatine (Cr), and N-acetylaspartate (NAA). Using shorter echo times – 20 to 30 milliseconds – allows the observation of peaks corresponding to Myo-inositol, glutamine, and glutamate in normal brain tissue.[21,22] However, tumors are characterized by a significant reduction in the signal intensity of NAA,[23–26] reportedly because of a low density of neuronal cells, and increased Cho, compared with normal brain tissue.[27,28]

Advanced imaging modalities, including diffusion tensor imaging (DTI), functional MRI (fMRI), and perfusion weighted imaging (PWI) play an increasingly more important role in the management of GBMs. DTI and fMRI allow a noninvasive method of brain mapping that, despite being inferior to the current gold standard, intraoperative mapping, can be of extraordinary value in planning surgical approaches.[29]

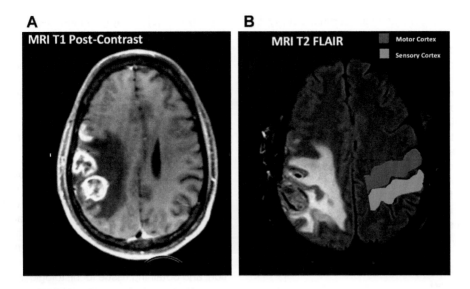

Fig. 1. MRI of a 55-year-old patient who presented with left-sided weakness and difficulty articulating speech, demonstrating a lesion located in eloquent cortex of the right cerebral hemisphere. (*A*) Axial T1-weighted image with contrast reveals a heterogeneously enhancing mass in the right ventral sensorimotor region. (*B*) Axial T2-FLAIR image identifies extensive surrounding vasogenic edema involving extensive subcortical white matter tracts. Given the location of the lesion, the patient underwent an awake craniotomy with brain mapping and surgical resection of the lesion.

DTI, developed from diffusion-weighed imaging (DWI), allows the surgeon to understand the anatomy of white matter tracts, including the corticospinal tracts and arcuate fasciculus, providing fundamental information to protect eloquent white matter tracts, while seeking maximal resection of the lesion (**Fig. 2**A, B).[30] However, tumors can change the architecture of white matter tracts, contributing to a potential underestimation of the presence of functional white matter tracts in the presence of tumor.[31] Furthermore, brain shifting during the course of surgery from positioning, anesthesia, retractions, and cerebrospinal fluid (CSF) leak can limit the accuracy of the anatomic information conveyed by DTI.[32]

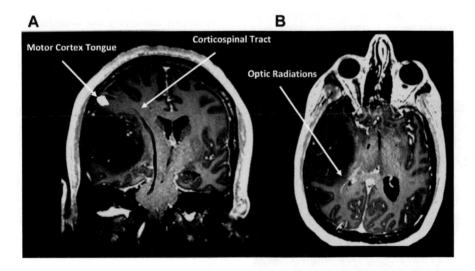

Fig. 2. (*A*) Coronal tractography view demonstrating the corticospinal tract and the motor tongue activation in yellow; (*B*) Axial tractography reveals the optic radiations traversing near the deep margin of the tumor.

fMRI indirectly measures neuronal activity by evaluating areas of increased blood flow through a pulse sequence that takes into account the ratio of oxyhemoglobin to deoxyhemoglobin as a contrast agent, also known as blood oxygen level-dependent (BOLD) imaging.[33] Functional motor mapping has a high correlation with direct cortical stimulation, while language mapping is less robust.[34–36] Nevertheless, it has become the study of first resort in establishing the patient's language dominance in preoperative surgical planning. Although fMRI cannot pinpoint which area is needed for a specific function, it can guide the surgical intraoperative mapping, potentially improving surgical efficiency (**Fig. 3**).[29]

Pathologic Diagnosis of Patients with Glioblastomas

Once tissue is obtained, pathologic diagnosis is usually made through formalin-fixed, paraffin-embedded tissue, with the tumor assuming a characteristically infiltrative aspect, with marked pleomorphism, brisk mitotic activity, microvascular proliferation, and necrosis, which can be geographic or pseudopalisading. Although the cellular morphology is predominantly astrocytic, in some cases a subset of tumor cells displays oligodendroglial or primitive neuroectodermal features. In these cases, molecular analysis can help clarify the diagnosis.[37]

Isocitrate dehydrogenases (IDH) are enzymes that catalyze the oxidative decarboxylation of isocitrate to α-ketoglutarate. IDH 1 and 2 mutations, which can be detected in the most cases by using the IDH-R132H antibody, and DNA sequencing in antibody-negative cases, are important prognosis factors, whereby mutant GBMs are associated with a significantly better prognosis than the wild-type variant.

MGMT (O[6]-methylguanine-DNA methyltransferase) is a DNA repair enzyme that rescues tumor cells from alkylating agent-induced damage. Epigenetic silencing of the MGMT gene by promoter methylation is an independent favorable prognostic factor and a predictor of responsiveness to alkylating chemotherapy.

Surgical and Medical Management of Patients with Glioblastomas

Patients with suspected GBM should be considered for surgical resection and referred, whenever possible, to tertiary care facilities with optimized surgical tools such as advanced intraoperative monitoring, awake mapping, and functional and intraoperative MRI. The goals of surgery include relieving mass effect, accomplishing cytoreduction, and obtaining tissue for histologic and molecular characterization. In inoperable tumors, stereotactic biopsy might be performed for histologic diagnosis.

Corticosteroids in Glioblastoma Patients

Corticosteroids have been widely used in GBM patients to reduce peritumoral edema and increased intracranial pressure and help with the associated neurologic deficits. Corticosteroids are also widely used during radiation therapy to help with the associated edema. The vasogenic edema surrounding brain tumors contributes to the morbidity experienced by patients. Edema results from the flow of fluid into the extracellular space of the brain through an altered blood–brain barrier (BBB). In high-grade gliomas, the BBB is typically disrupted, allowing passage of fluid into the extracellular space.[38] The exact mechanism underlying the antiedema effects of corticosteroids is not known, although it is widely believed that they suppress inflammation and decreases vasogenic edema through restoration of BBB integrity.

Dexamethasone is commonly the drug of choice in neuro-oncology because of its long half-life and low mineralocorticoid activity. Despite its common use, there have only been a few prospective clinical trials to determine the optimal dose of dexamethasone in brain cancer patients. Dexamethasone is most commonly used in a dose range of 2 to 16 mg daily (divided dosing of 2 or more times daily) depending on symptom severity. In emergent situations, higher doses of dexamethasone may be used, and mannitol may also be used.

Steroids are associated with a large number of potential adverse effects. Severity of adverse effects correlates with the daily dose and duration

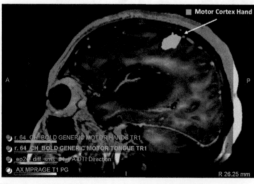

Fig. 3. Sagittal functional MRI highlighting cortical motor cortex hand activation (*bright green*).

of steroid treatment, with most complications resolving after cessation of steroid use. Systemic adverse effects include a cushingoid appearance, truncal obesity, hirsutism, acne, impaired wound healing, easy bruising, immunosuppression, hypertension, glucose intolerance, increased appetite, gastrointestinal bleeding, osteoporosis, cataracts, and glaucoma.

SEIZURES IN GLIOBLASTOMA PATIENTS

Seizures are a well-recognized symptom of primary brain tumors, regardless of tumor type or location, and they can occur at any point during the disease course. Seizures often herald the diagnosis or progression but can also occur in patients when there is no evidence of tumor growth. Although the underlying pathophysiology is not clearly understood, seizures may be provoked by a combination of factors including the impact of the tumor on peritumoral cortex, brain edema, increased intracranial pressure, and metabolic derangements. In GBM patients, the incidence of seizures has been reported to be between 30% and 62%, with two-thirds of seizures occurring at presentation.[39,40] Brain tumor-related seizures may be focal seizures with or without altered awareness, generalized tonic-clonic, or focal seizures with secondary generalization. Postoperative seizure control is correlated directly with the extend of resection.[39] The evidence to support prophylactic perioperative antiepileptic drugs in GBM patients is limited, and no clear recommendations are currently available.

Levetiracetam is the most commonly used drug in brain tumor patients because of its lack of drug-drug interactions (because of fact that it does not induce the cytochrome P450) and excellent tolerability. It has a rapid onset of action, does not require blood-level monitoring, and is effective in treating focal and generalized seizures.

REHABILITATION

The physical and psychosocial capacities of glioma patients are frequently impaired, resulting in a diminished capacity to cope. Importantly, patients often emerge from surgery with significant functional deficits, with inpatient rehabilitation to restore function and symptom control being often necessary.[41]

The rehabilitation team conventionally includes the physiatrist, rehabilitation nurse, physical and occupational therapist, respiratory therapist, speech pathologist, rehabilitation psychologist, and social worker or case manager. Rehabilitation focuses on restoring or supporting function in an effort to increase the quality of life of the patient and re-establish as much as possible a normal living routine.

Mobility strategies will include gait training, fall prevention, strengthening or reconditioning, and compensatory approaches for visual or other perceptual deficits. Deficits in cognition, speech, language, and swallowing should be addressed. Further, skin integrity, nutrition, and bowel or bladder function should also be addressed.

There is ample evidence supporting the impact of comprehensive inpatient rehabilitation programs in the functional capacity of GBM patients,[41–47] even when corrected for age, extent of resection, or the administration of radiotherapy during inpatient rehabilitation.[48]

Symptomatic corticosteroid myopathy is particularly common in patients receiving dexamethasone for more than 2 weeks, occurring in approximately 10% of brain tumor patients, with an onset between weeks 9 and 12.[49] Because of its unspecific findings on electrodiagnostic and laboratory testing, it is often difficult to distinguish from other causes of weakness. However, it is an important entity to recognize, given its potential impact on the monitoring of the functional recovery of patients undergoing rehabilitation.

ADJUVANT THERAPIES

After surgery, adjuvant radio and chemotherapy should be considered in all patients. Radiotherapy is usually administered in an intensity-modulated fashion with a typical dose of 60 Gy divided in 30 fractions. The use of this regimen is supported by a phase 3 randomized clinical trial[3] that found a substantial increase in median survival when compared with radiotherapy alone. Patients with promoter methylation of the DNA repair enzyme MGMT are more likely to benefit from the addition of temozolomide to radiotherapy.[50] Intraoperative ^{125}I seed implantation for brachytherapy has been showing promising results for patients with recurrent GBM.[51] The use of BCNU-impregnated biodegradable polymer wafers has been recommended by some authors in recurrent glioblastoma as an adjunct to cytoreductive surgery. In a double blinded, randomized prospective multicenter trial, Brem and colleagues[52] reported a 64% overall survival rate at 6 months following wafer implantation compared with 44% in patients receiving placebo polymer ($P=.002$). Tumor treating fields are a noninvasive antimitotic therapy that delivers alternating electric fields via the Optune system.[53] A Phase III trial in newly diagnosed GBM showed significantly improved progression-free, overall, and long-term survival when Optune was used together with maintenance TMZ compared with TMZ alone. Patients with a compliance of wearing the device over 90% of the time had a median overall survival of 24.9 months and a 5-year survival rate of 29.3%.[54]

SUMMARY

In GBM, statistically significant prognostic advantage begins at a level of volumetric resection of 70% to 78% and steadily increases as it approaches 100%. Because of its infiltrative nature, it is not always possible to achieve gross total resection while preserving neurologic function. Obtaining maximal resection with the least amount of morbidity is the goal of surgery. Several strategies can be used to achieve this goal, including IMRI, DTI, 5-ALA, and performing the surgery with the patient awake and continuous mapping. Given the complexity of the care needed for the perioperative management of patients with GBM, a multidisciplinary team is needed.[55]

CLINICS CARE POINTS

- The aim of glioma surgery is to maximize the extent of the resection, while minimizing the risk of neurologic deficit. Interindividual differences in function location exist. Awake brain mapping provides a personalized, safe approach to lesion resection.
- Corticosteroids are widely used in GBM patients to reduce peritumoral edema and increased intracranial pressure and help with the associated neurologic deficits. In GBM patients, the incidence of seizures has been reported to be between 30% and 62%, with two-thirds of seizures occurring at presentation.
- The evidence to support prophylactic perioperative antiepileptic drugs in GBM patients is limited, and no clear recommendations are currently available. Multidisciplinary teams are crucial to produce a successful outcome intraoperatively and postoperatively.

DISCLOSURE

The authors have nothing to disclose.

REFERENCES

1. Selby R. The surgical treatment of cerebral glioblastoma multiforme: an historical review. J Neurooncol 1994;18(3):175–82.
2. Bender MB, Elizan T. The non-surgical management of brain tumor. Trans Am Neurol Assoc 1962;87: 20–4.
3. Stupp R, Hegi ME, Mason WP, et al. Effects of radiotherapy with concomitant and adjuvant temozolomide versus radiotherapy alone on survival in glioblastoma in a randomised phase III study: 5-year analysis of the EORTC-NCIC trial. Lancet Oncol 2009;10(5):459–66.
4. Sabha N, Knobbe CB, Maganti M, et al. Analysis of IDH mutation, 1p/19q deletion, and PTEN loss delineates prognosis in clinical low-grade diffuse gliomas. Neuro Oncol 2014;16(7):914–23.
5. Chaichana KL, Jusue-Torres I, Navarro-Ramirez R, et al. Establishing percent resection and residual volume thresholds affecting survival and recurrence for patients with newly diagnosed intracranial glioblastoma. Neuro Oncol 2014;16(1): 113–22.
6. Lacroix M, Abi-Said D, Fourney DR, et al. A multivariate analysis of 416 patients with glioblastoma multiforme: prognosis, extent of resection, and survival. J Neurosurg 2001;95(2):190–8.
7. Sanai N, Polley MY, McDermott MW, et al. An extent of resection threshold for newly diagnosed glioblastomas. J Neurosurg 2011;115(1):3–8.
8. McGirt MJ, Mukherjee D, Chaichana KL, et al. Association of surgically acquired motor and language deficits on overall survival after resection of glioblastoma multiforme. Neurosurgery 2009;65(3):463–9 [discussion: 469–70].
9. Rahman M, Abbatematteo J, De Leo EK, et al. The effects of new or worsened postoperative neurological deficits on survival of patients with glioblastoma. J Neurosurg 2017;127(1):123–31.
10. Forsyth PA, Posner JB. Headaches in patients with brain tumors: a study of 111 patients. Neurology 1993;43(9):1678–83.
11. Omuro A, DeAngelis LM. Glioblastoma and other malignant gliomas: a clinical review. JAMA 2013; 310(17):1842–50.
12. Kreth FW, Warnke PC, Scheremet R, et al. Surgical resection and radiation therapy versus biopsy and radiation therapy in the treatment of glioblastoma multiforme. J Neurosurg 1993;78(5):762–6.
13. Laws ER, Parney IF, Huang W, et al. Survival following surgery and prognostic factors for recently diagnosed malignant glioma: data from the glioma outcomes project. J Neurosurg 2003; 99(3):467–73.
14. Glantz MJ, Cole BF, Forsyth PA, et al. Practice parameter: anticonvulsant prophylaxis in patients with newly diagnosed brain tumors. Report of the quality standards subcommittee of the American academy of neurology. Neurology 2000;54(10): 1886–93.
15. Bradley WG Jr, Waluch V, Yadley RA, et al. Comparison of CT and MR in 400 patients with suspected disease of the brain and cervical spinal cord. Radiology 1984;152(3):695–702.

16. Omuro AM, Leite CC, Mokhtari K, et al. Pitfalls in the diagnosis of brain tumours. Lancet Neurol 2006; 5(11):937–48.

17. Nelson SJ, Cha S. Imaging glioblastoma multiforme. Cancer J 2003;9(2):134–45.

18. Rydberg JN, Hammond CA, Grimm RC, et al. Initial clinical experience in MR imaging of the brain with a fast fluid-attenuated inversion-recovery pulse sequence. Radiology 1994;193(1):173–80.

19. De Coene B, Hajnal JV, Gatehouse P, et al. MR of the brain using fluid-attenuated inversion recovery (FLAIR) pulse sequences. AJNR Am J Neuroradiol 1992;13(6):1555–64.

20. Epstein FH, Mugler JP 3rd, Cail WS, et al. CSF-suppressed T2-weighted three-dimensional MP-RAGE MR imaging. J Magn Reson Imaging 1995;5(4): 463–9.

21. Chang L, McBride D, Miller BL, et al. Localized in vivo 1H magnetic resonance spectroscopy and in vitro analyses of heterogeneous brain tumors. J Neuroimaging 1995;5(3):157–63.

22. Castillo M, Smith JK, Kwock L. Correlation of myoinositol levels and grading of cerebral astrocytomas. AJNR Am J Neuroradiol 2000;21(9):1645–9.

23. Negendank WG, Sauter R, Brown TR, et al. Proton magnetic resonance spectroscopy in patients with glial tumors: a multicenter study. J Neurosurg 1996;84(3):449–58.

24. Heesters MA, Kamman RL, Mooyaart EL, et al. Localized proton spectroscopy of inoperable brain gliomas. Response to radiation therapy. J Neurooncol 1993;17(1):27–35.

25. Shimizu H, Kumabe T, Tominaga T, et al. Noninvasive evaluation of malignancy of brain tumors with proton MR spectroscopy. AJNR Am J Neuroradiol 1996;17(4):737–47.

26. Segebarth CM, Baleriaux DF, Luyten PR, et al. Detection of metabolic heterogeneity of human intracranial tumors in vivo by 1H NMR spectroscopic imaging. Magn Reson Med 1990;13(1):62–76.

27. Luyten PR, Marien AJ, Heindel W, et al. Metabolic imaging of patients with intracranial tumors: H-1 MR spectroscopic imaging and PET. Radiology 1990;176(3):791–9.

28. Fulham MJ, Bizzi A, Dietz MJ, et al. Mapping of brain tumor metabolites with proton MR spectroscopic imaging: clinical relevance. Radiology 1992;185(3):675–86.

29. Salama GR, Heier LA, Patel P, et al. Diffusion weighted/tensor imaging, functional MRI and perfusion weighted imaging in glioblastoma-foundations and future. Front Neurol 2017;8:660.

30. Potgieser AR, Wagemakers M, van Hulzen AL, et al. The role of diffusion tensor imaging in brain tumor surgery: a review of the literature. Clin Neurol Neurosurg 2014;124:51–8.

31. Spena G, Nava A, Cassini F, et al. Preoperative and intraoperative brain mapping for the resection of eloquent-area tumors. A prospective analysis of methodology, correlation, and usefulness based on clinical outcomes. Acta Neurochir (Wien) 2010; 152(11):1835–46.

32. Nimsky C, Ganslandt O, Hastreiter P, et al. Preoperative and intraoperative diffusion tensor imaging-based fiber tracking in glioma surgery. Neurosurgery 2005; 56(1):130–7 [discussion: 138].

33. Matthews PM, Honey GD, Bullmore ET. Applications of fMRI in translational medicine and clinical practice. Nat Rev Neurosci 2006;7(9):732–44.

34. Tate MC, Herbet G, Moritz-Gasser S, et al. Probabilistic map of critical functional regions of the human cerebral cortex: Broca's area revisited. Brain 2014; 137(Pt 10):2773–82.

35. Trinh VT, Fahim DK, Maldaun MV, et al. Impact of preoperative functional magnetic resonance imaging during awake craniotomy procedures for intraoperative guidance and complication avoidance. Stereotact Funct Neurosurg 2014;92(5): 315–22.

36. Ottenhausen M, Krieg SM, Meyer B, et al. Functional preoperative and intraoperative mapping and monitoring: increasing safety and efficacy in glioma surgery. Neurosurg Focus 2015;38(1):E3.

37. Alexander BM, Cloughesy TF. Adult Glioblastoma. J Clin Oncol 2017;35(21):2402–9.

38. Wen PY, Schiff D, Kesari S, et al. Medical management of patients with brain tumors. J Neurooncol 2006;80(3):313–32.

39. Kerkhof M, Vecht CJ. Seizure characteristics and prognostic factors of gliomas. Epilepsia 2013; 54(Suppl 9):12–7.

40. van Breemen MS, Wilms EB, Vecht CJ. Epilepsy in patients with brain tumours: epidemiology, mechanisms, and management. Lancet Neurol 2007;6(5): 421–30.

41. Bartolo M, Zucchella C, Pace A, et al. Early rehabilitation after surgery improves functional outcome in inpatients with brain tumours. J Neurooncol 2012; 107(3):537–44.

42. Fu JB, Parsons HA, Shin KY, et al. Comparison of functional outcomes in low- and high-grade astrocytoma rehabilitation inpatients. Am J Phys Med Rehabil 2010;89(3):205–12.

43. Marciniak CM, Sliwa JA, Heinemann AW, et al. Functional outcomes of persons with brain tumors after inpatient rehabilitation. Arch Phys Med Rehabil 2001;82(4):457–63.

44. Geler-Kulcu D, Gulsen G, Buyukbaba E, et al. Functional recovery of patients with brain tumor or acute stroke after rehabilitation: a comparative study. J Clin Neurosci 2009;16(1):74–8.

45. Greenberg E, Treger I, Ring H. Rehabilitation outcomes in patients with brain tumors and acute stroke: comparative study of inpatient rehabilitation. Am J Phys Med Rehabil 2006;85(7):568–73.

46. O'Dell MW, Barr K, Spanier D, et al. Functional outcome of inpatient rehabilitation in persons with brain tumors. Arch Phys Med Rehabil 1998;79(12):1530–4.

47. Huang ME, Wartella JE, Kreutzer JS. Functional outcomes and quality of life in patients with brain tumors: a preliminary report. Arch Phys Med Rehabil 2001;82(11):1540–6.

48. Roberts PS, Nuno M, Sherman D, et al. The impact of inpatient rehabilitation on function and survival of newly diagnosed patients with glioblastoma. PM R 2014;6(6):514–21.

49. Dropcho EJ, Soong SJ. Steroid-induced weakness in patients with primary brain tumors. Neurology 1991;41(8):1235–9.

50. Hegi ME, Diserens AC, Gorlia T, et al. MGMT gene silencing and benefit from temozolomide in glioblastoma. N Engl J Med 2005;352(10):997–1003.

51. Larson DA, Suplica JM, Chang SM, et al. Permanent iodine 125 brachytherapy in patients with progressive or recurrent glioblastoma multiforme. Neuro Oncol 2004;6(2):119–26.

52. Brem H, Piantadosi S, Burger PC, et al. Placebo-controlled trial of safety and efficacy of intraoperative controlled delivery by biodegradable polymers of chemotherapy for recurrent gliomas. The polymer-brain tumor treatment group. Lancet 1995; 345(8956):1008–12.

53. Kinzel A, Ambrogi M, Varshaver M, et al. Tumor treating fields for glioblastoma treatment: patient satisfaction and compliance with the second-generation Optune((R)) system. Clin Med Insights Oncol 2019;13. 1179554918825449.

54. Toms SA, Kim CY, Nicholas G, et al. Increased compliance with tumor treating fields therapy is prognostic for improved survival in the treatment of glioblastoma: a subgroup analysis of the EF-14 phase III trial. J Neurooncol 2019;141(2): 467–73.

55. Mahato D, De Biase G, Ruiz-Garcia HJ, et al. Impact of facility type and volume on post-surgical outcomes following diagnosis of WHO grade II glioma. J Clin Neurosci 2018;58:34–41.

Role of Resection in Glioblastoma Management

Mark W. Youngblood, MD, PhD[a], Roger Stupp, MD[a,b,c,d], Adam M. Sonabend, MD[a,d,*]

KEYWORDS

- Glioblastoma resection • Resectability • Survival • Supratotal resection • Operative adjuncts
- Cytoreduction

KEY POINTS

- There is extensive retrospective evidence that extent of resection is an independent predictor of survival in glioblastoma.
- Maximal resection may influence clinical course via cytoreduction, relief of mass effect, and palliation.
- Numerous technical innovations have been demonstrated to improve extent of resection, including advanced imaging and monitoring methods.
- Resectability also may play a role in survival and is an important variable to consider during clinical trial design.

INTRODUCTION

Optimal clinical management of glioblastoma (GBM) is ever-evolving, fueled by intensive research efforts and widespread enrollment of patients in clinical trials. Notwithstanding important progress in deciphering glioma pathogenesis, pharmacologic sensitivities, and optimization of medical and radiation therapies, surgical excision continues to play a paramount role. Surgery is essential for accurate pathologic and molecular diagnosis and may confer direct benefit to patients by reducing tumor burden (termed, *cytoreduction*) and alleviating mass effect. The evidence supporting the benefit of cytoreduction in long-term outcome is supported by extensive literature, yet the interpretation of these studies is nuanced. Although numerous studies have confirmed an association between resection and survival,[1–3] this relationship likely is more complex than it seems,

and the presence of confounding variables is an area of continued investigation (**Table 1**).

The success of an operation is graded in part by extent of resection (EOR), which measures the proportion of tumor removed during the procedure. As previous studies suggest prolonged survival with greater EOR, surgeons aim to maximally resect tumor tissue that can be safely separated from critical neurovascular structures. Complete resection of detectable tumor (CRDT) is the ultimate the goal of these surgeries, which includes all enhancing tumor as well as additional regions of T2/fluid-attenuate inversion recovery (FLAIR) abnormalities.[4] Maximal resection is accomplished in many cases, and rarely do surgeons perform a second procedure to remove small amounts of residual. Although removing as much tumor as possible makes sense in principle, the causal effect of extensive resection on survival derives mostly from retrospective, or post hoc

[a] Department of Neurological Surgery, Northwestern University, Northwestern Medicine, 676 North Saint Clair Street, Suite 2210, Chicago, IL 60611, USA; [b] Department of Neurology, Northwestern University, 676 North Saint Clair Street, Suite 2210, Chicago, IL 60611, USA; [c] Department of Medicine, Division of Hematology and Oncology, Northwestern University, 676 North Saint Clair Street, Suite 2210, Chicago, IL 60611, USA; [d] Lou and Jean Malnati Brain Tumor Institute, Robert H. Lurie Comprehensive Cancer Center, Northwestern University, 676 North Saint Clair Street, Suite 2210, Chicago, IL 60611, USA
* Corresponding author. 676 North Saint Clair Street, Suite 2210, Chicago, IL 60611.
E-mail address: adam.sonabend@nm.org

Neurosurg Clin N Am 32 (2021) 9–22
https://doi.org/10.1016/j.nec.2020.08.002
1042-3680/21/© 2020 Elsevier Inc. All rights reserved.

Table 1
Independent factors associated with survival in glioblastoma

	Oppenlander et al,[50] 2014	Stummer et al,[68] 2008	Lacroix et al,[1] 2001	Capellades et al,[80] 2018
Age	$P<.01$; HR = 1.04 (1.03–1.05)	$P<.01$; HR = 1.54 (1.11–2.12)	$P<.01$; HR = 2.5 (1.8–3.6)	$P = .04$; HR = 1.50 (1.02–2.20)
KPS	$P<.01$; HR = 0.96 (0.95–0.98)	$P = .02$; HR = 0.62 (0.42–0.92)	$P = .01$; HR = 1.4 (1.1–1.8)	$P = .05$; HR = 1.65 (1.01–2.69)
EOR	$P<.01$; HR = 0.97 (0.96–0.98)	$P<.01$; HR = 1.75 (1.26–2.44)	$P<.1$; HR = 1.6 (1.3–2.0)	$P<.01$; HR = 2.25 (1.34–3.78)
Volume	Unreported	$P = .48$; HR = 1.00 (1.0–1.01)	Unreported	$P<.01$; HR = 1.77 (1.24–2.52)

Numerous studies have identified age, KPS, tumor volume and EOR as independent factors associated with overall survival. The significance (P) and hazard ratio (HR) with 95% Confidence Interval (CI) are listed for each variable as obtained in the associated study. The directionality tested in both KPS and EOR varied among some studies, resulting in HRs less than 1 in those cases.

analyses. This has led to a range of philosophies regarding the importance of CRDT, often driven by surgical experience as well as patient demographics and disease burden. Most recently, the concept of supratotal resection has been advocated in GBM, including near-complete resection of FLAIR-signal regions, in an effort to further-eradicate infiltrative disease.[5–9]

As evidence suggests that maximally resected tumors are associated with better outcome, it follows that patients predicted amenable to CRDT should be expected to have a superior prognosis. Consideration of *resectability*, or the amount of tumor tissue that can be safely removed relative to the total tumor burden, therefore plays an important role in management of GBM patients. In many cases, this metric is the deciding factor in determining the appropriate goals of a surgery and is simultaneously considered with other variables, such as patient demographics, disease burden, and previous medical history. Resectability is not an entirely objective metric, however, because disagreement often exists among experts evaluating a given patient.[10,11] Thus, there are patient and surgeon factors that influence resectability and EOR for GBM.

This review discusses the role of resection in operative management of GBM. Resectability (potential for excision) is distinguished from EOR (change in disease burden), while noting overlap in the features that determine both. Finally, the evidence relating EOR and resectability to patient outcome is discussed, with

particular attention to variables that may confound these associations. The authors propose that resectability could be an important prognostic correlate, often independent of EOR, and should be afforded preeminent consideration in therapeutic planning. Whereas some scales have attempted to measure resectability, it is difficult to measure this variable reliably, and thus this potential confounder of survival often is ignored in the GBM literature.

MEASURING AND PREDICTING EXTENT OF RESECTION

EOR plays an important role in postoperative management decisions, as this feature is predictive of long-term survival and occasionally, clinical trial eligibility. However, precise quantification of this metric is difficult. Before the advent of neuroimaging, estimates of EOR relied on intraoperative evaluation of tumor bulk and thus were influenced by tumor location, histology, and level of experience.[12] The ability to detect remaining tumor in situ is variable among surgeons, and, even when gross total resection (GTR) is perceived, there may be residual tumor apparent on postoperative magnetic resonance imaging (MRI).[10,12,13] A previous study suggested that GTR is incorrectly assigned to as many as 69.6% of cases based on intraoperative judgment,[10] whereas radiographic evidence indicates that true GTR may be achieved in as few as one-third of high-grade gliomas.[14] With widespread adaptation of preoperative and postoperative MRI, quantitative methods have emerged that aim to improve the accuracy of EOR. These techniques use semiautomated approaches to segment contrast-enhancing lesions and calculate tumor burden after intervention, which then can be compared with preoperative scans to determine EOR.[2] Nonetheless, diffuse penetration of malignant glioma cells remains invisible to contemporary imaging technologies, and thus is not possible to obtain an exact quantification of remaining disease burden.

Extensive efforts have been undertaken to understand the factors associated with optimal EOR, with the goal of predicting which patients harbor lesions amenable to CRDT (**Fig. 1**). Tumor-related factors, such as accessibility, proximity of eloquent structures, invasion, and disease burden, can be useful in understanding the risks associated with aggressive excision as well as predicting the surgical outcome.[10,15] Tumors located in less accessible regions, such as the basal ganglia, often have reduced EOR, as do those adjacent to eloquent cortex. Tumor molecular features, such as *IDH1* mutation status, also may play a role in EOR, although results have been mixed among studies.[16,17] Patient factors, including age, Karnofsky performance scale score (KPS), medical comorbidities, and history of previous surgeries also might independently influence EOR. These contextual variables can determine the perceived benefit from extensive cytoreduction and thus affect the balance between aggressive intervention and operative morbidity. For example, previous studies have suggested a limited benefit to tumor volume reduction in elderly patients.[18,19] Consequently, surgeons may be directed to more conservative resections in some cases, thus minimizing surgical risk and optimizing quality of life.

In addition to these intrinsic factors, the experience and skill of individual surgeons also play an important role in achieving CRDT.[10] Previous studies have noted variability in surgeons' ability to detect residual disease,[10,12,13] which could prevent accurate determination of CRDT intraoperatively. Institutional factors may further dictate the extent of surgical intervention. Highly specialized centers with advanced imaging capabilities, experienced tumor surgeons, fluorescence-guided resection (ie, 5-aminolovelulinic acid [5-ALA] and sodium fluorescein), intraoperative monitoring teams, and multispecialty tumor boards, are better poised to achieve CRDT. Previous studies confirm that the case volume at a given institution may be an important covariate in patient clinical course.[20,21]

METHODS FOR OPTIMIZING EXTENT OF RESECTION

The association of EOR with survival has prompted technical advances aimed at improving EOR while minimizing risks to eloquent regions. A pivotal milestone was the development of sophisticated intraoperative visualization techniques, which have enabled more precise identification and dissection of tumor from normal tissue. For example, high-resolution ultrasound is an effective method to confirm completeness of resection, because this modality can readily distinguish tumor boundaries[22] (although it remains subject to imaging artifacts that result in reduced identification of residual disease[23]). Leveraging high-resolution preoperative MRI data, neuronavigation also has become a near ubiquitous tool for in situ tumor localization.[24] Although a previous prospective trial indicated no difference in EOR with use of navigation,[25] a large study group with more homogeneous features may be needed to conclusively evaluate the benefits of this modality.[26] A particular challenge with neuronavigation is the occurrence of anatomic shifts during a procedure, resulting in unreliable accuracy as the case

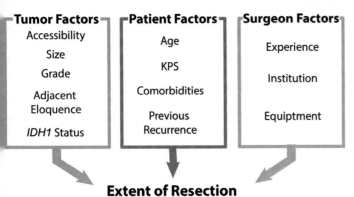

Tumor Factors	Patient Factors	Surgeon Factors
Accessibility	Age	Experience
Size	KPS	
Grade		Institution
Adjacent Eloquence	Comorbidities	
IDH1 Status	Previous Recurrence	Equiptment

Extent of Resection

Fig. 1. Selected factors associated with EOR. Various tumor-related, patient-related, and surgeon-related features may play a role in determining (and possibly predicting) EOR.

advances.[27,28] In some institutions, this limitation has been circumvented with the use of intraoperative MRI (iMRI), which provides updated anatomic data for neuronavigation as well as real-time information regarding EOR.[29,30] Previous studies have validated the role of this modality for improvement of resection rates[31–34] and also noted that surgeons frequently resect additional tissue after an intraoperative scan is performed.[14,32,35] However, iMRI remains an expensive and cumbersome undertaking, requiring considerable institutional investment, extra time in the operating room, as well as expertise that is developed over many cases.

In situ visualization of neoplastic tissue has gained recent popularity, using administration of tumor-enhancing fluorescent compounds that distinguish cancerous lesions from nontumor tissue. Oral administration of 5-ALA, a prodrug that results in intratumoral accumulation of fluorescent porphyrins, has shown particular promise.[36] In a randomized clinical trial, use of 5-ALA resulted in an increase in complete resection rate and 6-month progression-free survival, without a significant difference in adverse events.[37] This result was consistent with an earlier phase II study by the same group.[38] Although the study did not show a difference in overall survival related to the use of 5-ALA, this result could conceivably be explained by the proportion of patients in the white-light group that received GTR. Sodium fluorescein is an alternative tool for intraoperative visualization of tumor tissue. This dye labels the region of tumor that corresponds to enhancement on an MRI done with contrast. Intravenous administration leads to in situ fluorescence due to leakage of dye in regions where the blood-brain barrier is deficient,[39] and previous studies suggest that this approach improves the rate of GTR.[40] The effects of fluorescein may be further augmented using intraoperative confocal microscopy,[41] allowing direct visualization of tumor cytoarchitecture during resection. Relative to 5-ALA, fluorescein is inexpensive[42] and carries a low rate of associated side effects. Prospective trials, however, have yet to demonstrate a survival effect associated with fluorescein use in GBM patients.

Neurophysiologic monitoring techniques provide intraoperative feedback and have improved EOR by decreasing the risk associated with resection near eloquent cortex and white matter tracts. These approaches address the functional anatomic variability that exists between patients[43] and provide immediate functional validation that a given region is "silent" prior to removal of tissue. A common technique in glioma surgery is cortical and subcortical stimulation during an awake craniotomy, which can be performed under local anesthesia.[44] During these procedures, direct electrical stimulation of neural structures allows real-time detection of functional regions, resulting in fewer long-term neurologic deficits and more extensive EOR.[45] Preoperative brain mapping also can provide benefit and is used to identify functional cortical areas (functional MRI) or white matter tracts (diffusion tensor imaging). The resulting data typically are mapped onto preoperative scans within neuronavigation systems, thus providing patient-specific information to guide resection boundaries. The accuracy of these modalities, however, is subject to technical aspects of imaging acquisition, the possibility of false-negative results and false-positive results, and anatomic shifts (discussed previously). Thus, this modality should not be used as an alternative to intraoperative brain mapping.

RELATIONSHIP BETWEEN EXTENT OF RESECTION AND SURVIVAL

Surgical goals are shaped by the expected net benefit of the procedure for the patient, and the delicate balance between disease eradication and operative morbidity must be considered thoughtfully. Because GBM is an infiltrative disease, it is expected that even GTR is a contemporizing measure. Nonetheless, numerous studies have demonstrated increased survival with greater EOR, even when accounting for covariates, such as histology and previous recurrence[1,3,46–50] (Table 2). Although evidence supports an association between surgical intervention and survival, debate remains about the proportional nature of this relationship. An all-or-none benefit to EOR has been suggested in some studies, whereby a near-complete resection is associated with prolonged clinical course,[1,13] whereas the effects of subtotal resections are diminished or absent. It is possible that limited sample size might cloud the association of a modest resection with modest survival on these studies. One investigation on GBMs found a survival benefit after 98% resection, which conferred a median of 4 additional months.[1] Studies using a more granular approach have shown a stepwise improvement in progression-free survival with greater EOR,[49] with some suggesting an effect threshold of 70% to 80% in both primary[3,51] and recurrent GBM.[50] The relative importance of specific resection thresholds likely depends on additional tumor and patient features (such as histology, grade, genomics, location, age, and KPS), which dictate the biological behavior and clinical aggressiveness of residual disease. For example, evidence in low-grade

Table 2
Selected studies investigating the role of extent of resection in glioblastoma survival

First Author, Year	Cohort	Key Findings	Comments
Lacroix et al,[1] 2001	416 GBM; 233 previously untreated	A survival advantage is found among previously untreated patients when 98% or more of the tumor is resected. Age, KPS, and imaging features also are predictive of survival.	A large proportion of untreated patients had EOR >98%, which may decrease sensitivity to detect significance of lower thresholds.
Keles et al,[49] 1999	92 Hemispheric GBM	Survival was affected by age, KPS, EOR, and volume of residual disease. All patients had KPS >70; a subset of patients did not receive adjuvant chemotherapy.	Greater resections did not have an impact on quality of life. EOR affects both survival and time to progression
Sanai et al,[3] 2011	500 Consecutive, newly diagnosed, supratentorial GBM	All patients received standard chemotherapy and radiation. Age, KPS, postoperative tumor volume and EOR were independent predictors of survival. EOR demonstrated a stepwise benefit beginning at 78%, with improvement up to 100%.	Challenged the all-or-nothing paradigm for GBM resection.
Stummer et al,[68] 2008	243 GBM	Reallocation of the phase III 5-ALA study group data into complete vs incomplete resection cohorts, which otherwise were balanced (or stratified) for covariates relevant to outcome. A 4.9-mo survival benefit was observed in the GTR group, with a hazard ratio that was greater than age and KPS.	Based on enrollment protocol of original study and validated balancing of other prognostic factors, this study provides level IIB evidence associating EOR with survival.
Li et al,[6] 2016	1229 GBM that underwent >78% EOR	Patients undergoing complete resection of contrast-enhancing lesion (or better) survived longer that sub-total resection, even after correction for other prognostic factors. Resection of >53.2% of the FLAIR region provided additional benefit.	Supports the value of supratotal resection when safe, although effects may have been constrained by heterogeneous EOR across cohort.
Chaichana et al,[51] 2014	259 Supratentorial GBM	EOR was associated with both survival and recurrence after correcting for other prognostic values. Similarly, tumor residual volume also was found to be related to survival.	Demonstrated that residual volume also plays a prognostic role.

(continued on next page)

Table 2
(continued)

First Author, Year	Cohort	Key Findings	Comments
Molinaro et al,[17] 2020	761 GBM newly diagnosed; validation with 206 additional GBM	Younger patients benefited from maximal resection of both enhancing and nonenhancing tumor, which resulted in similar outcomes regardless of *IDH1* status. Older patients with *IDH* wild-type benefited from complete resection of contrast-enhancing lesion.	Stratification by molecular subgroup (*IDH1*) controls for an important confounder that often is ignored.

Numerous studies have reported an association between EOR and survival, with variable consideration of relevant covariates and patient populations.

gliomas has suggested thresholds that affect outcome ranging from 50% to 90%.[52–54] In addition to EOR, the volume of residual tumor also has been shown to play an independent role in survival,[51,54,55] further complicating the use of precise resection thresholds.

If a causal association between EOR and survival is assumed, aggressive resections of GBM, when safe, should represent the optimal surgical intervention. Furthermore, as tumor cell infiltration has been shown to extend well beyond contrast-enhancing region,[56] resection of surrounding FLAIR signal and even normal-appearing tissue may be advantageous. This approach, known as supratotal resection,[5,6] has been associated with longer survival in GBM[6] and also may delay malignant transformation of diffuse low-grade lesions.[57,58] Evidence suggests its effects may be manifold in patients with already favorable prognosis, such as younger patients or those with *IDH1* mutations[16,17,59] (although mutation status typically is not known intraoperatively). A recent study found that maximal resection of non–contrast-enhancing tumor in younger patients resulted in similar survival profiles between *IDH* mutant and wild-type lesions.[17] Although surgeons historically have defined resection margins according to preoperative imaging boundaries, the success of supratotal resections argues that functional boundaries may be more appropriate in some cases, whereby the maximal amount of tissue that can be removed safely is targeted (**Fig. 2**).[7,60] Intraoperative brain mapping is essential when eloquent cortex or circuits are presumed to be involved, as FLAIR positive regions that do not enhance often remain capable of neurologic function in spite of tumor infiltration.

Despite an increasing number of well-designed studies (see **Table 2**), some skepticism persists regarding a causal relationship between EOR and survival in GBM. Several earlier studies have failed to find an association between these variables,[61–64] although most acknowledge cohort limitations (sample size, heterogeneity, and so forth) or technical factors. Conflicting data regarding the benefits of EOR has arisen in part due to the retrospective nature of almost all studies, which introduces variation and bias, such as differing inclusion criteria and survivorship bias in the case of resection in the recurrence setting as well as diverse statistical and classification methods.[65] To the authors' knowledge, only a single prospective trial randomizing for resection has been performed in a controlled manner,[66] and this often-cited work was limited to an elderly population and with limited recruitment. As a result, studies must be relied on that may be subject to preoperative confounders affecting both EOR and survival, as well as postoperative treatment bias between groups. For example, GBMs located in surgically accessible regions may be naturally slower to cause disease-related mortality, thus obfuscating a causal relationship with resection.[67] Although many studies correct for location and other well-established confounders (such as age, tumor volume, previous treatments, KPS, and histology),[65] it is impossible to conclusively eliminate this bias in a retrospective analysis. Similarly, studies rarely consider *IDH1* status as a cofactor for survival, although this feature results in a protracted clinical course and typically earlier diagnosis (due to seizures associated with 2-hydroxygluterate metabolite). An

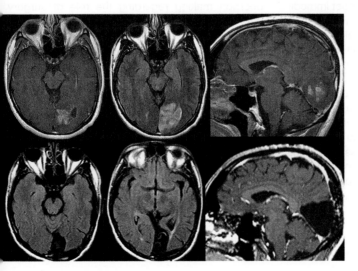

Fig. 2. Supratotal resection. Upper panels show preoperative imaging of a left occipital GBM. From left to right, these panels show axial T1 (with contrast), axial FLAIR, and sagittal T1 (with contrast) sequences. Bottom panels are after supratotal resection, including all FLAIR-positive signal. The sequences are shown in the same order as above. (*From* Duffau H. Is supratotal resection of glioblastoma in noneloquent areas possible? World Neurosurg. 2014;82(1-2):e102; with permission.)

additional factor is survivorship bias, which refers to the fact that people who remain alive, or who are doing well at recurrence, are likely to undergo surgery, which confounds the association between surgery and survival at recurrence. Thus, it may appear that surgery at recurrence prolongs survival, but in fact the converse also is true: survival makes surgery more likely.

In the absence of large-cohort prospective studies, insights may be gleaned from well-controlled surrogate investigations in which EOR highly was correlated with the variable under study. A randomized trial evaluating the intraoperative use of 5-ALA observed a significantly higher complete resection rate in the treatment group (65% complete resection in the treatment group, vs. 35% in the control group)[37] without improvement in overall survival. In a subsequent study, the authors restratified these data according to EOR[68] and reported level IIb evidence that complete excision is associated with survival of GBM patients (with a median benefit of 4.9 months), although a specific resection threshold of was not established.[68] A small German randomized study with 49 evaluable patients compared the use of iMRI during glioma surgery versus standard navigation techniques[33] and found a significant increase in GTR rate but without improvement in overall survival.

MECHANISMS BY WHICH EXTENT OF RESECTION MIGHT AFFECT SURVIVAL

Assuming a causal relationship between EOR and survival does exist, the reason for this association is a topic of much debate. Surgical excision is not curative of diffuse glioma, and after GTR, GBM recurrence occurs after a median of 13 months.[69] However, tumor excision undoubtedly alters disease course, even if transiently. The most immediate consequence of resection is reduction of mass effect, which relieves the risk of neurologic symptoms due to brain compression by the tumor, and in some cases, imminent death due to herniation or other fatal sequalae. Patients presenting with an urgent need for life-preserving surgery thus will have an associated increase in survival after a successful operation, and this benefit can be achieved with partial resection. The impact of reducing mass effect on outcome is instantaneous and powerful, but it also is temporary. This is a scenario in which resection might prolong survival, but this benefit stems from brain decompression rather than cytoreduction.

Extensive resections that result in reduced tumor burden (termed, *cytoreduction*) may alter disease course further. GBMs are poorly circumscribed lesions with extensive infiltration, and residual lesions are expected to eventually grow and replace empty resection cavity. This process, however, may not be immediate, and a small portion of patients may experience a prolonged disease-free window prior to progression.[69] Furthermore, extensive cytoreduction alters tumor architecture, resulting in microenvironmental changes that can stall tumor growth. For example, central hypoxic regions of GBM, which frequently are targeted during surgery, are associated with greater proliferation and aggressive features.[70] The patient's long-term outcome thus is determined by the biology of the residual disease, which is distinct from the primary lesion that underwent resection. Finally, cytoreduction also may enhance efficacy of adjuvant therapies, such as radiation or chemotherapeutics.[71]

In addition to survival, tumor debulking as a palliative measure also can benefit patients in some scenarios. Tumor mass effect frequently is associated with debilitating sequelae, such as nausea, visual changes, headache, weakness, and seizures, among other neurologic symptoms. Reduction of volume may relieve these symptoms and improve quality of life,[72] albeit temporarily. Because excision itself may be associated with morbidity,[73] particularly with reoperation,[74] the benefits of palliation must be considered on an individual basis. In some cases, bevacizumab is a reasonable alternative to debulking with a palliative intent.[75] In the academic setting, resection also offers the opportunity for enrollment of patients into clinical trials that require an intraoperative intervention,[76,77] in which case, resection represents a window for a salvage therapy. The involvement of a multidisciplinary team, including neurosurgeons, neurooncologists, social workers, and palliative care specialists, can facilitate patient decision making regarding the role of surgery, particularly in the recurrent setting.

PREOPERATIVE ASSESSMENT OF RESECTABILITY

Careful consideration of resectability has become a routine part of preoperative evaluation of GBM, because it plays an integral role in shaping surgical planning and in some cases may argue against a procedure. Although evidence suggests that surgical excision improves outcomes in most cases, this intervention can be associated with morbidity,[73] and the advanced presentation of some patients may mitigate the benefits of treatment. Resectability thus provides insights into the balance between operative risks and benefits and often can tilt the scale in one direction or the other. Furthermore, it also may serve as an independent predictor of outcome, because patients with poorly resectable lesions (ie, diffuse), regardless of operative intervention, are expected to have reduced survival.

Resectability measures the degree to which a particular lesion is amenable to surgical excision, and often represents a gestalt formed from simultaneous consideration of numerous features. Imaging plays a key (but not complete) role in assessing this variable, because it identifies proximal eloquent structures and denotes the surgical accessibility. As discussed previously, tumor location is predictive of EOR, and this relationship undoubtedly depends in part on resectability. Contrast-enhanced MRI is the most common preoperative imaging modality used to determine resectability, because it conveys key structural relationships that affect surgical planning.[10,78] Further studies, including functional MRI and DTI, can provide additional insights by identifying hazardous regions, such as eloquent cortex and white matter tracts. In addition to eloquent areas proximal to the tumor, surgeons also must consider the overall accessibility of a lesion to excision. For example, previous studies have observed decreased EOR associated with periventricular and subcortical tumors, likely owing to the technical difficulty of safely accessing these regions.[10]

Whereas imaging plays a central role in resectability, patient demographics also are an important consideration in determining the extent of an operation. Those with significant comorbidities (eg, obesity and diabetes, coronary artery disease and heart failure, respiratory insufficiency, and renal impairment) may tolerate an extended operative intervention poorly and require prolonged postoperative recovery. Furthermore, patients with extensive infiltrative disease may derive limited benefit from partial resection and could spend a significant portion of their remaining life recovering from a morbid procedure. However, previous work has suggested that patient factors may not affect EOR once the decision has been made for surgical intervention.[10]

The complex and multivariate nature of resectability adds an element of subjectivity in its assessment, because the relative weights of each factor depends on the experiences of the evaluating surgeon. Consequently, previous studies have noted disagreement on resectability among common cohorts of patients, even among seasoned experts (**Fig. 3**).[10,11,79] An analysis of concordance between 2 experienced surgeons on whether a lesion could safely undergo GTR found agreement in only 72% of cases.[10] A more recent study (conducted by the senior author of this review) found comparable variation when a larger number of experts was consulted.[11] Using a panel of 13 board-certified academic brain tumor neurosurgeons, the latter report indicated more than 80% of experts agreed in a surgical goal (resection vs biopsy) in more than 80% of the lesions assessed. Collectively, these results indicate that in some cases, resectability can be observer-dependent, which results in important changes in a patient's clinical management.

ROLE OF RESECTABILITY IN CLINICAL TRIALS

Given a likely independent effect of resectability on outcome, this feature may be a relevant covariate

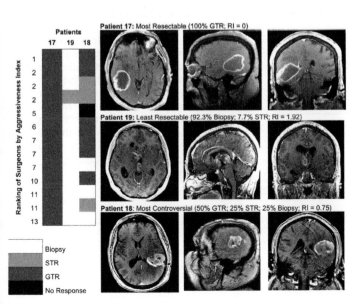

Fig. 3. Varying levels of resectability among GBM. Shown are radiographic examples of highly resectable, poorly resectable, and controversial GBMs according to expert opinion. The decision to pursue biopsy (white), subtotal resection (light gray), GTR (dark gray), or undecided (black) for each lesion is shown in the adjacent heatmap, with surgeons ranked from most aggressive (1) to least aggressive (13) based on evaluation of 20 cases. (*From* Sonabend AM, Zacharia BE, Cloney MB, et al. Defining glioblastoma resectability through the wisdom of the crowd: a proof-of-principle study. Neurosurgery. 2017;80(4):598; with permission.)

to consider during clinical trial design. It is conceivable that stratification by EOR, tumor location, and/or patient demographics may incompletely capture a potential bias that arises from differences in resectability, which may affect response to a therapeutic intervention. Such an imbalance may be difficult to detect and correct for post hoc. A recent search of clinicaltrials.gov indicates that resectability is a cofactor commonly considered in gastrointestinal, lung and pancreatic cancers but rarely mentioned in trials involving primary brain tumors, such as glioma (search performed June, 2020). To account for this confounder, preoperative measures of resectability should be recorded and used as a covariate in randomization algorithms. In retrospective studies, there also may be benefit to inclusion of resectability as a covariate, because this more accurately models and tests the independence of other features under study. Integration of resectability into clinical trials, however, will require a standardized, objective, and reproducible method for measuring this variable, which currently does not exist.

MEASURING RESECTABILITY

Although GBM resectability is intertwined with several objective features, it remains, in part, a subjective assessment by the treating surgeon.

Nonetheless, several scales previously designed for other purposes may offer insights into resectability,[80–84] because they harbor overlap in a portion of the relevant variables. The National Institute of Health (NIH) Recurrent GBM Scale was developed to predict postoperative survival after resection of recurrent GBM and considered involvement of eloquent brain regions, KPS ($\leq$80), and tumor volume ($\geq$50 cm^3).[81] Based on the selected variables, this scale gives insights into the benefit derived from surgery as well as the probability of achieving a CRDT. It does not include, however, additional features that may be independent predictors of resectability, such as surgeon experience. An additional preoperative scale has been reported to predict long-term outcome in low-grade gliomas.[82] Similar to the NIH Recurrent GBM Scale, the authors selected eloquent location and KPS ($\leq$80) as score components but substituted tumor diameter (>4 cm) for tumor volume and also included patient age (>50 years). Several components of their score were found to associate with EOR, thus suggesting relevancy of the scale for preoperative assessment of resectability. Because the proximity of contrast-enhancing lesion to functional regions often dictates the EOR, algorithms based on preoperative imaging also may be predictive of EOR and can provide probabilistic maps of likely residual tissue. For example, a previous study found an

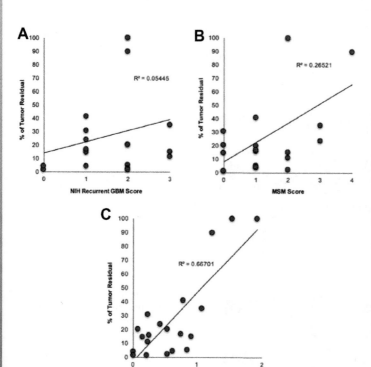

Fig. 4. Comparison of methods for measuring resectability, including (A) NIH Recurrent GBM Score, (B) motor-speech-middle cerebral artery (MSM) component of NIH GBM Score, and (C) the Resectability Index (a composite of crowdsourced expert opinion). A previous study found that resectability index exhibited higher correlation with percent of residual contrast-enhancing lesion than the other two clinical scales. (*From* Sonabend AM, Zacharia BE, Cloney MB, et al. Defining glioblastoma resectability through the wisdom of the crowd: a proof-of-principle study. Neurosurgery. 2017;80(4):600; with permission.)

32% success rate in preoperative prediction of resection amount based on imaging of grade II gliomas.[85] The difficulty in objectively defining resectability has limited the predictive value of preoperative scales. A previous study demonstrated that crowd-sourcing among experienced neurosurgeons led to higher concordance between predicted resectability and residual enhancing disease than 2 radiographic scales (**Fig. 4**).[11]

SUMMARY AND FURTHER CONSIDERATIONS

Surgery remains a cornerstone of GBM management and is a standard component of the multimodal treatment regimens now in practice. When safe, evidence suggests that increasing EOR (thereby decreasing residual disease) is associated with a better outcome, and this assumption is validated by numerous retrospective studies as well as a small number of prospective surrogate studies in which EOR was balanced against other covariates. Controversy, however, remains regarding the level of benefit, the appropriate safety threshold, whether the EOR and survival simply are associated or have a causal relationship, and whether this is explained by cytoreduction or brain decompression from tumor debulking. It is probable that additional covariates may stratify the efficacy of EOR for improving survival, such as patient age, comorbidities, tumor molecular features, and invasiveness. Thus, patients who otherwise are healthy, lack genomic alterations associated with poor prognosis, and have well-circumscribed disease may benefit most from CRDT. Studies with higher granularity are needed to confidently ascertain these relationships and will provide important insight into which patients warrant aggressive resections at the risk of surgical morbidity.

CLINICS CARE POINTS

- Maximal resection of abnormal tissue (including FLAIR signal), when safe, optimizes patient survival.
- Use of intraoperative adjuncts, such as 5-ALA, neuromonitoring, and MRI, improve EOR.
- Resectability depends on tumor-specific, patient-specific, and surgeon-specific factors, and its assessment can differ among a panel of experts.

DISCLOSURE

The authors have nothing to disclose.

REFERENCES

1. Lacroix M, Abi-Said D, Fourney DR, et al. A multivariate analysis of 416 patients with glioblastoma multiforme: prognosis, extent of resection, and survival. J Neurosurg 2001;95(2):190–8.
2. Sanai N, Berger MS. Glioma extent of resection and its impact on patient outcome. Neurosurgery 2008; 62(4):753–64 [discussion: 264–6].
3. Sanai N, Polley MY, McDermott MW, et al. An extent of resection threshold for newly diagnosed glioblastomas. J Neurosurg 2011;115(1):3–8.
4. Vogelbaum MA, Jost S, Aghi MK, et al. Application of novel response/progression measures for surgically delivered therapies for gliomas: Response Assessment in Neuro-Oncology (RANO) Working Group. Neurosurgery 2012;70(1):234–43 [discussion: 243–4].
5. de Leeuw CN, Vogelbaum MA. Supratotal resection in glioma: a systematic review. Neuro Oncol 2019; 21(2):179–88.
6. Li YM, Suki D, Hess K, et al. The influence of maximum safe resection of glioblastoma on survival in 1229 patients: can we do better than gross-total resection? J Neurosurg 2016;124(4):977–88.
7. Yordanova Y, Duffau H. Supratotal resection of diffuse gliomas–an overview of its multifaceted implications. Neurochirurgie 2017;63(3):243–9.
8. Pessina F, Navarria P, Cozzi L, et al. Maximize surgical resection beyond contrast-enhancing boundaries in newly diagnosed glioblastoma multiforme: is it useful and safe? A single institution retrospective experience. J Neurooncol 2017;135(1):129–39.
9. Sanai N, Berger MS. Surgical oncology for gliomas: the state of the art. Nat Rev Clin Oncol 2018;15(2): 112–25.
10. Orringer D, Lau D, Khatri S, et al. Extent of resection in patients with glioblastoma: limiting factors, perception of resectability, and effect on survival. J Neurosurg 2012;117(5):851–9.
11. Sonabend AM, Zacharia BE, Cloney MB, et al. Defining glioblastoma resectability through the wisdom of the crowd: a proof-of-principle study. Neurosurgery 2017;80(4):590–601.
12. Lau D, Hervey-Jumper SL, Han SJ, et al. Intraoperative perception and estimates on extent of resection during awake glioma surgery: Overcoming the learning curve. J Neurosurg 2018;128(5):1410–8.
13. Albert FK, Forsting M, Sartor K, et al. Early postoperative magnetic resonance imaging after resection of malignant glioma: objective evaluation of residual tumor and its influence on regrowth and prognosis. Neurosurgery 1994;34(1):45–60 [discussion: 60–1].
14. Nimsky C, Fujita A, Ganslandt O, et al. Volumetric assessment of glioma removal by intraoperative high-field magnetic resonance imaging. Neurosurgery 2004;55(2):358–70 [discussion: 370–1].

15. Castellano A, Bello L, Michelozzi C, et al. Role of diffusion tensor magnetic resonance tractography in predicting the extent of resection in glioma surgery. Neuro Oncol 2011;14(2):192–202.

16. Beiko J, Suki D, Hess KR, et al. IDH1 mutant malignant astrocytomas are more amenable to surgical resection and have a survival benefit associated with maximal surgical resection. Neuro Oncol 2014;16(1):81–91.

17. Molinaro AM, Hervey-Jumper S, Morshed RA, et al. Association of maximal extent of resection of contrast-enhanced and non-contrast-enhanced tumor with survival within molecular subgroups of patients with newly diagnosed glioblastoma. JAMA Oncol 2020;6(4):495–503.

18. Whittle IR, Denholm SW, Gregor A. Management of patients aged over 60 years with supratentorial glioma: lessons from an audit. Surg Neurol 1991; 36(2):106–11.

19. Kelly PJ, Hunt C. The limited value of cytoreductive surgery in elderly patients with malignant gliomas. Neurosurgery 1994;34(1):62–6 [discussion: 66–7].

20. Barker FG, Curry WT Jr, Carter BS. Surgery for primary supratentorial brain tumors in the United States, 1988 to 2000: the effect of provider caseload and centralization of care. Neuro Oncol 2005;7(1): 49–63.

21. Cowan JA Jr, Dimick JB, Leveque J-C, et al. The impact of provider volume on mortality after intracranial tumor resection. Neurosurgery 2003;52(1): 48–54.

22. Hammoud MA, Ligon BL, elSouki R, et al. Use of intraoperative ultrasound for localizing tumors and determining the extent of resection: a comparative study with magnetic resonance imaging. J Neurosurg 1996;84(5):737–41.

23. Gerganov VM, Samii A, Akbarian A, et al. Reliability of intraoperative high-resolution 2D ultrasound as an alternative to high-field strength MR imaging for tumor resection control: a prospective comparative study. J Neurosurg 2009;111(3):512–9.

24. Wirtz CR, Albert FK, Schwaderer M, et al. The benefit of neuronavigation for neurosurgery analyzed by its impact on glioblastoma surgery. Neurol Res 2000;22(4):354–60.

25. Willems PW, Taphoorn MJ, Burger H, et al. Effectiveness of neuronavigation in resecting solitary intracerebral contrast-enhancing tumors: a randomized controlled trial. J Neurosurg 2006;104(3):360–8.

26. Vandertop WP. Neuronavigation in solitary intracerebral tumors. J Neurosurg 2006;105(5):802–3 [author reply: 803].

27. Roberts DW, Hartov A, Kennedy FE, et al. Intraoperative brain shift and deformation: a quantitative analysis of cortical displacement in 28 cases. Neurosurgery 1998;43(4):749–58 [discussion: 758–60].

28. Nimsky C, Ganslandt O, Cerny S, et al. Quantification of, visualization of, and compensation for brain shift using intraoperative magnetic resonance imaging. Neurosurgery 2000;47(5):1070–9 [discussion: 1079–80].

29. Black PM, Moriarty T, Alexander E 3rd, et al. Development and implementation of intraoperative magnetic resonance imaging and its neurosurgical applications. Neurosurgery 1997;41(4):831–42 [discussion: 842–5].

30. Sutherland GR, Kaibara T, Louw D, et al. A mobile high-field magnetic resonance system for neurosurgery. J Neurosurg 1999;91(5):804–13.

31. Knauth M, Wirtz CR, Tronnier VM, et al. Intraoperative MR imaging increases the extent of tumor resection in patients with high-grade gliomas. AJNR Am J Neuroradiol 1999;20(9):1642–6.

32. Senft C, Seifert V, Hermann E, et al. Usefulness of intraoperative ultra low-field magnetic resonance imaging in glioma surgery. Neurosurgery 2008;63(4 Suppl 2):257–66 [discussion: 266–7].

33. Senft C, Bink A, Franz K, et al. Intraoperative MRI guidance and extent of resection in glioma surgery: a randomised, controlled trial. Lancet Oncol 2011; 12(11):997–1003.

34. Senft C, Franz K, Ulrich CT, et al. Low field intraoperative MRI-guided surgery of gliomas: a single center experience. Clin Neurol Neurosurg 2010;112(3): 237–43.

35. Hatiboglu MA, Weinberg JS, Suki D, et al. Impact of intraoperative high-field magnetic resonance imaging guidance on glioma surgery: a prospective volumetric analysis. Neurosurgery 2009;64(6):1073–81 [discussion: 1081].

36. Stummer W, Stocker S, Wagner S, et al. Intraoperative detection of malignant gliomas by 5-aminolevulinic acid-induced porphyrin fluorescence. Neurosurgery 1998;42(3):518–25 [discussion: 525–6].

37. Stummer W, Pichlmeier U, Meinel T, et al. Fluorescence-guided surgery with 5-aminolevulinic acid for resection of malignant glioma: a randomised controlled multicentre phase III trial. Lancet Oncol 2006;7(5):392–401.

38. Stummer W, Novotny A, Stepp H, et al. Fluorescence-guided resection of glioblastoma multiforme utilizing 5-ALA-induced porphyrins: a prospective study in 52 consecutive patients. J Neurosurg 2000;93(6):1003–13.

39. Shinoda J, Yano H, Yoshimura S, et al. Fluorescence-guided resection of glioblastoma multiforme by using high-dose fluorescein sodium. Technical note. J Neurosurg 2003;99(3):597–603.

40. Koc K, Anik I, Cabuk B, et al. Fluorescein sodium-guided surgery in glioblastoma multiforme: a prospective evaluation. Br J Neurosurg 2008;22(1): 99–103.

41. Sankar T, Delaney PM, Ryan RW, et al. Miniaturized handheld confocal microscopy for neurosurgery: results in an experimental glioblastoma model. Neurosurgery 2010;66(2):410–7 [discussion: 417–8].

42. Eljamel MS, Mahboob SO. The effectiveness and cost-effectiveness of intraoperative imaging in high-grade glioma resection; a comparative review of intraoperative ALA, fluorescein, ultrasound and MRI. Photodiagnosis Photodyn Ther 2016;16: 35–43.

43. Ojemann GA. Individual variability in cortical localization of language. J Neurosurg 1979;50(2):164–9.

44. Hervey-Jumper SL, Li J, Lau D, et al. Awake craniotomy to maximize glioma resection: methods and technical nuances over a 27-year period. J Neurosurg 2015;123(2):325–39.

45. De Witt Hamer PC, Robles SG, Zwinderman AH, et al. Impact of intraoperative stimulation brain mapping on glioma surgery outcome: a meta-analysis. J Clin Oncol 2012;30(20):2559–65.

46. Chaichana KL, Zadnik P, Weingart JD, et al. Multiple resections for patients with glioblastoma: prolonging survival. J Neurosurg 2013;118(4):812–20.

47. Hervey-Jumper SL, Berger MS. Reoperation for recurrent high-grade glioma: a current perspective of the literature. Neurosurgery 2014;75(5):491–9 [discussion: 498–9].

48. Bloch O, Han SJ, Cha S, et al. Impact of extent of resection for recurrent glioblastoma on overall survival: clinical article. J Neurosurg 2012;117(6): 1032–8.

49. Keles GE, Anderson B, Berger MS. The effect of extent of resection on time to tumor progression and survival in patients with glioblastoma multiforme of the cerebral hemisphere. Surg Neurol 1999;52(4): 371–9.

50. Oppenlander ME, Wolf AB, Snyder LA, et al. An extent of resection threshold for recurrent glioblastoma and its risk for neurological morbidity. J Neurosurg 2014;120(4):846–53.

51. Chaichana KL, Jusue-Torres I, Navarro-Ramirez R, et al. Establishing percent resection and residual volume thresholds affecting survival and recurrence for patients with newly diagnosed intracranial glioblastoma. Neuro Oncol 2014;16(1):113–22.

52. Smith JS, Chang EF, Lamborn KR, et al. Role of extent of resection in the long-term outcome of low-grade hemispheric gliomas. J Clin Oncol 2008; 26(8):1338–45.

53. Ius T, Isola M, Budai R, et al. Low-grade glioma surgery in eloquent areas: volumetric analysis of extent of resection and its impact on overall survival. A single-institution experience in 190 patients: clinical article. J Neurosurg 2012;117(6):1039–52.

54. Capelle L, Fontaine D, Mandonnet E, et al. Spontaneous and therapeutic prognostic factors in adult hemispheric World Health Organization Grade II gliomas: a series of 1097 cases. J Neurosurg 2013;118(6):1157–68.

55. Grabowski MM, Recinos PF, Nowacki AS, et al. Residual tumor volume versus extent of resection: predictors of survival after surgery for glioblastoma. J Neurosurg 2014;121(5):1115–23.

56. Kelly PJ, Daumas-Duport C, Kispert DB, et al. Imaging-based stereotaxic serial biopsies in untreated intracranial glial neoplasms. J Neurosurg 1987; 66(6):865–74.

57. Yordanova YN, Moritz-Gasser S, Duffau H. Awake surgery for WHO Grade II gliomas within "noneloquent" areas in the left dominant hemisphere: toward a "supratotal" resection. Clinical article. J Neurosurg 2011;115(2):232–9.

58. Duffau H. Long-term outcomes after supratotal resection of diffuse low-grade gliomas: a consecutive series with 11-year follow-up. Acta Neurochir (Wien) 2016;158(1):51–8.

59. Kawaguchi T, Sonoda Y, Shibahara I, et al. Impact of gross total resection in patients with WHO grade III glioma harboring the IDH 1/2 mutation without the 1p/19q co-deletion. J Neurooncol 2016;129(3): 505–14.

60. Duffau H. Is supratotal resection of glioblastoma in noneloquent areas possible? World Neurosurg 2014;82(1–2):e101–3.

61. Nazzaro JM, Neuwelt EA. The role of surgery in the management of supratentorial intermediate and high-grade astrocytomas in adults. J Neurosurg 1990;73(3):331–44.

62. Kowalczuk A, Macdonald RL, Amidei C, et al. Quantitative imaging study of extent of surgical resection and prognosis of malignant astrocytomas. Neurosurgery 1997;41(5):1028–38.

63. Coffey RJ, Lunsford LD, Taylor FH. Survival after stereotactic biopsy of malignant gliomas. Neurosurgery 1988;22(3):465–73.

64. Pope WB, Sayre J, Perlina A, et al. MR imaging correlates of survival in patients with high-grade gliomas. AJNR Am J Neuroradiol 2005;26(10): 2466–74.

65. Hess KR. Extent of resection as a prognostic variable in the treatment of gliomas. J Neurooncol 1999;42(3):227–31.

66. Vuorinen V, Hinkka S, Farkkila M, et al. Debulking or biopsy of malignant glioma in elderly people - a randomised study. Acta Neurochir (Wien) 2003; 145(1):5–10.

67. Simpson JR, Horton J, Scott C, et al. Influence of location and extent of surgical resection on survival of patients with glioblastoma multiforme: results of three consecutive Radiation Therapy Oncology Group (RTOG) clinical trials. Int J Radiat Oncol Biol Phys 1993;26(2):239–44.

68. Stummer W, Reulen HJ, Meinel T, et al. Extent of resection and survival in glioblastoma multiforme:

identification of and adjustment for bias. Neurosurgery 2008;62(3):564–76 [discussion: 564–6].

69. Tykocki T, Eltayeb M. Ten-year survival in glioblastoma. A systematic review. J Clin Neurosci 2018; 54:7–13.

70. Giese A, Bjerkvig R, Berens ME, et al. Cost of migration: invasion of malignant gliomas and implications for treatment. J Clin Oncol 2003;21(8):1624–36.

71. Nelson DF, Nelson JS, Davis DR, et al. Survival and prognosis of patients with astrocytoma with atypical or anaplastic features. J Neurooncol 1985;3(2):99–103.

72. Ammirati M, Vick N, Liao YL, et al. Effect of the extent of surgical resection on survival and quality of life in patients with supratentorial glioblastomas and anaplastic astrocytomas. Neurosurgery 1987; 21(2):201–6.

73. Chang SM, Parney IF, McDermott M, et al. Perioperative complications and neurological outcomes of first and second craniotomies among patients enrolled in the Glioma Outcome Project. J Neurosurg 2003;98(6):1175–81.

74. Dützmann S, Geßler F, Bink A, et al. Risk of ischemia in glioma surgery: comparison of first and repeat procedures. J Neurooncol 2012;107(3):599–607.

75. Narita Y. Bevacizumab for glioblastoma. Ther Clin Risk Manag 2015;11:1759.

76. Chiocca EA, Lukas RV, Chen CC, et al. Controlled IL-12 in combination with a PD-1 inhibitor subjects with recurrent glioblastoma. American Society of Clinical Oncology; 2020. https://ascopubs.org/doi/abs/10.1200/JCO.2020.38.15_suppl.2510.

77. Carpentier A, Canney M, Vignot A, et al. Clinical trial of blood-brain barrier disruption by pulsed ultrasound. Sci Transl Med 2016;8(343):343re342.

78. Southwell DG, Birk HS, Han SJ, et al. Resection of gliomas deemed inoperable by neurosurgeons based on preoperative imaging studies. J Neurosurg 2018;129(3):567–75.

79. Capellades J, Teixidor P, Villalba G, et al. Results of a multicenter survey showing interindividual variability among neurosurgeons when deciding on the radicality of surgical resection in glioblastoma highlight the need for more objective guidelines. Clin Transl Oncol 2017;19(6):727–34.

80. Capellades J, Puig J, Domenech S, et al. Is a pretreatment radiological staging system feasible for suggesting the optimal extent of resection and predicting prognosis in glioblastoma? An observational study. J Neurooncol 2018;137(2):367–77.

81. Park JK, Hodges T, Arko L, et al. Scale to predict survival after surgery for recurrent glioblastoma multiforme. J Clin Oncol 2010;28(24):3838–43.

82. Chang EF, Smith JS, Chang SM, et al. Preoperative prognostic classification system for hemispheric low-grade gliomas in adults. J Neurosurg 2008; 109(5):817–24.

83. Shinoda J, Sakai N, Murase S, et al. Selection of eligible patients with supratentorial glioblastoma multiforme for gross total resection. J Neurooncol 2001;52(2):161–71.

84. Hervey-Jumper SL, Li J, Osorio JA, et al. Surgical assessment of the insula. Part 2: validation of the Berger-Sanai zone classification system for predicting extent of glioma resection. J Neurosurg 2016; 124(2):482–8.

85. Mandonnet E, Jbabdi S, Taillandier L, et al. Preoperative estimation of residual volume for WHO grade II glioma resected with intraoperative functional mapping. Neuro Oncol 2007;9(1):63–9.

Extent of Resection of Glioblastoma
A Critical Evaluation in the Molecular Era

Daniel P. Cahill, MD, PhD

KEYWORDS

• Glioma • Surgery • IDH1 mutation

KEY POINTS

- The evidence base for surgery differs for the 3 most common gliomas of adults.
- For patients with Glioblastoma IDH wild-type, the evidence supports a surgical strategy aiming for complete resection of enhancing disease.
- For patients with Astrocytoma IDH mutant, the evidence supports a maximal surgical strategy aiming for complete resection of enhancing and non-enhancing disease.
- For patients with Oligodendroglioma IDH mutant 1p19q-codeleted, the overall outcome is favorable due to an indolent natural history and effective radio-chemotherapeutic treatment; more-extensive resection may provide additional benefit.

INTRODUCTION

What is the goal of surgery for glioma? In the routine neurosurgical oncology practice there are 2 intertwined goals: diagnostic tissue acquisition and therapeutic cytoreduction. Although scant "level I" evidence exists, accumulating data support the proposal that more-extensive surgical resection has a pivotal role in improving survival in adults with glioma. With recent discoveries in glioma genetics now incorporated into the 2016 World Health Organization (WHO) Revised Classification of Tumors of the Central Nervous System,[1] a key conceptual advance has been recognition that gliomas segregate into distinct molecular groups; as a consequence, legacy WHO grading alone does not provide sufficient guidance for optimized surgical technique. Borrowing from the language of statistics, rather than considering the relationship between differently-graded tumors to be "ordinal" (ie, grades 2, 3, 4) as a stepwise progression, WHO2016 has underscored the need to transition to "nominal" consideration of these gliomas as distinct disease processes. Simply put, IDH mutant gliomas do not progress to become wild-type glioblastomas, and the evidence base for surgical resection of these different tumor types needs to be reevaluated separately. Herein, we consider the evidence base (**Table 1**) for surgical resection and treatment in the molecular era, with a focus on the 3 most common diffuse gliomas of adults: Glioblastoma IDH wild-type (which represents approximately 65%–70% of adult glioma), Astrocytoma IDH mutant (representing approximately 20%–25%), and Oligodendroglioma IDH mutant (5%–7%).

DIAGNOSTIC ACCURACY

For the initial surgical procedure in a patient with suspected adult diffuse glioma, accurate diagnosis is paramount. Before WHO2016, the existing dogma driving neurosurgical strategy was that accurate histologic grading was the most important goal of the surgical diagnostic procedure. However, the extent of surgery and histologic grading of

Funding: The author is supported by the NIH R01CA227821 and P50165862. The author also acknowledges support from the Tawingo Fund, the Loglio Foundation and OligoNation.
Department of Neurosurgery, Massachusetts General Hospital, Harvard Medical School, 55 Fruit Street, Yawkey 9E, Boston, MA 02114, USA
E-mail address: cahill@mgh.harvard.edu

neurosurgery.theclinics.com

Table 1
The three most common diffuse gliomas of adults

WHO Diagnosis	Typical Age	Co-Mutations	Evidenced Therapy
Astrocytoma, IDH mutant	20–40s	TP53, ATRX	Maximal surgery, PCV or TMZ + RT
Oligodendroglioma, IDH mutant, 1p/19q-codeleted	40–50s	TERT, CIC	PCV + RT
Glioblastoma, IDH wild-type	50–70s	TERT mutation, EGFR amplification, Chr 9p and 10 loss, Chr 7 gain	Resect enhancing disease, TMZ + RT

These 3 gliomas differ in typical age-of-presentation, and co-mutations, as indicated. Glioblastoma IDH wild-type represent approximately 65%-70% of adult gliomas. Astrocytoma IDH mutant represent approximately 20%-25%. Oligodendroglioma IDH mutant 1p/19q-codeleted only 5%-7%. The evidence for optimal therapy differs between these different tumors.
Abbreviations: CCNU, vincristine; Chr, chromosome; PCV, procarbazine; RT, radiation therapy; TMZ, temozolomide.

an adult diffuse glioma had been shown to be tightly linked. In a seminal paper, Dr Glantz and colleagues[2] examined 262 patients undergoing resection for suspected high-grade malignant glioma, and found that 214 (82%) were ultimately diagnosed with WHO grade IV glioblastomas and 48 (18%) with WHO grade III anaplastic astrocytoma (AA). Conversely, in a cohort of 67 comparable patients with suspected high-grade malignant glioma undergoing stereotactic biopsy, 33 (49%) were diagnosed with glioblastomas and 34 (51%) had AAs. The investigators concluded that "some AAs diagnosed by stereotactic biopsy are actually glioblastomas,"[2] underscoring the issues associated with undersampling that provide insufficient tissue for neuropathologic review to identify the presence of specific histopathological features diagnostic of grade IV disease, namely pseudopalisading necrosis and microvascular proliferation. Taking this a step further, Dr Jackson and his colleagues[3] from the MD Anderson Cancer Center evaluated biopsy and subsequent surgical resection diagnoses derived from the same patient, without intervening therapy. They noted that diagnoses based on biopsy and then subsequent resection in the same patient differed in 40 (49%) of 82 cases. These investigators concluded that stereotactic biopsy was therefore frequently inaccurate in providing a correct diagnosis.[3]

Thus, in the prior era, a convincing argument could be made for a more-extensive surgical procedure as a strategy to avoid the known limitation on accurate diagnosis imposed by surgical sampling error with limited biopsies. Patients who underwent biopsy-only could unfortunately too often have inaccurate grading by the legacy histologic criteria, suffering from so-called "undergrading," as there would be insufficient material sampled via a core needle biopsy for pathologic assessment of the entire tumor mass. Fear of this inaccuracy motivated substantial effort among the neurosurgical oncology community to improve radiographic imaging and stereotactic targeting of "more enhancing" areas of a suspected glioma, to improve the accuracy of grading by biopsy.

With the advent of modern molecular genomic analyses, this scenario occurs much less frequently,[4] because vastly smaller amounts of tissue are required for molecular testing. There are active efforts in the neuropathology community, led by the cIMPACT-NOW working group,[5] to advance the practical application of these molecular classifiers, freeing diagnosis and grading from dependency on volumetric sampling constraints. For instance, this working group has now identified at least 3 separate categories of glioma, which are grade 4 (transitioning to Arabic numerals in this updated classifier) - diffuse midline gliomas which are H3K27M-mutant,[6] progressive IDH mutant astrocytomas (formerly "secondary" glioblastomas),[7] and IDH wild-type gliomas containing either histologic features (microvascular proliferation or palisading necrosis) or molecular features (EGFR amplification, chromosome 7 gain or 10 loss, or TERT promoter mutation) of glioblastoma.[8] In the modern era with molecular classifiers, the demand for more-extensive surgery (or so-called "second look" procedures) to obtain a correct diagnosis has lessened. This has in turn highlighted the therapeutic role of surgery for different molecular categories of disease; for instance, it can be appreciated how the impact of aggressive surgery on survival could be different when comparing diffuse midline gliomas to glioblastoma IDH wild-type, despite both being grade 4 lesions.

THERAPEUTIC CYTOREDUCTION

Indeed, the second and perhaps most important goal of surgery, is to perform therapeutic cytore-duction to secure a prolonged survival and preservation of neurologic function for the patient. In the era preceding WHO2016, for glioblastoma this has traditionally meant that "complete resection of enhancement" was the intended surgical goal,[9,10] whereas for low-grade lesions, which are characteristically nonenhancing, this has meant "complete resection of T2/FLAIR hyper-in-tensity."[11,12] The evidence base that supports these surgical strategies requires updating in the context of the new WHO2016 diagnostic criteria.

Given the infiltrative biology of diffuse gliomas, no surgery can completely remove all tumor cells from the surrounding cortex. Surgical procedures should be guided by the evidence detailing what the optimal surgical result is for each patient, to extend survival and preserve neurologic function. The optimal amount of surgery is determined by the molecular diagnosis, not the WHO grade. Legacy terms like "glioblastoma" or "low-grade glioma" lack precision, and only serve to cloud careful consideration of the evidence. Furthermore, the thresholds of postoperative MRI residual disease for how we can measure surgical results also depend on this underlying diagnosis, and prior studies that form the evidence base for clinical decision-making need to be reassessed with an eye toward the updated WHO2016 molecular categories of tumor.

Importantly, undergrading in pre-WHO2016 studies complicated any retrospective analysis of surgical treatment, because biopsy-only diagnoses were more frequently "molecularly incorrect," and therefore not reflective of the more aggressive natural history of these tumors; resulting in a selection bias that made biopsy-only cohorts appear to have worse outcome when compared with more-extensively resected grade-matched cohorts. This diagnostic inaccuracy leads to an inherent flaw of pre-WHO2016 diagnoses in retrospective studies of surgical resection of lower-grade glioma (grades II and III), since the control groups, which were less-extensively resected, invariably included more grade IV tumors than the more-extensively resected group (as an example, potentially confounding the interpretation of the initial results from the Norwegian glioma study[13]).

When considering the evidence base from prior eras, it is critically important to keep in mind the relative frequency of the different molecular groups in these legacy cohorts, and whether the outcomes observed could be explained by "contamination" with mixed molecularly-heterogeneous cohorts. Notwithstanding these caveats, the evidence has shown that extensive resection is associated with a survival benefit in histologically defined glioblastoma (IDH wild-type) and also low-grade glioma (most frequently IDH mutant), but with important nuances with regards to the definition of disease assessment.

Glioblastoma IDH Wild-Type

There has been a small nonblinded randomized study that enrolled 30 elderly (age >65 years old) patients with suspected malignant glioma[14] for comparison of survival outcome with surgery versus biopsy. This randomized study under-scored the importance of prospective study design, as in 7 of these patients (23%) diagnoses of stroke, metastases, central nervous system lymphoma, and 1 nondiagnostic result were obtained. Nevertheless, the remaining cohort of 23 patients diagnosed with grade III or grade IV glioma were statistically likely to all have disease categorized as WHO 2016 glioblastoma IDH wild-type, given their older age at presentation. Conclusively for this randomized study, the patients who underwent surgical resection experienced prolonged survival. This element of survival benefit from surgery seems to be derived from the relief of mass effect, and prevention thereby of demise due to hydrocephalus or ischemia of deep brain structures from herniation. A more difficult question to answer in a randomized fashion has been whether small amounts of residual disease, so-called "near total" resection, is associated with worse outcome.

The signature study of surgery for grade IV gliomas was authored by Dr Lacroix and colleagues[9] from MD Anderson Cancer Center, who analyzed the extent-of-surgical resection and survival outcomes of 420 consecutive patients undergoing surgery for malignant glioma. This work is the most highly cited paper of the modern neurosurgical oncology literature. To briefly review this study given its importance, the investigators enrolled 420 consecutive patients diagnosed with GBM at MD Anderson Cancer Center between the years of 1993 and 1999. They prospectively recorded clinical and radiographic outcome data, and only 4 patients excluded due to incomplete imaging data. Within this cohort, 233 of 416 were previously untreated. The investigators used computer software to calculate enhancing tumor volume from axial T1-post contrast MRI images obtained preop and postop. From a statistical standpoint, most patients had aggressive surgery, but there was an otherwise good distribution of extent of resection (EOR, defined as [preoperative volume − postoperative volume]/preoperative volume) of enhancing disease at the extreme of near-complete resection, 47% of patients had greater-than-or-equal-to 98% EOR compared with 53% who had less than 98% EOR. In multivariate analysis using a Cox proportional hazards model: Age (<45, 45–64, >64), performance score (<80), necrosis, enhancement, and EOR (≥98%) were associated with survival. Similar results found in the previously untreated subset: age, Karnofsky performance status (KPS), necrosis, EOR, where more-extensive resection was associated with a 13.0-month versus 10.1-month survival for less-extensive resection.

In the era after the introduction of routine use of temozolomide for patients with glioblastoma, Dr Stummer and colleagues[15] performed a randomized study of 270 newly diagnosed glioblastoma patients who were deemed eligible for complete resection. Patients were assigned to surgical resection with either the fluorescent adjunct 5-ALA or the control arm of "white-light only." The outcome of this study demonstrated that complete resection was achieved in 65% of ALA cases versus 36% of white-light cases.[15] As noted by Drs Barker and Chang,[16] this trial likely represents the first large multicenter study that randomly allocated patients eligible for a complete resection between 2 types of surgical methodology (5-ALA guidance vs white-light only). Subsequent reanalysis of survival between patients who received gross-total resection compared subtotal resection demonstrated an approximate 5-month survival benefit (16.7 vs 11.8 months) associated with gross-total resection,[10] which stands at the current best level of evidence for complete resection of enhancing disease as a surgical goal for Glioblastoma IDH wild-type.

Intriguingly, in one of the first surgical analyses to perform molecular stratification by IDH status, the results of Beiko and colleagues[17] largely mirrored these results by dividing grade III and IV astrocytic gliomas into IDH wild-type and IDH mutant cohorts. In patients with IDH wild-type gliomas, absence of residual postoperative enhancement was associated with a median survival of 17.4 months, compared with 9.9 months in patients with residual enhancement. This survival benefit was significant after controlling for other factors in multivariate analysis. It was also significant in legacy (histologic) glioblastomas, essentially mirroring the findings of Lacroix and colleagues[9] and Stummer and colleagues.[15] Importantly however, residual nonenhancing disease had no observable impact on survival in patients with IDH wild-type tumors, when scored as continuous volumetric measure (95% confidence interval [CI] 0.99–1.01, $P = .608$).[17]

Astrocytoma IDH Mutant

To capture historical cohorts likely to be IDH mutant, we look to studies of strictly defined low-grade glioma (grade II) from prior eras, as they are likely to have cohorts that are 80% or more IDH mutant. Grade III cohorts of anaplastic tumors are often an even mixture of the IDH mutant and wild-type tumors, and therefore difficult to interpret in the modern era. In an important observational study, Dr Shaw and colleagues[12] followed the outcomes of 111 patients from the RTOG 9802 study of low-grade glioma assigned to observation after surgeon-determined gross-total resection. They assessed clinical factors associated with better outcome in these patients. The most favorable risk cohort shared 3 factors: less than 1 cm residual tumor (as postoperative MRI would, on occasion, identify residual tumor even in surgeon-determined gross-total resection cases), preoperative tumor diameter <4 cm, and oligodendroglioma histologic type, with resulting 2-year and 5-year progression-free survival rates of 100% and 70%. The favorable natural history of this cohort suggested that more-extensive surgical resection may be causally associated with better outcome. In a notable single institution study, Dr Smith and colleagues[11] from the University of California San Francisco demonstrated an association between gross-total resection and survival in low-grade gliomas, with a median survival of approximately 10 years in subtotally resected cases, which was significantly exceeded by the median of "not reached" in patients who underwent gross-total resection of disease.

Intriguingly, in the study of Beiko and colleagues,[17] patients with IDH1-mutant malignant astrocytic glioma also displayed a substantial survival benefit in association with more-extensive resection of nonenhancing disease. These patients had impressively favorable prognosis, despite putative malignant grading (grades III and IV); indeed, the survival of more-extensively resected T2-weighted-fluid-attenuated inversion recovery (T2/FLAIR) cohort largely matched the results from the study by Smith and colleagues[11] of grade II gliomas, suggesting that the common feature driving "surgical responsiveness" was their IDH mutant classification, and not their WHO grading. Several subsequent studies have demonstrated consistent results pointing toward extended survival with more-extensive resection of nonenhancing disease

n the astrocytoma IDH mutant subgroup of pa-
ients.[18–20] Thus, for patients with astrocytoma
DH mutant, these findings suggest that extensive
esection of both enhancing and nonenhancing
(T2/FLAIR hyperintense) disease should be pursued, regardless of WHO grade.[21] Consideration
should be given to staging of second surgical procedures, using advanced assessment techniques
such as intraoperative MRI or ultrasound, to pursue
these radical resections.

Of note, IDH mutant gliomas have characteristic
anatomic location of presentation, more
commonly arising in the frontal lobe, with a more
frequent unilateral pattern of growth, sharp tumor
margin, and less contrast enhancement.[22] These
anatomic features suggest that IDH mutant gliomas could be relatively more feasible for resection, when compared with their wild-type
counterparts. Also, patients with IDH mutant gliomas also display relatively preserved neurocognitive function (NCF) and better performance
scores than those with similarly sized IDH wild-
type gliomas.[23] Because IDH mutant gliomas are
predominantly located in frontal lobe and cause
less disturbance of adjacent normal brain, these
tumors may also be intrinsically more amenable
to maximal resection.[17]

Oligodendroglioma, IDH Mutant, 1p/19q Codeleted

Comprising approximately 5% to 7% of adult
diffuse gliomas, oligodendroglioma IDH mutant
1p/19q-codeleted tumors represent perhaps the
first molecularly defined glioma.[24] Somewhat sur-
prisingly, it is difficult to demonstrate a survival
benefit for more-extensive surgery in this cohort,[25]
likely due to 2 factors. First, these patients often
present at older age compared with astrocytoma
IDH mutant,[20] presumably reflecting their more
slow-growing natural history. As such, a prolonged
survival in many cases will start to extend into decades of life when more common systemic diseases become life-limiting. In addition, the
prolonged natural history of oligodendroglioma
can require an extensive follow-up of 1 or more decades to determine the survival benefit of an effective therapy.[27] Thus, although it is likely that more-
extensive surgery provides a survival benefit to
these patients, and indeed in some cases offers
a result that is, effectively a "cure" by bridging patients into the more routine health scenarios of the
elderly, it remains to be well demonstrated by the
existing evidence.

For the clinical scenario of patients who present with suspected IDH mutant disease, but
with question as to whether the tumor is likely

to be astrocytoma or oligodendroglioma, it is
worthwhile to note that a recently discovered
radiographic biomarker, termed "T2/FLAIR
mismatch" can be a highly specific marker of
astrocytic glioma.[28] This sign is positive when
the T2-weighted image demonstrates complete
or near-complete hyperintense signal throughout
the lesion, and comparatively the FLAIR
sequence displays the central majority of lesion
to be relatively hypointense signal when
compared with T2 image, with the exception of
a peripheral rim of hyperintense signal. Although
not highly sensitive, this mismatch sign has
been shown to be highly specific, when scored
correctly, for astrocytoma IDH mutant and might
therefore have utility to prompt more aggressive
resection in this tumor type.[29]

Less Frequent Tumor Molecular Subtypes

There are 2 minor frequency (~1% each) tumor
subtypes worthy of mention: BRAF-mutant glioma,
and histone H3.3 mutant diffuse midline glioma.
These gliomas are more commonly found in
younger adults, with the age of presentation
extending into the older pediatric cohorts as well.
The diffuse midline gliomas, understandably due
to their typical anatomic localization at presentation
within the spinal cord, brainstem or thalamus, do
not have evidence of benefit from more-extensive
surgical resection. The prognosis of these tumors
is dismal, worse than glioblastoma IDH wild-type
in most studies. On the other hand, the BRAF-
altered gliomas are an emerging subclass that harbors diverse legacy histologic correlates, including
pilocytic astrocytoma, gangliogliomas, pleomor-
phic xanthoastrocytoma, diffuse glioma, and
epithelioid malignant glioma. Regrouping and
refinement of these interrelated legacy histologies
is under way[30]; however, the well-established historical benefit of aggressive surgical resection for
pilocytic astrocytoma seems to be at least partially
reflected in studies of "pediatric-type" BRAF-
mutant diffuse gliomas.[31] These gliomas warrant
close neurosurgical study in the future.

Last, intraoperative technologies to rapidly
assess for signature mutations (IDH1, IDH2,
BRAF, TERT, H3F3A) have been preliminarily pro-
visioned.[32–34] Combined with preoperative radiologic biomarkers, advances in these technologies
may allow the surgical strategy to determine the
degree of resection to be adjusted intraoperatively
during a surgical procedure.

SUMMARY

In conclusion, with the 2016 revision of the WHO
diagnostic criteria, surgery for adult diffuse

gliomas has become even more tightly integrated with radiology and pathology, in both the diagnostic phase as well as the surgical treatment of these diseases. Certain classes of glioma, such as astrocytoma IDH mutant, display a substantial survival benefit in association with maximal resection, regardless of tumor grade under the legacy criteria. Thus, individualization of surgical strategy for patients with gliomas has advanced significantly in the modern era.

CLINICS CARE POINTS

- For patients with Glioblastoma IDH wild-type, the evidence supports a surgical strategy aiming for complete resection of enhancing disease. For the rare non-enhancing glioblastoma IDH wild-type, debulking can be pursued if safe, but there is scant evidence to indicate that this practice confers a survival benefit.
- For patients with Astrocytoma IDH mutant, the evidence supports a maximal surgical strategy of complete resection of enhancing and non-enhancing disease. There is an impressive prolongation of survival associated with minimization of residual disease burden in this cohort of patients.
- For patients with Oligodendroglioma IDH mutant 1p19q-codeleted, the overall outcome is favorable due to an indolent natural history and effect adjuvant treatment regimens; as such, more-extensive resection may provide additional benefit, but has been difficult to definitively link with further improvement in outcome, in part due to the need for prolonged follow-up (>decade) for any potential survival difference to become apparent.

DISCLOSURE

D.P. Cahill has received honoraria and travel reimbursement from Merck and has served as a consultant for Lilly and Boston Pharmaceuticals.

REFERENCES

1. Louis DN, Ohgaki H, Wiestler OD, et al, editors. World Health Organization histological classification of tumours of the central nervous system. Lyon, France: International Agency for Research on Cancer; 2016.
2. Glantz MJ, Burger PC, Herndon JE 2nd, et al. Influence of the type of surgery on the histologic diagnosis in patients with anaplastic gliomas. Neurology 1991;41(11):1741–4.
3. Jackson RJ, Fuller GN, Abi-Said D, et al. Limitations of stereotactic biopsy in the initial management of gliomas. Neuro Oncol 2001;3(3):193–200.
4. Kim BY, Jiang W, Beiko J, et al. Diagnostic discrepancies in malignant astrocytoma due to limited small pathological tumor sample can be overcome by IDH1 testing. J Neurooncol 2014;118(2):405–12.
5. Louis DN, Aldape K, Brat DJ, et al. Announcing cIMPACT-NOW: the consortium to inform molecular and practical approaches to CNS Tumor Taxonomy. Acta Neuropathol 2017;133(1):1–3.
6. Louis DN, Giannini C, Capper D, et al. cIMPACT-NOW update 2: diagnostic clarifications for diffuse midline glioma, H3 K27M-mutant and diffuse astrocytoma/anaplastic astrocytoma, IDH-mutant. Acta Neuropathol 2018;135(4):639–42.
7. Brat DJ, Aldape K, Colman H, et al. cIMPACT-NOW update 5: recommended grading criteria and terminologies for IDH-mutant astrocytomas. Acta Neuropathol 2020;139(3):603–8.
8. Brat DJ, Aldape K, Colman H, et al. cIMPACT-NOW update 3: recommended diagnostic criteria for "Diffuse astrocytic glioma, IDH-wildtype, with molecular features of glioblastoma, WHO grade IV. Acta Neuropathol 2018;136(5):805–10.
9. Lacroix M, Abi-Said D, Fourney DR, et al. A multivariate analysis of 416 patients with glioblastoma multiforme: prognosis, extent of resection, and survival. J Neurosurg 2001;95(2):190–8.
10. Stummer W, Reulen HJ, Meinel T, et al. Extent of resection and survival in glioblastoma multiforme: identification of and adjustment for bias. Neurosurgery 2008;62(3):564–76 [discussion: 564–6].
11. Smith JS, Chang EF, Lamborn KR, et al. Role of extent of resection in the long-term outcome of low-grade hemispheric gliomas. J Clin Oncol 2008; 26(8):1338–45.
12. Shaw EG, Berkey B, Coons SW, et al. Recurrence following neurosurgeon-determined gross-total resection of adult supratentorial low-grade glioma: results of a prospective clinical trial. J Neurosurg 2008;109(5):835–41.
13. Jakola AS, Myrmel KS, Kloster R, et al. Comparison of a strategy favoring early surgical resection vs a strategy favoring watchful waiting in low-grade gliomas. JAMA 2012;308(18):1881–8.
14. Vuorinen V, Hinkka S, Farkkila M, et al. Debulking or biopsy of malignant glioma in elderly people - a randomised study. Acta Neurochir (Wien) 2003; 145(1):5–10.
15. Stummer W, Pichlmeier U, Meinel T, et al. Fluorescence-guided surgery with 5-aminolevulinic acid for resection of malignant glioma: a randomised controlled multicentre phase III trial. Lancet Oncol 2006;7(5):392–401.

16. Barker FG 2nd, Chang SM. Improving resection of malignant glioma. Lancet Oncol 2006;7(5): 359–60.

17. Beiko J, Suki D, Hess KR, et al. IDH1 mutant malignant astrocytomas are more amenable to surgical resection and have a survival benefit associated with maximal surgical resection. Neuro Oncol 2014;16(1):81–91.

18. Kawaguchi T, Sonoda Y, Shibahara I, et al. Impact of gross total resection in patients with WHO grade III glioma harboring the IDH 1/2 mutation without the 1p/19q co-deletion. J Neurooncol 2016;129(3): 505–14.

19. Jakola AS, Skjulsvik AJ, Myrmel KS, et al. Surgical resection versus watchful waiting in low-grade gliomas. Ann Oncol 2017;28(8):1942–8.

20. Wijnenga MMJ, French PJ, Dubbink HJ, et al. The impact of surgery in molecularly defined low-grade glioma: an integrated clinical, radiological, and molecular analysis. Neuro Oncol 2018;20(1):103–12.

21. Taylor JW, Chi AS, Cahill DP. Tailored therapy in diffuse gliomas: using molecular classifiers to optimize clinical management. Oncology (Williston Park) 2013;27(6):504–14.

22. Lai A, Kharbanda S, Pope WB, et al. Evidence for sequenced molecular evolution of IDH1 mutant glioblastoma from a distinct cell of origin. J Clin Oncol 2011;29(34):4482–90.

23. Wefel JS, Noll KR, Rao G, et al. Neurocognitive function varies by IDH1 genetic mutation status in patients with malignant glioma prior to surgical resection. Neuro Oncol 2016;18(12):1656–63.

24. Cahill DP, Louis DN, Cairncross JG. Molecular background of oligodendroglioma: 1p/19q, IDH, TERT, CIC and FUBP1. CNS Oncol 2015;4(5):287–94.

25. Ding X, Wang Z, Chen D, et al. The prognostic value of maximal surgical resection is attenuated in oligodendroglioma subgroups of adult diffuse glioma: a multicenter retrospective study. J Neurooncol 2018;140(3):591–603.

26. Killela PJ, Pirozzi CJ, Healy P, et al. Mutations in IDH1, IDH2, and in the TERT promoter define clinically distinct subgroups of adult malignant gliomas. Oncotarget 2014;5(6):1515–25.

27. Cairncross JG, Wang M, Jenkins RB, et al. Benefit from procarbazine, lomustine, and vincristine in oligodendroglial tumors is associated with mutation of IDH. J Clin Oncol 2014;32(8):783–90.

28. Patel SH, Poisson LM, Brat DJ, et al. T2-FLAIR mismatch, an imaging biomarker for IDH and 1p/19q status in lower-grade gliomas: A TCGA/TCIA Project. Clin Cancer Res 2017;23(20):6078–85.

29. Jain R, Johnson DR, Patel SH, et al. Real world" use of a highly reliable imaging sign: "T2-FLAIR mismatch" for identification of IDH mutant astrocytomas. Neuro Oncol 2020;22(7):936–43.

30. Ellison DW, Hawkins C, Jones DTW, et al. cIMPACT-NOW update 4: diffuse gliomas characterized by MYB, MYBL1, or FGFR1 alterations or BRAF(V600E) mutation. Acta Neuropathol 2019;137(4):683–7.

31. Lassaletta A, Zapotocky M, Mistry M, et al. Therapeutic and prognostic implications of BRAF V600E in pediatric low-grade gliomas. J Clin Oncol 2017; 35(25):2934–41.

32. Santagata S, Eberlin LS, Norton I, et al. Intraoperative mass spectrometry mapping of an oncometabolite to guide brain tumor surgery. Proc Natl Acad Sci U S A 2014;111(30):11121–6.

33. Shankar GM, Francis JM, Rinne ML, et al. Rapid intraoperative molecular characterization of glioma. JAMA Oncol 2015;1(5):662–7.

34. Diplas BH, Liu H, Yang R, et al. Sensitive and rapid detection of TERT promoter and IDH mutations in diffuse gliomas. Neuro Oncol 2019;21(4):440–50.

Advancing Imaging to Enhance Surgery
From Image to Information Guidance

Marco Riva, MD[a,b,*], Egesta Lopci, MD, PhD[c], Lorenzo G. Gay, MD[b,d], Marco Conti Nibali, MD[b,d], Marco Rossi, MD[b,d], Tommaso Sciortino, MD[b,d], Antonella Castellano, MD, PhD[e], Lorenzo Bello, MD[b,d]

KEYWORDS

- Glioblastoma • Surgery • Magnetic resonance imaging (MRI) • PET • Presurgical planning
- Image guidance • Radiomics

KEY POINTS

- Glioblastomas have tissue heterogeneity and an infiltrative nature beyond the contrast-enhanced region that cannot be fully resolved with conventional imaging.
- Radiomics and radiogenomics are transforming images into mineable data, contributing to identifying biomarkers of molecular features with clinical relevance and leading a paradigm shift from image guidance to information guidance.
- Advanced imaging can optimize diagnostic workflow and therapeutic strategies.

INTRODUCTION
Background

The continuous advancements of scanning procedures and processes for the extraction of quantitative features have revolutionized the traditional view of medical images as pictures intended solely for visual interpretation. These ongoing improvements are toggling images into mineable data that can be analyzed to support clinical decisions; this practice has been termed, *radiomics*.[1]

The improved understanding of the genomic signatures underlying gliomas[2–4] led to a new brain tumor classification.[5] Intense efforts have been undertaken to make imaging capable of depicting distinct phenotypes, of identifying biomarkers of molecular features, and of providing a quantitative report of the findings. This effort has been referred to as *radiogenomics*.[6,7]

Imaging is essential in the management of gliomas, providing morphologic, functional, and metabolic data that support the diagnosis, treatment planning, and follow-up of patients and response to therapies.

A Paradigm Shift: From Image Guidance to Information Guidance in Brain Surgery

Image guidance is a term used to identify the use of imaging in brain surgery. The power of scanning and analytical methods has rendered images an invaluable source of data, leading to a paradigm shift[8,9]: from image-guided surgery to information-guided surgery.

a Department of Medical Biotechnology and Translational Medicine, Università degli Studi di Milano, Via Festa del Perdono 7, Milan 20122, Italy; b IRCCS Istituto Ortopedico Galeazzi, U.O. Neurochirurgia Oncologica, Milan, Italy; c Unit of Nuclear Medicine, Humanitas Clinical and Research Center - IRCCS, Via Manzoni 56, Rozzano, Milan 20089, Italy; d Department of Oncology and Hemato-Oncology, Via Festa del Perdono 7, Milan 20122, Italy; e Neuroradiology Unit and CERMAC, Vita-Salute San Raffaele University, IRCCS San Raffaele Scientific Institute, Via Olgettina 60, Milan 20123, Italy
* Corresponding author.
E-mail address: marco.riva@unimi.it
Twitter: @mriva_eu (M.R.); @LopciEgesta (E.L.); @dr_mcn (M.C.N.); @antocastella (A.C.)

Neurosurg Clin N Am 32 (2021) 31–46
https://doi.org/10.1016/j.nec.2020.08.003
1042-3680/21/

The brain surgeon can employ refined imaging to guide the management of gliomas within an integrated analysis of various data regarding anatomic, functional, and histopathologic characteristics. In the pursuit of precision medicine,[10] validated biomarkers are essential to enable a tailored care.

It also is currently acknowledged that most solid tumors, including glioblastoma multiforme (GBM), have both spatial and temporal heterogeneity.[11–15] This heterogeneity cannot be fully resolved accurately, timely, and noninvasively. Such a lack of information can hamper the choice of the right type of treatment, including surgery, especially, the targeted therapies available and under clinical development and validation.[16]

This review analyzes the shift from image guidance to information guidance and the limitations that are still are challenging, with a distinct emphasis on the role and benefits for brain surgery of GBMs.

CURRENT EVIDENCE
Conventional Magnetic Resonance Imaging

Conventional magnetic resonance imaging (cMRI) is the elective neuroradiological technique for the study of GBMs.[16] The cMRI assesses the T2/fluid-attenuated inversion recovery (FLAIR) abnormality and the enhancement on postcontrast T1-weighted images, due to the extravasation of contrast agents through the abnormal tumor blood-brain barrier. cMRI typically depicts an enhancing, necrotic-appearing mass surrounded by nonenhancing signal abnormalities. Hemorrhage, cystic changes, or multicentric enhancements also frequently are present.[17,18]

cMRI is accurate in providing essential morphologic details of the tumor and of its adjacent neural and vascular structures. cMRI also assesses the disease burden, that is, whether the tumor changes are restricted to 1 anatomic site or appear at a macroscopic level[19] as a multicentric disease. Considering the rapid growth and expansion and the infiltrative behavior of GBMs,[20,21] cMRI also depicts the displacement of brain structures resulting from the mass effect. These features confidentially lead to a radiological diagnosis of GBMs in the vast majority of cases. Differential diagnosis still should be considered, however, with other intra-axial (metastasis, lower-grade gliomas, and lymphoma) and non-neoplastic lesions (abscess and demyelinating diseases) that can have overlapping imaging findings and eventually may require further diagnostic work-up.

The Contribution of Conventional Magnetic Resonance Imaging to Brain Surgery

The information that cMRI conveys is pivotal for the initial therapeutic management, to establish the indication and the type of surgery, the surgical planning of the resection, and the assessment of the potential risks of the procedure.[22] cMRI also is advised within 48 hours from surgery to assess the extent of resection (EOR).[23] EOR is among the most relevant prognostic factors for GBMs, because the maximal resection of the contrast-enhancing tumor (CET) on T1-weighted magnetic resonance imaging (MRI) has been consistently associated with more prolonged survival in both newly diagnosed[24–32] and recurrent[33–37] GBMs. This evidence argues for surgery to pursue the gross total resection of the enhancing solid tumor mass in patients with GBMs, whenever feasible and safe.[16] Preventing new neurologic deficits is a crucial priority because postoperative complications are a negative prognostic factor.[38,39] In the postoperative cMRI, diffusion-weighted imaging (DWI) is essential to detect possible cytotoxic edema, reflecting ischemic alterations at the margins of the resection that eventually enhance after 48 hours. If imaging is performed after 48 hours, contrast enhancement may be misinterpreted as a residual tumor, potentially having an impact on future evaluations.

cMRI is essential for the accurate diagnosis. It contributes to guiding therapeutic decisions and monitoring disease status.[40,41] As such, cMRI consistently has been advocated as a crucial disease parameter in both clinicosurgical practice and clinical trials.[16] In this context, efforts to develop a standardized imaging protocol also have been made to reduce variability and increase reliability.[42]

CLINICAL RELEVANCE

The progress in the treatment of GBMs has been slower than that observed in the majority of the extracranial malignancies. GBMs inexorably develop ultimate treatment resistance. Before new therapeutics options and delivery strategies become clinically available, it is essential, therefore, to optimize current therapies to improve overall survival and progression-free survival, to preserve the quality of life throughout the disease and, with longer survival, to eventually benefit the patients with new emerging therapeutic options.[16,43]

Conventional Magnetic Resonance Imaging, Contrast Enhancement, and the Extent of Resection

The primary therapeutic management of GBMs consists of the surgical resection of the CET followed by adjuvant therapies.[16,44] The gross total resection of the enhancing tumor is associated with longer survival in both adult and elderly subjects.[32,45,46] Gross total resection thus can be regarded as the neurosurgical standard of care. Despite extensive efforts to reach a total resection of the CET components with several intraoperative technologies and adjuncts, the potential gains from improved resection of the CET currently seem plateauing.

Resection with clear margins is a common concept in surgical oncology. It is virtually unfeasible, however, for GBMs because the neoplastic cells remain in the macroscopically normal-appearing brain tissue due to their highly infiltrative nature.[19,47,48] GBMs are highly infiltrative tumors, with neoplastic cells extending beyond the contrast-enhancing lesion. Retrospective case series studies also reported an improved survival of patients who received resection of the non-CET (nCET) of GBMs as depicted by the T2/FLAIR sequence.[49–53] These studies reported an additional prognostic benefit of 5 months to 13 months over patients who received resection merely of the CET. Although the quality of evidence is not yet robust due to the number of enrolled subjects and the retrospective mono-institutional study design, these initial results claims for reconsidering the definition of the EOR. In particular, what can be considered a total resection? Has a so-called supratotal or supramaximal resection[54–56] to be pursued in patients with GBMs[57]?

Collaterally, different studies employed slightly different thresholds for defining the resection; as a result, qualitative definitions of subtotal, gross-total and near-total resections are found, arbitrarily corresponding, respectively, to 90%, 95%, and 99% EOR. Therefore, caution must be used when comparing different studies using qualitative definitions. A precise quantitative measure for the EOR or alternative reporting methods, such as the residual tumor volume (RTV),[30,58] are advocated for agreeing on the measure that most reliably describes the disease burden of pathobiological relevance. Although most studies focused on the prognostic impact of the preoperative tumor volume and of the EOR, fewer[24,30,58] analyzed the RTV as a volumetric measurement of postoperative MRI-detectable abnormalities, either CET or nCET, to assess the impact of surgery and the relevance of eventual tumor burden to be targeted by adjuvant treatments. Nevertheless, available studies[24,30,58] provided meaningful data to argue that the RTV of both nonenhancing and enhancing components of GBM can stratify patients into distinct survival groups better than the EOR before the start of the medical therapies. Because it is a ratio, EOR is not an absolute measure and, as such, its biological impact is strongly dependent on the preoperative lesion volume. Also, regarding the RTV, given that tumor-infiltrated brain tissue does not invariably enhance on MRI, controversy persists about which measure better depicts the actual extent of the tumor burden between the enhancing or the nonenhancing (ie, T2/FLAIR) RTV.[58] Both measurements also could suffer from methodological limitations[30]: differential diagnoses among true pathologic and nonpathologic signal abnormalities are not trivial, because brain shift, hemostatic agents, hemosiderin deposits, surgical damage of the blood-brain barrier, and hypoxic-ischemic injuries make the evaluation of the immediate postoperative MRI scans user dependent and experience dependent, thus calling for more automated and reproducible methods. Although the acknowledged value of the EOR is not diminished, the benefit yielded by extensive resection could be attributed to smaller RTVs that have been neglected in previous studies focusing merely on EOR. The RTV thus could be used in clinical practice to differently convey the pathobiological impact and meaning of surgical resection to clinicians and patients before adjuvant treatments.

It also is essential to tailor the definition of supratotal when applied to GBMs to find a shared definition that can be employed for a multi-institutional confirmation of the initial clinical evidence. To precisely define the extent of disease beyond the pathologic enhancement also is mandatory for avoiding unnecessary risks to the patients and for improving the prognostic impact of surgery.

As a result, it thus is a strong priority to enhance the radiological detection of residual tissue in postoperative cMRIs, to also discriminate vital tumor from postsurgical abnormalities.[59] It is further relevant to investigate the nCET components,[60,61] to accurately depict and monitor them noninvasively with imaging. The nCET components have overlapping signal features with non-neoplastic abnormalities, such as edema, on T2/FLAIR sequences, hampering an accurate differential diagnosis. The nCET subregions of GBMs are not habitually resected, but they often are the primary site of recurrence or progression.[62]

These arguments also must be framed within a clear understanding of the association of the maximal EOR with the molecular subgroups for survival, which is essential for counseling patients and clinical-surgical decision making.

In this regard, a recent retrospective multi-institutional study reported a median survival of 37.3 months of subjects, younger than 65 years, receiving complete CET resection with less than

5.4 mL residual nCET, as measured on postoperative T2/FLAIR cMRI, of pathologically proved GBMs. The younger patients with complete CET, near-total (median 90% resection) nCET resection, and isocitrate dehydrogenase (IDH) wild-type tumor showed an overlapping survival with patients with IDH-mutant tumors within the first 3 years of treatments. These results were confirmed after adjusting for other clinical and molecular prognostic variables and with 2 validation sets from different institutes. This study thus represents a new robust source of evidence that the surgical resection of both CET and nCET on cMRI has a prognostic impact in the management of younger (<65 years) patients with GBMs, independently from IDH and O(6)-methylguanine-DNA methyltransferase (MGMT) status. These results set the momentum for the proposal for an updated surgical strategy. This strategy keeps as a priority to maximize the EOR to the morpho-functional limits and to avoid postoperative morbidity, with the aid of advanced preoperative and intraoperative imaging modalities and intraoperative stimulation mapping.[63–67]

As for what imaging is concerned, given the survival benefit that is emerging from aggressive surgery, a better characterization of signal abnormalities additional to the CET and accurate differential diagnosis of these from other pathologic entities is of paramount relevance to optimize the available therapeutic strategies. cMRI is limited in resolution for such a characterization to guide a more aggressive resection. Therefore, it is needed to improve the delineation of nCET from edema and of tumor parts with an intact blood-brain barrier that, lacks enhancement.[68,69] A better characterization of eloquent subcortical structures also can be beneficial for the preoperative risk assessment and to contribute to safety. Advanced imaging is advocated to overcome current limitations of cMRI in depicting the actual tumor extent, additional to the CET, and the eloquent white matter structures. It is essential to avoid both false-negative and false-positive radiological reports, which can be detrimental for safety (not halting the resection before morpho-functional eloquent landmarks) and for the EOR (halting the resection before it can be considered complete), respectively. To develop better methods to detect nonenhancing lesion burden would optimize surgical and radiation planning while minimizing risks to the truly healthy parenchyma.

ADVANCED IMAGING FOR IMPROVING INFORMATION GUIDANCE

Advanced imaging is asked to address distinct unmet challenges in neurosurgical oncology to increase the amount and quality of information that cMRI can convey to surgery for better guidance: (1) to improve the spatial resolution of the lesion tissue heterogeneity and microstructural features (tumor core, infiltrative areas, and microenvironment), including a thorough characterization of nCET; (2) to better describe eloquent white matter structures[70,71]; (3) to investigate and validate imaging surrogates of molecular features (radiogenomics); (4) to develop computational analytical methods (radiomics), testing sensitivity, specificity, and accuracy in detecting signal abnormalities that are not discernible to the human eye; and (5) to research acquisition and evaluation methods to identify and quantify the tumor changes in response to the different types of therapies (ie, surgery, radiation therapy, chemotherapy, immunotherapy, and targeted therapies). It also will be beneficial to match eventual findings of advanced features with cMRI for the clinical practice and to develop standardized protocols. These efforts could ease widespread use across centers and multi-institutional studies, individualize the acquisition to the specific needs and clinical queries about the patient at a given time, and optimize examination time to be clinically feasible, with a reduction in patient discomfort for repeated scans over time.

The available imaging armamentarium and expected developing pipelines are (1) the application of quantitative imaging approaches, such as the analysis of texture features (ie, a pattern of local variations in image intensity) on cMRI images[72]; (2) advanced MRI techniques; and (3) different imaging modalities, such as PET.

Advanced Magnetic Resonance Imaging

Advanced MRI techniques, such as diffusion MRI (dMRI), perfusion-weighted imaging (PWI), and proton magnetic resonance spectroscopy (^{1}H-MRS) can provide a visual depiction and quantitative measurement of the pathophysiologic characteristics of the tumor.

Diffusion Magnetic Resonance Imaging

The dMRI-derived mean diffusivity, or apparent diffusion coefficient, is considered a measure of tumor cellularity, because the diffusion of extracellular water is abnormally restricted when tumor cells proliferate and disrupt the normal tissue architecture.[73] Quantitative apparent diffusion coefficient measurements in GBMs have been reported to predict the methylation status of the MGMT promoter and patients' survival.[74–76] Other metrics derived from diffusion tensor imaging may help characterizing the extent of tumor infiltration beyond the apparent margins on cMRI, thus reflecting glioma cells' invasion[77] according to the GBM molecular phenotype.[78]

Functional magnetic resonance imaging and diffusion magnetic resonance imaging tractography

Functional MRI and dMRI tractography have become an integral part of the preoperative assessment and intraoperative guidance for brain gliomas. These techniques provide information on the anatomical-functional organization of eloquent cortical areas and subcortical connections near or within a tumor to aid the maximal safe resection. Classical diffusion tensor imaging tractography approaches were proved valid and highly sensitive tools for localizing eloquent subcortical areas in glioma patients.[68] Newer diffusion models and tractography techniques, based on high angular resolution DWI (HARDI), have been developed to enhance the accuracy of magnetic resonance tractography for glioma surgery[68] (Fig. 1).

Perfusion-weighted imaging

PWI allows to measure changes associated with neoangiogenesis in GBMs both at first diagnosis (see Fig. 1; Fig. 2) and after treatment.[79–82] The dynamic susceptibility contrast (DSC)-derived relative cerebral blood volume (rCBV) is the most validated parameter,[83] with a reliable correlation with microvascular changes induced by neoangiogenesis, such as the increase of microvessel density.[84,85] Dynamic contrast-enhanced (DCE) is a further PWI technique that reflects a combination of tissue intravascular compartment volume (fractional volume of the intravascular compartment), microvessel permeability (volume transfer constant [K^{trans}]), and extravascular-extracellular space).[80,86,87] DCE allows a multiparametric quantification of tumor microvascular features. Notably, PWI-derived metrics have been shown to predict key molecular signatures, such EGFRvIII status in EGFR-amplified GBMs, with high accuracy, both alone or in combination with other conventional and advanced MRI features (cMRI, DWI, DSC, susceptibility-weighted imaging,[88,89] and PWI).[90–93] Finally, in the setting

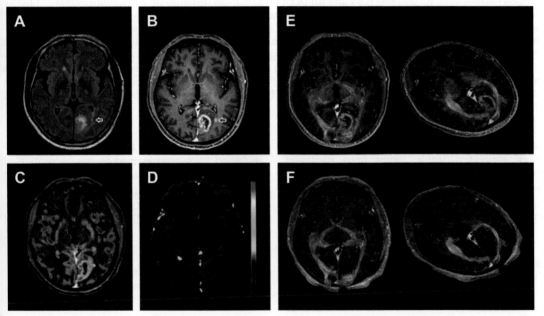

Fig. 1. Advanced MRI of a 64-year-old man with GBM (grade IV), IDH1 wild-type, and MGMT promoter methylation. Axial FLAIR (A) and T1-weighted postgadolinium (B) images demonstrate an inhomogeneous lesion in the left occipital lobe with strong but irregular ring enhancement surrounding a central nonenhancing necrotic core. A satellite, small enhancing nodule also is evident (open arrows). (C) DSC PWI rCBV and (D) DCE PWI K^{trans} maps demonstrate significantly increased perfusion and leakiness along the enhancing margins of the lesion. (E) Preoperative, 3-dimensional HARDI Q-ball tractography reconstructions superimposed on postgadolinium T1-weighted images demonstrate with high resolution the entire course of the optic pathways (orange) and their relationships with the tumor tissue: the left optic radiation runs very closely to the lateral margin of the lesion and of the satellite nodule. Surgery was performed with intraoperative visual-evoked potentials and tractography reconstructions available on the neuronavigation platform. (F) Postoperative contrast-enhanced T1-weighted images with superimposed preoperative tractography show a complete resection of both the lesions, with the left optic radiation aligned to the functional limits of resection along the border of the surgical cavity.

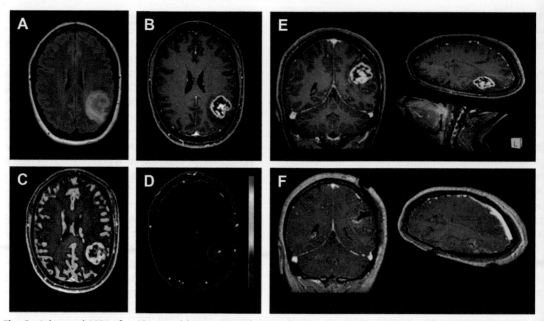

Fig. 2. Advanced MRI of a 42-year-old woman with GBM (grade IV), IDH2 mutated without MGMT promoter methylation. Axial FLAIR (*A*) and T1-weighted postgadolinium (*B*) images demonstrate an inhomogeneous lesion in the left parietal lobe with intense, irregular enhancement with a peripheral rim surrounding a central nonenhancing necrotic core. (*C*) DSC PWI rCBV and (*D*) DCE PWI *K^tran* maps demonstrate a moderate increase of perfusion and permeability along the enhancing margins of the lesion. (*E*) Three-dimensional rendering of preoperative HARDI Q-ball tractography reconstruction of the arcuate fascicle (red) superimposed on postgadolinium T1-weighted images show the relationship of this tract with the lesion: the deep portion of the tract runs in close contiguity to the deep margin of the lesion. Surgery was performed with intraoperative neurophysiological and neuropsychological monitoring and mapping techniques under the asleep-awake-asleep anesthesia regimen.[66] (*F*) Postoperative contrast-enhanced T1-weighted images with superimposed preoperative tractography show a complete resection of the lesion, with the left arcuate fascicle lining the border of the surgical cavity, thus aligned to the functional limits of resection.

of GBM follow-up, PWI-derived quantitative parameters separating viable tumor from treatment changes demonstrate relatively good accuracy in individual studies, with pooled sensitivities and specificities of 90% and 88%, respectively, for DSC and 89% and 85%, respectively, for DCE.[82]

Magnetic resonance spectroscopy

^{1}H-MRS provides metabolic biomarkers that complement MRI anatomic and physiologic information in gliomas.[94] ^{1}H-MRS has been used to detect in vivo the intratumoral accumulation of 2-hydroxyglutarate (2HG), a metabolite that is present at high levels in IDH-mutant GBMs.[95–98] Although still technically challenging, 2HG-MRS has demonstrated excellent diagnostic performance in the prediction of IDH-mutant glioma, with pooled sensitivity and specificity of 95% and 91%, respectively.[99] These findings open a new scenario for the noninvasive monitoring of the biological effects of new targeted therapies, such as inhibitors in IDH1-mutant gliomas.[100]

Specific studies are available that thoroughly reviewed each step leading to the generation of quantitative radiomics output from conventional and advanced MRI data (ie, image acquisition, processing, segmentation of tumor regions of interest, features extraction, data analyses, and validation).[1,6,72,101]

Advanced Magnetic Resonance Imaging and Tumor Microenvironment: Spatial Habitat Imaging

Applying advanced mathematical modeling, it also is possible to segment tumors into subregions containing clusters of voxels with similar quantitative radiomics features that represent and quantify tumor microenvironment heterogeneity.[102] Imaging of the tumor microenvironment, or spatial habitat imaging, has been applied mainly on cMRIs. Nevertheless, it can be virtually extended to any imaging modality, including PWI and dMRI, to scrutinize specific features to infer tumor behavior from imaging characteristics.

Intratumoral heterogeneity of oxygen metabolism combined with variable patterns of neovascularization, as depicted by advanced MRI, has been shown to affect the landscape of tumor microenvironments in GBM and correlate with prognosis.[103,104]

Molecular Imaging with Amino Acid PET

Molecular imaging based on nuclear medicine compounds retains 3 amino acid (AA) tracers as principal representatives for glioma assessment[105,106]: [11C-methyl]-methionine (11C-METH); O-(2-[18F]fluoroethyl)-L-tyrosine (18F-FET); and 3,4-dihydroxy-6-[18F]fluoro-L-phenylalanine (18F-FDOPA). Their mechanism of uptake is related to the L-AA transport system and their application in brain tumor imaging relies on the acknowledged enhancement of AA transport and protein synthesis in cancer cells, which are crucial for cell proliferation and growth as well as extracellular matrix production in gliomas.[107–109]

Evidence-based recommendations on the use of AA tracers in glioma imaging with PET[105] and practice guidelines about the procedure standards[106] recently have been released. In principal, AA-PET is utilized at primary glioma diagnosis, allowing tumor differentiation, glioma grading, and prognostication as well as definition of tumor delineation (**Fig. 3**) and can guide targeting optimal biopsy sites (**Fig. 4**) thanks to the definition of hot spots or areas with maximum tracer uptake.[110–116]

The role of AA-PET has been maintained also in the light of the new World Health Organization classification 2016 for brain tumors,[117] thanks to the significant differences observed in imaging variables obtained from 11C-METH PET and 18F-FET PET in gliomas with different mutational status or molecular characteristics.[113,114,118,119] Conversely, more contradictory results have been reported for 18F-FDOPA PET,[120,121] which might present with paradoxically increased uptake in IDH1-positive diffuse gliomas.

The use of imaging parameters to detect intrinsic glioma characteristics noninvasively largely has involved PET radiomics and more recently it has implicated artificial intelligence.[122,123] Although investigated at a lower extent compared with corresponding MRI radiomics, encouraging results on AA-PET suggest an accuracy of 93% in predicting grade-based texture features in GBM[124] and an accuracy of 90.66% in predicting glioma overall survival.[125]

Overall, 90% of primary brain tumors are detectable by AA-PET as hypermetabolic lesions, with a small proportion of cases resulting isometabolic or even hypometabolic compared with normal brain uptake.[126,127] Regardless of morphologic characteristics, the information provided by PET still proves valuable and clear photopenic (ie, hypometabolic) areas defined in negative 18F-FET PET scans correspond to different prognostic outcomes in grade III and grade IV gliomas.[127]

In comparison to conventional and advanced MRI, AA-PET retains a complementary role and allows a more precise distinction of gliomas due to the improved specificity and metabolic characterization,[114,128] even in cases of recurrence or when assessing the response from pseudoprogression or other treatment-related changes. For presumed recurrent glioma, the modality performs with a high sensitivity (range 96%–100%) and diagnostic accuracy (range 82%–94%).[126,129] Applying hybrid 11C-METH PET/MRI, AA-PET outperformed MRI and differentiated progression versus pseudoprogression with a 97.1% sensitivity and 93.3% specificity compared with 86.1% sensitivity and 71.4% specificity for MRI.[128,129]

DISCUSSION

Neurosurgery can take the momentum of advanced imaging to improve surgical practice and match the oncological needs of patients in a multidisciplinary context. Neurosurgery also can represent an essential validation ground of these techniques, linking noninvasive biomarkers to histomolecular data from targeted tissue samples.

An accurate and precise integrated histomolecular diagnosis at a given time is mandatory for treatment decisions and prognosis, especially in a time claiming for precision medicine,[130,131] because therapeutic options become increasingly depending on molecular features for both clinical and experimental management.[132,133]

The Information Yield of Advance Imaging to Brain Surgery

The molecular features currently relevant (ie, IDH mutation and MGMT methylation) for integrated diagnosis generally are homogeneously represented throughout the tumor tissue.[115,134,135] Therefore, a sampling error resulting in misclassification of acknowledged tumor molecular features that have current therapeutic and prognostic relevance[5] is unlikely both during open surgery and bioptic procedures if adequately performed. cMRI guides the appropriate site for sampling, targeting areas of enhancement likely containing viable tumor cells, preferably avoiding necrotic areas or adjacent nonneoplastic brain. Metabolic PET imaging also can support the targeting, increasing the diagnostic yield of stereotactic biopsies.[110,115,134]

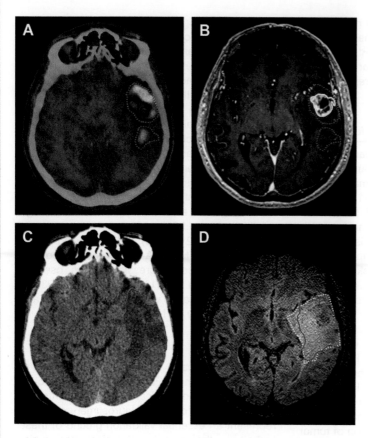

Fig. 3. Imaging findings of a 75-year-old man with GBM (grade IV), IDH1 wild-type, MGMT promoter methylation and 11p/19q codeletion. The coregistered 11C-METH PET/CT (*A*), gadolinium-enhanced MRI (*B*), axial low-dose CT (*C*), and FLAIR (*D*) are shown. The areas with intense PET tracer accumulation (maximum standardized uptake value 4.9; standardized uptake value ratio 3.5) are defined with red dotted lines (*A*, *B*) and superimposed on the corresponding region on MRI (*B*), in comparison to the extent of the enhanced area (*yellow line* [*B*]). Similarly, the hypodense/edematous area on localization CT (*red line* [*C*]) is placed in comparison to the altered FLAIR signal (*white dotted line* [*D*]).

Spatial and temporal heterogeneity of GBMs, however, is increasingly characterized and considered from the genomic to the phenotypic level.[13,15,48,132,136,137] The potential translation of these discoveries into improved patient outcomes is yet to come. Validated and reproducible methods thus are needed to resolve both intralesional (spatial) and longitudinal (temporal) heterogeneity of these tumors that is related to both tumor natural history and the treatment-related

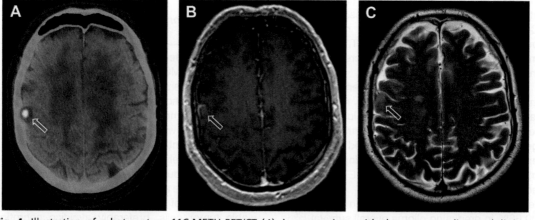

Fig. 4. Illustration of a hot-spot on 11C-METH PET/CT (*A*), in comparison with the corresponding gadolinium-enhanced MRI (*B*) and T2-weighted views (*C*). The lesion indicated with the arrows corresponds to an anaplastic astrocytoma (grade III), IDH1 wild-type, not methylated and not codeleted. The focal uptake on PET (maximum standardized uptake value 5.5; standardized uptake value ratio 5) is clearly visible, whereas a faint signal is seen on gadolinium-enhanced (*B*) or T2-weighted MRI (*C*).

effects. In particular, advanced imaging methods can contribute effectively to target sampling to areas with biological relevance for an impactful clinical strategy.[138]

By clinical convention, current sampling still is guided by the enhancement of cMRI. This policy assumes a homogeneous representation that summarizes the tumor as a whole with a single representative profile and imaging signature of the instead heterogeneous features of the tumor.[139,140] This surgical strategy lacks specific information to distinguish many of the genetically distinct tumor populations that can reside within a single tumor.[141]

Favoring the CET, the surgical targeting neglects the clonal populations and the heterogeneity of nCET areas.[141] Both cMRI and surgical targeting currently underdiagnose these areas, despite that they represent the primary targets of adjuvant therapies, the main site of recurrence[62] and they likely harbor therapeutic targets remaining elusive after resection or biopsy of the CET.[69,139] Because both tumor and nontumoral pathophysiological changes coexist within the nCET area, caution still must be taken to claim surgical targeting of both normal-appearing (on cMRI) or nontumoral white matter.

The lack of discriminative power of cMRI is evident particularly when a differential diagnosis between recurrence and treatment-induced changes mimicking progression is requested. Such signal abnormalities (ie, pseudoprogression and radiation-induced necrosis[142]) can occur in up to 36% of patients with high-grade gliomas.[143,144] In this circumstance, the agreement among pathologists for diagnosing a recurrent disease is far from being optimal, with a reported agreement rate of 36% to 58%.[145,146] This reported rate is partially due to tissue heterogeneity and a mixture of viable tumor cells and treatment-related changes that cMRI cannot correctly discriminate. This lack of information leaves surgery a target, with a likely low confidence of being representative of the driving tumor populations, which, however, share identical conventional radiological phenotypes with nontumor changes.[147] Increasing the quality and quantity of noninvasive presurgical data can influence the decision-making with enhanced information and, eventually, lead to a better outcome.

Brain surgery must and can take advantage of advanced imaging to tailor the surgical targeting of representative tumor areas that are biologically and clinically relevant. Instead of a cloud targeting of abnormal areas of cMRI, an information-guided surgical strategy avoids both unneeded risk exposure and a low diagnostic yield. It also supports treatment decisions at a given time throughout the disease course more robustly. The multidisciplinary management of these subjects also must agree on consistent radiological protocols, comprehensive of cMRI and selected advanced magnetic resonance sequences. Such standardized adaptive protocols should match the oncological need at a given time point and, at the same time, constrain scanning and analytical times. Standardization also will be essential to increase study comparisons and reproducibility and to pursue and validate cutoff values of quantitative measures.

FINAL REMARKS

A subject with GBM undergoes serial magnetic resonance scans, from clinical presentation, through the perioperative time, to the adjuvant therapeutic stage. Histomolecular characterization of the tumor is essential for effective and timely decision making. Current limitations exist in resolving the intratumoral spatial heterogeneity and the longitudinal evolving mutational landscape over time, because their determination depends on the analysis of invasive tissue sampling through surgery. Such invasive sampling results are limited to the time and site, when and where, respectively, the tissue is collected from a highly heterogeneous tumor.

Acknowledging that the role of cMRI as established, advanced imaging is building a consistent momentum for noninvasive profiling of tissue composition in addition to known pathologic landmarks. Brain surgery thus can benefit from enhanced information to tailor surgical indication and to guide sampling, within multidisciplinary management. Targeting the tumor areas with the more relevant biological features and, thus, with a likely more meaningful clinical impact will be essential to address oncological needs more adequately. A better-informed surgical strategy is expected to lower sampling errors further and to represent the validation benchmark of radiogenomic findings, while keeping patient safety a critical priority. Leaving the role of liquid biopsy of the central nervous system's tumors apart,[148] advanced imaging can be regarded as a watchful noninvasive sentinel aiding the clinical surveillance in patrolling the disease status and providing the clinician with the enhanced information needed for an improved individualized care.

CLINICS CARE POINTS

- MRI is essential in the management of gliomas, supporting diagnosis, surgical planning, treatment assessment, and follow-up.

- The current neurosurgical standard of care of GBMs aims at total resection of the contrast-enhancing lesion, as depicted by cMRI.
- cMRI cannot fully resolve the spatial and temporal heterogeneity and the highly infiltrative nature beyond the contrast-enhanced region of GBMs.
- Advance MRI and PET contribute to improving the understanding, the characterization, and the differential diagnosis of distinct tumor habitats and the non–contrast-enhanced regions.
- Neurosurgery can benefit from enhanced information from imaging to target the tumor areas with the most relevant biological features.
- Advanced imaging can support multidisciplinary decision making to precisely address oncologic needs with an individualized approach, pursuing a meaningful clinical impact.

DISCLOSURE

The MRI protocol reported in **Figs. 1** and **2** has been performed in the context of the Enhanced Delivery Ecosystem for Neurosurgery in 2020 (EDEN2020) project, which received funding from the European Union's EU Research and Innovation programme Horizon 2020 under Grant Agreement no. 688279.

REFERENCES

1. Gillies RJ, Kinahan PE, Hricak H. Radiomics: Images Are More than Pictures, They Are Data. Radiology 2016;278(2):563–77.
2. Cancer Genome Atlas Research Network., Brat Daniel J, Verhaak Roel GW, Aldape KD, et al. Comprehensive, Integrative Genomic Analysis of Diffuse Lower-Grade Gliomas. N Engl J Med 2015;372(26):2481–98.
3. Yan H, Parsons DW, Jin G, et al. *IDH1* and *IDH2* Mutations in Gliomas. N Engl J Med 2009;360(8): 765–73.
4. Hegi ME, Diserens AC, Gorlia T, et al. MGMT gene silencing and benefit from temozolomide in glioblastoma. N Engl J Med 2005;352(10):997–1003.
5. Louis DN, Perry A, Reifenberger G, et al. The 2016 World Health Organization Classification of Tumors of the Central Nervous System: a summary. Acta Neuropathol 2016;131(6):803–20.
6. Castellano A, Falini A. Progress in neuro-imaging of brain tumors. Curr Opin Oncol 2016;28(6):484–93.
7. Pope Whitney B. Genomics of Brain Tumor Imaging. Neuroimaging Clin N Am 2015;25(1):105–19.
8. Muragaki Y, Iseki H, Maruyama T, et al. Information-guided surgical management of gliomas using low-field-strength intraoperative MRI. Acta Neurochir Suppl 2011;109:67–72.
9. Fukuya Y, Ikuta S, Maruyama T, et al. Tumor recurrence patterns after surgical resection of intracranial low-grade gliomas. J Neurooncol 2019; 144(3):519–28.
10. Collins Francis S, Varmus H. A new initiative on precision medicine. N Engl J Med 2015;372(9): 793–5.
11. Patel AP, Tirosh I, Trombetta JJ, et al. Single-cell RNA-seq highlights intratumoral heterogeneity in primary glioblastoma. Science 2014;344(6190): 1396–401.
12. Neftel C, Laffy J, Filbin Mariella G, et al. An Integrative Model of Cellular States, Plasticity, and Genetics for Glioblastoma. Cell 2019;178(4):835–49. e21.
13. Sottoriva A, Spiteri I, Piccirillo SG, et al. Intratumor heterogeneity in human glioblastoma reflects cancer evolutionary dynamics. Proc Natl Acad Sci U S A 2013;110(10):4009–14.
14. Johnson BE, Mazor T, Hong C, et al. Mutational analysis reveals the origin and therapy-driven evolution of recurrent glioma. Science 2014;343(6167): 189–93.
15. Barthel Floris P, Johnson KC, Varn Frederick S, et al. Longitudinal molecular trajectories of diffuse glioma in adults. Nature 2019;576(7785):112–20.
16. Wen PY, Weller M, Lee EQ, et al. Glioblastoma in Adults: A Society for Neuro-Oncology (SNO) and European Society of Neuro-Oncology (EANO) Consensus Review on Current Management and Future Directions. Neuro Oncol 2020. https://doi.org/10.1093/neuonc/noaa106.
17. Henson JW, Paola G, Gilberto GR. MRI in treatment of adult gliomas. Lancet Oncol 2005;167–75. https://doi.org/10.1016/S1470-2045(05)01767-5.
18. Ly KI, Wen PY, Huang RY. Imaging of Central Nervous System Tumors Based on the 2016 World Health Organization Classification. Neurol Clin 2020;95–113. https://doi.org/10.1016/j.ncl.2019.08.004.
19. Sahm F, Capper D, Jeibmann A, et al. Addressing diffuse glioma as a systemic brain disease with single-cell analysis. Arch Neurol 2012;69(4):523–6.
20. Giese A, Westphal M. Glioma invasion in the central nervous system. Neurosurgery 1996;235–52. https://doi.org/10.1097/00006123-199608000-00001.
21. Cuddapah VA, Robel S, Watkins S, et al. A neurocentric perspective on glioma invasion. Nat Rev Neurosci 2014;455–65. https://doi.org/10.1038/nrn3765.
22. Riva M, Bello L. Low-grade glioma management: A contemporary surgical approach. Curr Opin Oncol

2014;26(6). https://doi.org/10.1097/CCO.0000000000000120.

23. Vogelbaum Michael A, Jost S, Aghi Manish K, et al. Application of novel response/progression measures for surgically delivered therapies for gliomas: Response Assessment in Neuro-Oncology (RANO) working group. Neurosurgery 2012;70(1):234–43.

24. Chaichana KL, Jusue-Torres I, Navarro-Ramirez R, et al. Establishing percent resection and residual volume thresholds affecting survival and recurrence for patients with newly diagnosed intracranial glioblastoma. Neuro Oncol 2013;16(1):113–22.

25. Sanai N, Polley MY, McDermott MW, et al. An extent of resection threshold for newly diagnosed glioblastomas: Clinical article. J Neurosurg 2011; 115(1):3–8.

26. Stummer W, Reulen HJ, Meinel T, et al. Extent of resection and survival in glioblastoma multiforme: Identification of and adjustment for bias. Neurosurgery 2008;62(3):564–74.

27. Stummer W, Pichlmeier U, Meinel T, et al. Fluorescence-guided surgery with 5-aminolevulinic acid for resection of malignant glioma: a randomised controlled multicentre phase III trial. Lancet Oncol 2006;7(5):392–401.

28. Marko Nicholas F, Weil Robert J, Schroeder Jason L, et al. Extent of Resection of Glioblastoma Revisited: Personalized Survival Modeling Facilitates More Accurate Survival Prediction and Supports a Maximum-Safe-Resection Approach to Surgery. J Clin Oncol 2014;32(8):774–82.

29. Lacroix M, Abi-Said D, Fourney DR, et al. A multivariate analysis of 416 patients with glioblastoma multiforme: Prognosis, extent of resection, and survival. J Neurosurg 2001;95(2):190–8.

30. Grabowski Matthew M, Recinos PF, Nowacki AS, et al. Residual tumor volume versus extent of resection: Predictors of survival after surgery for glioblastoma. J Neurosurg 2014;121(5):1115–23.

31. Kreth FW, Thon N, Simon M, et al. Gross total but not incomplete resection of glioblastoma prolongs survival in the era of radiochemotherapy. Ann Oncol 2013;24:3117–23.

32. Brown Timothy J, Brennan Matthew C, Li M, et al. Association of the extent of resection with survival in glioblastoma a systematic review and meta-Analysis. JAMA Oncol 2016;2(11):1460–9.

33. Oppenlander Mark E, Wolf Andrew B, Snyder Laura A, et al. An extent of resection threshold for recurrent glioblastoma and its risk for neurological morbidity: Clinical article. J Neurosurg 2014; 120(4):846–53.

34. Ringel F, Pape H, Sabel M, et al. Clinical benefit from resection of recurrent glioblastomas: results of a multicenter study including 503 patients with recurrent glioblastomas undergoing surgical resection. Neuro Oncol 2015;18(1):96–104.

35. Bloch O, Han Seunggu J, Cha S, et al. Impact of extent of resection for recurrent glioblastoma on overall survival: Clinical article. J Neurosurg 2012; 117(6):1032–8.

36. Suchorska B, Weller M, Tabatabai G, et al. Complete resection of contrast-enhancing tumor volume is associated with improved survival in recurrent glioblastoma—results from the DIRECTOR trial. Neuro Oncol 2016;18(4): 549–56.

37. Pessina F, Navarria P, Cozzi L, et al. Role of surgical resection in recurrent glioblastoma: prognostic factors and outcome evaluation in an observational study. J Neurooncol 2017;131(2):377–84.

38. Stummer W, Tonn J-C, Mehdorn HM, et al. Counterbalancing risks and gains from extended resections in malignant glioma surgery: a supplemental analysis from the randomized 5-aminolevulinic acid glioma resection study. Clinical article. J Neurosurg 2011;114(3):613–23.

39. Gulati S, Jakola Asgeir S, Nerland Ulf S, et al. The risk of getting worse: Surgically acquired deficits, perioperative complications, and functional outcomes after primary resection of glioblastoma. World Neurosurg 2011;572–9. https://doi.org/10.1016/j.wneu.2011.06.014.

40. Wen Patrick Y, Macdonald David R, Reardon David A, et al. Updated response assessment criteria for high-grade gliomas: Response assessment in neuro-oncology working group. J Clin Oncol 2010;1963–72. https://doi.org/10.1200/JCO.2009.26.3541.

41. Okada H, Weller M, Huang R, et al. Immunotherapy response assessment in neuro-oncology: A report of the RANO working group. Lancet Oncol 2015; e534–42. https://doi.org/10.1016/S1470-2045(15)00088-1.

42. Ellingson BM, Bendszus M, Boxerman J, et al. Consensus recommendations for a standardized Brain Tumor Imaging Protocol in clinical trials. Neuro Oncol 2015;17(9):1188–98.

43. Lim M, Xia Y, Bettegowda C, et al. Current state of immunotherapy for glioblastoma. Nat Rev Clin Oncol 2018;422–42. https://doi.org/10.1038/s41571-018-0003-5.

44. Stupp R, Mason Warren P, Van Den Bent MJ, et al. Radiotherapy plus concomitant and adjuvant temozolomide for glioblastoma. N Engl J Med 2005; 352(10):987–96. https://doi.org/10.1056/NEJMoa043330.

45. Molinaro Annette M, Hervey-Jumper S, Morshed Ramin A, et al. Association of Maximal Extent of Resection of Contrast-Enhanced and Non-Contrast-Enhanced Tumor with Survival within Molecular Subgroups of Patients with Newly Diagnosed Glioblastoma. JAMA Oncol 2020;6(4). https://doi.org/10.1001/jamaoncol.2019.6143.

46. Nibali MC, Lorenzo G, Sciortino T, et al. Surgery For Glioblastoma in Elderly Patients. Neurosurg Clin N Am 2020.

47. Daubon T, Céline L, Clarke K, et al. Deciphering the complex role of thrombospondin-1 in glioblastoma development. Nat Commun 2019;10(1). https://doi.org/10.1038/s41467-019-08480-y.

48. Boyé K, Pujol N, Alves I D, et al. The role of CXCR3/LRP1 cross-talk in the invasion of primary brain tumors. Nat Commun 2017;8(1). https://doi.org/10.1038/s41467-017-01686-y.

49. Li YM, Suki D, Hess K, et al. The influence of maximum safe resection of glioblastoma on survival in 1229 patients: Can we do better than gross-total resection? J Neurosurg 2016;124(4):977–88.

50. Pessina F, Navarria P, Cozzi L, et al. Maximize surgical resection beyond contrast-enhancing boundaries in newly diagnosed glioblastoma multiforme: is it useful and safe? A single institution retrospective experience. J Neurooncol 2017;135(1):129–39.

51. Beiko J, Suki D, Hess KR, et al. IDH1 mutant malignant astrocytomas are more amenable to surgical resection and have a survival benefit associated with maximal surgical resection. Neuro Oncol 2013;16(1):81–91.

52. Jain R, Poisson Laila M, Gutman D, et al. Outcome prediction in patients with glioblastoma by using imaging, clinical, and genomic biomarkers: Focus on the nonenhancing component of the tumor. Radiology 2014;272(2):484–93.

53. Shah AH, Mahavadi A, Di L, et al. Survival benefit of lobectomy for glioblastoma: moving towards radical supramaximal resection. J Neurooncol 2020. https://doi.org/10.1007/s11060-020-03541-5.

54. Yordanova YN, Moritz-Gasser S, Duffau H. Awake surgery for WHO grade II gliomas within "nonelo-quent" areas in the left dominant hemisphere: Toward a "supratotal" resection - Clinical article. J Neurosurg 2011;115(2):232–9.

55. de Leeuw CN, Vogelbaum MA. Supratotal resection in glioma: a systematic review. Neuro Oncol 2019;21(2):179–88.

56. Rossi M, Ambrogi F, Gay L, et al. Is supratotal resection achievable in low-grade gliomas? Feasibility, putative factors, safety, and functional outcome. J Neurosurg 2019;1–14. https://doi.org/10.3171/2019.2.jns183408.

57. Jackson C, Choi J, Khalafallah Adham M, et al. A systematic review and meta-analysis of supratotal versus gross total resection for glioblastoma. J Neurooncol 2020. https://doi.org/10.1007/s11060-020-03556-y.

58. Kotrotsou A, Elakkad A, Sun J, et al. Multi-center study finds postoperative residual non-enhancing component of glioblastoma as a new determinant of patient outcome. J Neurooncol 2018;139(1):125–33.

59. Ellingson Benjamin M, Abrey Lauren E, Nelson Sarah J, et al. Validation of postoperative residual contrast-enhancing tumor volume as an independent prognostic factor for overall survival in newly diagnosed glioblastoma. Neuro Oncol 2018;20(9):1240–50.

60. Navarria P, Reggiori G, Pessina F, et al. Investigation on the role of integrated PET/MRI for target volume definition and radiotherapy planning in patients with high grade glioma. Radiother Oncol 2014;112(3):425–9.

61. Lasocki XA, Gaillard XF. Non-Contrast-Enhancing Tumor: A New Frontier in Glioblastoma Research. AJNR Am J Neuroradiol 2019;40(5):758–65.

62. John F, Bosnyák E, Robinette Natasha L, et al. Multimodal imaging-defined subregions in newly diagnosed glioblastoma: impact on overall survival. Neuro Oncol 2018;21(2):264–73.

63. De Witt Hamer PC, Robles SG, Zwinderman Aeilko H, et al. Impact of intraoperative stimulation brain mapping on glioma surgery outcome: A meta-analysis. J Clin Oncol 2012;2559–65. https://doi.org/10.1200/JCO.2011.38.4818.

64. Bello L, Riva M, Fava E, et al. Tailoring neurophysiological strategies with clinical context enhances resection and safety and expands indications in gliomas involving motor pathways. Neuro Oncol 2014;16(8). https://doi.org/10.1093/neuonc/not327.

65. Riva M, Fava E, Gallucci M, et al. Monopolar high-frequency language mapping: Can it help in the surgical management of gliomas? A comparative clinical study. J Neurosurg 2016;124(5). https://doi.org/10.3171/2015.4.JNS14333.

66. Bello L, Rossi M, Nibali MC, et al. Neurophysiology of language and cognitive mapping. In: Neurophysiology in Neurosurgery. Elsevier; 2020. p. 101–12.

67. Bello L, Rossi M, Nibali MC, et al. Functional approach to brain tumor surgery: awake setting. In: Neurophysiology in Neurosurgery. Elsevier; 2020. p. 257–69.

68. Sarkaria Jann N, Hu Leland S, Parney Ian F, et al. Is the blood–brain barrier really disrupted in all glioblastomas? A critical assessment of existing clinical data. Neuro Oncol 2017;20(2):184–91.

69. Price SJ, Jena R, Burnet NG, et al. Improved Delineation of Glioma Margins and Regions of Infiltration with the Use of Diffusion Tensor Imaging: An Image-Guided Biopsy Study. AJNR Am J Neuroradiol 2006;27(9):1969–74.

70. Castellano A, Cirillo S, Bello L, et al. Functional MRI for Surgery of Gliomas. Curr Treat Options Neurol 2017;19(10). https://doi.org/10.1007/s11940-017-0469-y.

71. Sanvito F, Caverzasi E, Riva M, et al. fMRI-Targeted High-Angular Resolution Diffusion MR Tractography to Identify Functional Language Tracts in Healthy Controls and Glioma Patients. Front Neurosci 2020;14. https://doi.org/10.3389/fnins.2020.00225.

72. Fathi Kazerooni A, Bakas S, Saligheh Rad H, et al. Imaging signatures of glioblastoma molecular characteristics: A radiogenomics review. J Magn Reson Imaging 2019. https://doi.org/10.1002/jmri.26907.

73. Hygino da Cruz LC, Vieira IG, Domingues RC. Diffusion MR Imaging: An Important Tool in the Assessment of Brain Tumors. Neuroimaging Clin N Am 2011;27–49. https://doi.org/10.1016/j.nic.2011.01.010.

74. Romano A, Calabria LF, Tavanti F, et al. Apparent diffusion coefficient obtained by magnetic resonance imaging as a prognostic marker in glioblastomas: Correlation with MGMT promoter methylation status. Eur Radiol 2013;23(2):513–20.

75. Sunwoo L, Choi SH, Park CK, et al. Correlation of apparent diffusion coefficient values measured by diffusion MRI and MGMT promoter methylation semiquantitatively analyzed with MS-MLPA in patients with glioblastoma multiforme. J Magn Reson Imaging 2013;37(2):351–8.

76. Moon WJ, Choi JW, Gee RH, et al. Imaging parameters of high grade gliomas in relation to the MGMT promoter methylation status: The CT, diffusion tensor imaging, and perfusion MR imaging. Neuroradiology 2012;54(6):555–63.

77. Sternberg EJ, Lipton ML, Burns J. Utility of diffusion tensor imaging in evaluation of the peritumoral region in patients with primary and metastatic brain tumors. Am J Neuroradiol 2014;439–44.

78. Price SJ, Allinson K, Liu H, et al. Less invasive phenotype found in isocitrate dehydrogenase-mutated glioblastomas than in isocitrate dehydrogenase wild-type glioblastomas: A diffusion-tensor imaging study. Radiology 2017;283(1):215–21.

79. Shiroishi Mark S, Boxerman Jerrold L, Pope Whitney B. Physiologic MRI for assessment of response to therapy and prognosis in glioblastoma. Neuro Oncol 2015;18(4):467–78.

80. Anzalone N, Castellano A, Cadioli M, et al. Brain Gliomas: Multicenter Standardized Assessment of Dynamic Contrast-enhanced and Dynamic Susceptibility Contrast MR Images. Radiology 2018;287(3):933–43.

81. Del Mar Álvarez-Torres M, Juan-Albarracín J, Fuster-Garcia E, et al. Robust association between vascular habitats and patient prognosis in glioblastoma: An international multicenter study. J Magn Reson Imaging 2020;51(5):1478–86.

82. Patel P, Baradaran H, Delgado D, et al. MR perfusion-weighted imaging in the evaluation of high-grade gliomas after treatment: a systematic review and meta-analysis. Neuro Oncol 2017;19(1):118–27.

83. Shiroishi MS, Castellazzi G, Boxerman JL, et al. Principles of T2*-weighted dynamic susceptibility contrast MRI technique in brain tumor imaging. J Magn Reson Imaging 2015;296–313.

84. Barajas RF Jr, Phillips RJ, Parvataneni RJ, et al. Regional variation in histopathologic features of tumor specimens from treatment-naive glioblastoma correlates with anatomic and physiologic MR Imaging. Neuro Oncol 2012;14(7):942–54.

85. Sadeghi N, D'Haene N, Decaestecker C, et al. Apparent diffusion coefficient and cerebral blood volume in brain gliomas: Relation to tumor cell density and tumor microvessel density based on stereotactic biopsies. Am J Neuroradiol 2008;29(3):476–82.

86. Essig M, Nguyen TB, Shiroishi MS, et al. Perfusion MRI: The five most frequently asked clinical questions. Am J Roentgenol 2013. https://doi.org/10.2214/AJR.12.9544.

87. Heye Anna K, Culling Ross D, Valdés Hernández Mdel C, et al. Assessment of blood-brain barrier disruption using dynamic contrast-enhanced MRI. A systematic review. Neuroimage Clin 2014;262–74. https://doi.org/10.1016/j.nicl.2014.09.002.

88. Kickingereder P, Radbruch A, Burth S, et al. Mr Perfusion-derived hemodynamic Parametric response Mapping of Bevacizumab efficacy in recurrent glioblastoma. Radiology 2016;279(2):542–52.

89. Ellingson BM, Gerstner ER, Smits M, et al. Diffusion MRI phenotypes predict overall survival benefit from Anti-VEGF monotherapy in recurrent glioblastoma: Converging evidence from phase II trials. Clin Cancer Res 2017;23(19):5745 56.

90. Arevalo-Perez J, Thomas AA, Kaley T, et al. T1-weighted dynamic contrast-enhanced MRI as a noninvasive biomarker of epidermal growth factor receptor VIII status. Am J Neuroradiol 2015;36(12):2256–61.

91. Politi LS, Brugnara G, Castellano A, et al. T1-weighted dynamic contrast-enhanced MRI is a noninvasive marker of epidermal growth factor receptor VIII status in cancer stem cell-derived experimental glioblastomas. Am J Neuroradiol 2016;E49–51. https://doi.org/10.3174/ajnr.A4774.

92. Akbari H, Bakas S, Pisapia Jared M, et al. In vivo evaluation of EGFRvIII mutation in primary glioblastoma patients via complex multiparametric MRI signature. Neuro Oncol 2018;20(8):1068–79.

93. Tykocinski Elana S, Grant Ryan A, Kapoor Gurpreet S, et al. Use of magnetic perfusion-weighted imaging to determine epidermal growth

factor receptor variant III expression in glioblastoma. Neuro Oncol 2012;14(5):613–23. https://doi.org/10.1093/neuonc/nos073.

94. Chaumeil Myriam M, Lupo Janine M, Ronen Sabrina M. Magnetic Resonance (MR) Metabolic Imaging in Glioma. Brain Pathol 2015;25(6): 769–80.

95. Andronesi Ovidiu C, Kim Grace S, Gerstner E, et al. Detection of 2-hydroxyglutarate in IDH-mutated glioma patients by in vivo spectral-editing and 2D correlation magnetic resonance spectroscopy. Sci Transl Med 2012;4(116). https://doi.org/10.1126/scitranslmed.3002693.

96. Choi C, Ganji Sandeep K, DeBerardinis RJ, et al. 2-Hydroxyglutarate detection by magnetic resonance spectroscopy in IDH-mutated patients with gliomas. Nat Med 2012;18(4):624–9.

97. Choi C, Raisanen Jack M, Ganji Sandeep K, et al. Prospective longitudinal analysis of 2-hydroxyglutarate magnetic resonance spectroscopy identifies broad clinical utility for the management of patients with IDH-mutant glioma. J Clin Oncol 2016;34(33):4030–9.

98. Branzoli F, Di Stefano AL, Capelle L, et al. Highly specific determination of IDH status using edited in vivo magnetic resonance spectroscopy. Neuro Oncol 2017;20(7):907–16.

99. Suh CH, Kim HS, Jung SC, et al. 2-Hydroxyglutarate MR spectroscopy for prediction of isocitrate dehydrogenase mutant glioma: a systemic review and meta-analysis using individual patient data. Neuro Oncol 2018;20(12):1573–83.

100. Andronesi OC, Arrillaga-Romany IC, Ly KI, et al. Pharmacodynamics of mutant-IDH1 inhibitors in glioma patients probed by in vivo 3D MRS imaging of 2-hydroxyglutarate. Nat Commun 2018;9(1). https://doi.org/10.1038/s41467-018-03905-6.

101. Smits M, Van Den Bent MJ. Imaging correlates of adult glioma genotypes. Radiology 2017;316–31. https://doi.org/10.1148/radiol.2017151930.

102. Gatenby Robert A, Grove O, Gillies Robert J. Quantitative imaging in cancer evolution and ecology. Radiology 2013;8–15. https://doi.org/10.1148/radiol.13122697.

103. Stadlbauer A, Zimmermann M, Doerfler A, et al. Intratumoral heterogeneity of oxygen metabolism and neovascularization uncovers 2 survival-relevant subgroups of IDH1 wild-type glioblastoma. Neuro Oncol 2018;20(11):1536–46.

104. Stadlbauer A, Oberndorfer S, Zimmermann M, et al. Physiologic MR imaging of the tumor microenvironment revealed switching of metabolic phenotype upon recurrence of glioblastoma in humans. J Cereb Blood Flow Metab 2020;40(3): 528–38.

105. Albert Nathalie L, Weller M, Suchorska B, et al. Response Assessment in Neuro-Oncology working group and European Association for Neuro-Oncology recommendations for the clinical use of PET imaging in gliomas. Neuro Oncol 2016;18(9): 1199–208.

106. Law I, Albert Nathalie L, Arbizu J, et al. Joint EANM/EANO/RANO practice guidelines/SNMMI procedure standards for imaging of gliomas using PET with radiolabelled amino acids and [18 F] FDG: version 1.0. Eur J Nucl Med Mol Imaging 2019;46(3):540–57.

107. Deykin D, Christine B, Isselbacher KJ. Sugar and Amino Acid Transport by Cells in Culture — Differences between Normal and Malignant Cells. N Engl J Med 1972;929–33.

108. Ishiwata K, Kubota K, Murakami M, et al. Re-evaluation of Amino Acid PET Studies: Can the Protein Synthesis Rates in Brain and Tumor Tissues Be Measured In Vivo? J Nucl Med 1993;34(11): 1936–43.

109. la Fougère C, Suchorska B, Bartenstein P, et al. Molecular imaging of gliomas with PET: Opportunities and limitations. Neuro Oncol 2011;13(8): 806–19.

110. Pirotte B, Goldman S, Massager N, et al. Combined use of 18F-fluorodeoxyglucose and 11C-methionine in 45 positron emission tomography-guided stereotactic brain biopsies. J Neurosurg 2004; 101(3):476–83.

111. Torii K, Tsuyuguchi N, Kawabe J, et al. Correlation of amino-acid uptake using methionine PET and histological classifications in various gliomas. Ann Nucl Med 2005;19(8):677–83.

112. Pöpperl G, Kreth Friedrich W, Mehrkens Jan H, et al. FET PET for the evaluation of untreated gliomas: Correlation of FET uptake and uptake kinetics with tumour grading. Eur J Nucl Med Mol Imaging 2007;34(12):1933–42.

113. Lopci E, Riva M, Olivari L, et al. Prognostic value of molecular and imaging biomarkers in patients with supratentorial glioma. Eur J Nucl Med Mol Imaging 2017;44(7):1155–64.

114. Riva M, Lopci E, Castellano A, et al. Lower Grade Gliomas: Relationships Between Metabolic and Structural Imaging with Grading and Molecular Factors. World Neurosurg 2019;126:e270–80.

115. Sciortino T, Fernandes B, Nibali MC, et al. Frameless stereotactic biopsy for precision neurosurgery: diagnostic value, safety, and accuracy. Acta Neurochir (Wien) 2019. https://doi.org/10.1007/s00701-019-03873-w.

116. Castello A, Riva M, Fernandes B, et al. The role of 11C-methionine PET in patients with negative diffusion-weighted magnetic resonance imaging. Nucl Med Commun 2020;1. https://doi.org/10.1097/MNM.0000000000001202.

117. Suchorska B, Giese A, Biczok A, et al. Identification of time-to-peak on dynamic 18F-FET-PET as a

prognostic marker specifically in IDH1/2 mutant diffuse astrocytoma. Neuro Oncol 2018;20(2): 279–88.

118. Verger A, Stoffels G, Bauer EK, et al. Static and dynamic 18F–FET PET for the characterization of gliomas defined by IDH and 1p/19q status. Eur J Nucl Med Mol Imaging 2018;45(3):443–51.

119. Bauer Elena K, Stoffels G, Blau T, et al. Prediction of survival in patients with IDH-wildtype astrocytic gliomas using dynamic O-(2-[18F]-fluoroethyl)-l-tyrosine PET. Eur J Nucl Med Mol Imaging 2020;47(6). https://doi.org/10.1007/s00259-020-04695-0.

120. Verger A, Metellus Ph, Sala Q, et al. IDH mutation is paradoxically associated with higher 18F-FDOPA PET uptake in diffuse grade II and grade III gliomas. Eur J Nucl Med Mol Imaging 2017;44(8): 1306–11.

121. Cicone F, Carideo L, Scaringi C, et al. 18 F-DOPA uptake does not correlate with IDH mutation status and 1p/19q co-deletion in glioma. Ann Nucl Med 2019;33(4):295–302. https://doi.org/10.1007/s12149-018-01328-3.

122. Lohmann P, Kocher M, Steger J, et al. Radiomics derived from amino-acid PET and conventional MRI in patients with high-grade gliomas. Q J Nucl Med Mol Imaging 2018;272–80. https://doi.org/10.23736/S1824-4785.18.03095-9.

123. Sotoudeh H, Shafaat O, Bernstock Joshua D, et al. Artificial intelligence in the management of glioma: Era of personalized medicine. Front Oncol 2019. https://doi.org/10.3389/fonc.2019.00768.

124. Li-Chun Hsieh K, Chen CY, Lo CM. Quantitative glioma grading using transformed gray-scale invariant textures of MRI. Comput Biol Med 2017; 83:102–8.

125. Nie D, Lu J, Zhang H, et al. Multi-Channel 3D Deep Feature Learning for Survival Time Prediction of Brain Tumor Patients Using Multi-Modal Neuroimages. Sci Rep 2019;9(1). https://doi.org/10.1038/s41598-018-37387-9.

126. Glaudemans Andor WJM, Enting Roelien H, Heesters Mart AAM, et al. Value of 11C-methionine PET in imaging brain tumours and metastases. Eur J Nucl Med Mol Imaging 2013;615–35. https://doi.org/10.1007/s00259-012-2295-5.

127. Galldiks N, Unterrainer M, Judov N, et al. Photopenic defects on O-(2-[18F]-fluoroethyl)-L-tyrosine PET: clinical relevance in glioma patients. Neuro Oncol 2019;21(10):1331–8.

128. Bonm AV, Ritterbusch R, Throckmorton P, et al. Clinical Imaging for Diagnostic Challenges in the Management of Gliomas: A Review. J Neuroimaging 2020;139–45. https://doi.org/10.1111/jon.12687.

129. Deuschl C, Kirchner J, Poeppel TD, et al. 11C–MET PET/MRI for detection of recurrent glioma. Eur J Nucl Med Mol Imaging 2018;45(4):593–601.

130. Weller M, Stupp R, Hegi ME, et al. Personalized care in neuro-oncology coming of age: Why we need MGMT and 1p/19q testing for malignant glioma patients in clinical practice. Neuro Oncol 2012;14(SUPPL.4). https://doi.org/10.1093/neuonc/nos206.

131. Prados Michael D, Byron Sara A, Tran Nhan L, et al. Toward precision medicine in glioblastoma: the promise and the challenges. Neuro Oncol 2015; 17(8):1051–63.

132. Ene Chibawanye I, Fine Howard A. Many Tumors in one: A daunting therapeutic prospect. Cancer Cell 2011;695–7. https://doi.org/10.1016/j.ccr.2011.11.018.

133. Snuderl M, Fazlollahi L, Le LP, et al. Mosaic amplification of multiple receptor tyrosine kinase genes in glioblastoma. Cancer Cell 2011;20(6):810–7.

134. Eigenbrod S, Trabold R, Brucker D, et al. Molecular stereotactic biopsy technique improves diagnostic accuracy and enables personalized treatment strategies in glioma patients. Acta Neurochir (Wien) 2014;156(8):1427–40.

135. Mader MM, Rotermund R, Martens T, et al. The role of frameless stereotactic biopsy in contemporary neuro-oncology: molecular specifications and diagnostic yield in biopsied glioma patients. J Neurooncol 2019;141(1):183–94.

136. Brennan Cameron W, Verhaak Roel GW, McKenna A, et al. The somatic genomic landscape of glioblastoma. Cell 2013;155(2):462.

137. Klughammer J, Kiesel B, Roetzer T, et al. The DNA methylation landscape of glioblastoma disease progression shows extensive heterogeneity in time and space. Nat Med 2018;24(10): 1611–24.

138. Rathore S, Akbari H, Rozycki M, et al. Radiomic MRI signature reveals three distinct subtypes of glioblastoma with different clinical and molecular characteristics, offering prognostic value beyond IDH1. Sci Rep 2018;8(1). https://doi.org/10.1038/s41598-018-22739-2.

139. Barajas RF, Hodgson JG, Chang JS, et al. Glioblastoma multiforme regional genetic and cellular expression patterns: Influence on anatomic and physiologic MR imaging. Radiology 2010;254(2): 564–76.

140. Itakura H, Achrol Achal S, Mitchell LA, et al. Magnetic resonance image features identify glioblastoma phenotypic subtypes with distinct molecular pathway activities. Sci Transl Med 2015;7(303). https://doi.org/10.1126/scitranslmed.aaa7582.

141. Hu LS, Ning S, Eschbacher JM, et al. Radiogenomics to characterize regional genetic heterogeneity in glioblastoma. Neuro Oncol 2016;19(1):128–37.

142. Leao DJ, Craig PG, Godoy LF, et al. Response assessment in neuro-oncology criteria for gliomas: Practical approach using conventional and

advanced techniques. Am J Neuroradiol 2020; 10–20. https://doi.org/10.3174/ajnr.A6358.

143. Abbasi AW, Westerlaan Henriette E, Holtman Gea A, et al. Incidence of Tumour Progression and Pseudoprogression in High-Grade Gliomas: a Systematic Review and Meta-Analysis. Clin Neuroradiol 2018;28(3):401–11.

144. Brandes AA, Franceschi E, Tosoni A, et al. MGMT promoter methylation status can predict the incidence and outcome of pseudoprogression after concomitant radiochemotherapy in newly diagnosed glioblastoma patients. J Clin Oncol 2008; 26(13):2192–7.

145. Holdhoff M, Ye X, Piotrowski AF, et al. The consistency of neuropathological diagnoses in patients undergoing surgery for suspected recurrence of glioblastoma. J Neurooncol 2019; 141(2):347–54.

146. Kim JH, Kim YB, Han JH, et al. Pathologic diagnosis of recurrent glioblastoma: Morphologic, immunohistochemical, and molecular analysis of 20 paired cases. Am J Surg Pathol 2012;36(4):620–8.

147. Prah Melissa A, Al-Gizawiy Mona M, Mueller Wade M, et al. Spatial discrimination of glioblastoma and treatment effect with histologically-validated perfusion and diffusion magnetic resonance imaging metrics. J Neurooncol 2018; 136(1):13–21.

148. Seoane J, De Mattos-Arruda L, Le Rhun E, et al. Cerebrospinal fluid cell-free tumour DNA as a liquid biopsy for primary brain tumours and central nervous system metastases. Ann Oncol 2019; 30(2):211–8.

Intraoperative Imaging for High-Grade Glioma Surgery

Thomas Noh, MD[a,b], Martina Mustroph, MD, PhD[a,c],
Alexandra J. Golby, MD[a,d],*

KEYWORDS

- Glioblastoma • High-grade glioma • Intraoperative imaging • Intraoperative MRI • Intraoperative CT

KEY POINTS

- Intraoperative imaging provides updated information which can identify brain shift and areas of residual tumor to guide intraoperative decision-making thereby increasing extent of resection.
- Intraoperative imaging techniques useful in surgery for gliomas include ultrasound, MRI, and CT each of which offers distinct advantages and limitations.
- Novel strategies to further develop intraoperative imaging are ongoing and include the use of MR thermometry to guide real time estimation of thermal damage during laser interstitial thermal ablation.

INTRAOPERATIVE IMAGING

Intraoperative imaging, by acquiring and displaying timely information during surgery, provides a beneficial adjunct to glioma surgery. Gliomas are difficult to differentiate from surrounding tissue making intraoperative estimates of residual tumor inaccurate. During surgical resection, brain shift of as much as 1 cm can occur after craniotomy and dural opening[1] because of cerebrospinal fluid egress, diminished mass effect, osmotic diuresis, edema, lesion resection, or intraoperative pneumocephalus.[2,3] These changes render preoperatively acquired images increasingly inaccurate as the surgery proceeds, limiting their usefulness in guiding intraoperative decision-making.

Intraoperative imaging allows visualization of brain shift and other changes that have occurred during tumor resection providing an updated set of images to guide additional tumor resection.

The opportunity to perform additional resection reduces the need for return to operating room (OR), because residual tumor can be taken after the intraoperative scan and before closure.[4] Intraoperative imaging can also identify intraoperative complications, such as hematoma, so that these are promptly managed while the patient is still in OR.[2,4] Through real-time monitoring, intraoperative imaging has led to the development of novel interventions for gliomas including laser interstitial thermal therapy (LITT) and focused ultrasound blood-brain barrier disruption.

Although beneficial, intraoperative imaging and intraoperative MRI (iMRI) in particular also presents several clinical challenges. Between patient set up, scanning time, moving the MRI into and out of the OR, instrument counts, and safety protocol procedures, iMRI can add more than 2 hours to craniotomy.[2] Solutions to some of these inherent problems have been mitigated by establishing

Grant Funding: National Center for Image Guided Therapy NIH P41 EB015898.
[a] Department of Neurosurgery, Brigham and Women's Hospital, 75 Francis Street, Boston, MA 02115, USA;
[b] Hawaii Pacific Health, John A Burns School of Medicine, Honolulu, Hawaii, USA; [c] Harvard Medical School, Boston, Massachusetts, USA; [d] Department of Radiology, Harvard Medical School, Boston, Massachusetts, USA
* Corresponding author.
E-mail address: agolby@bwh.harvard.edu

Neurosurg Clin N Am 32 (2021) 47–54
https://doi.org/10.1016/j.nec.2020.09.003
1042-3680/21/© 2020 Elsevier Inc. All rights reserved.

iMRI workflows and newer methods that shorten scanning times.[2] As newer technology becomes available, such as 5-aminolevulinic acid,[5] further studies are needed to establish the relative benefit costs of different intraoperative adjuncts.

INTRAOPERATIVE ULTRASOUND

The first report of interoperative ultrasound (iUS) for brain tumors was by Ballantine and colleagues[6] in 1950. Original ultrasound techniques were first developed using two-dimensional (2D) B-mode. This technology is based on pulsed acoustic waves that are reflected off the tissue of interest and detected at transducers to display their properties based on time and scattering. Most neurosurgical transducers operate within 1 to 25 MHz and provide up to 10 cm of depth penetration. A basic principle is that the higher the frequency, the better the resolution closer to the probe; however, higher frequencies have less penetration and hence less ability to image deeper structures (eg, 25 MHz can provide maximum resolutions only a few centimeters from the emitting source).[7] Most often, the transducer type is determined by tumor size, craniotomy, anatomy of interest, and surgeon preference. iUS has significant advantages in that it has a lower cost of purchase and upkeep, takes up less OR space, is less disruptive to workflow, and may be available in settings in which iMRI is not available.[8]

Integration with Neuronavigation and Brain Shift

iUS has been an effective tool in maximizing resection of brain tumors (**Fig. 1**).[9–11] Advances in technology have revitalized the use of iUS. Most ultrasound systems used in neurosurgical ORs use 2D B-mode ultrasound. One method of reconstructing a three-dimensional (3D) image is to acquire a "sweep" of 2D images while tracking the probe with neuronavigation and rebuilding these into a 3D dataset. This technique has provided powerful volumetric data that are typically collected by freehand sweeps, mechanical sweeps, or a phased array transducer.[12] 3D ultrasound data can then be integrated and fused with preoperative MRI scans for neuronavigaton.[13–17] Research groups have developed 3D ultrasound/MRI fusion-based neuronavigation and this approach has been commercialized recently.

Because iUS offers real-time imaging, it can help by giving updated information regarding brain shift. There are a variety of techniques that have been applied to compensate for brain shift including rigid registration using hyperechoic

structures,[18] automated nonrigid registration,[19–21] a "pseudoultrasound" technique,[22] and vessel registration.[23] iUS is often compared with iMRI because both can provide updated imaging in the OR. There are no randomized controlled trials comparing iUS with iMRI, but there are mixed reviews showing less sensitivity in detecting small residual tumor volumes.[10,11,24,25]

Artifacts in Intraoperative Ultrasound

Although iUS usefulness improves with surgeon experience, there are conditions present during surgery, such as blood products, that can make interpretation variable and challenging. For instance, sound waves transmit through air at 330 m/s, saline at 1480 m/s, and brain tissue around 1550 m/s.[26] This can produce errors in location of approximately 1.6 mm, 10 cm from the transducer. A clinically significant problem is that there is an artifactual hyperechoic signal because of changes in impedance at the margin of the fluid-filled resection cavity and the surrounding parenchyma, which makes interpretation of the images particularly challenging in the area of greatest clinical concern. Recently, a promising acoustic coupling fluid has been developed to

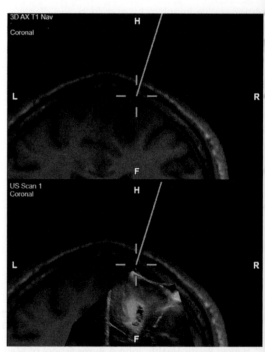

Fig. 1. Navigated iUS fused to a preoperative T1-weighted MRI image of a glioma. Navigated iUS allows for accommodation of brain shift showing shift of the hyperechoic tumor relative to the registered preoperative MRI.

reduce this artifact, and is currently in phase 1 clinical studies.[27]

Advanced Intraoperative Ultrasound Modalities

There are several advanced ultrasound modalities currently in development. One promising well-studied technique[28] is contrast-enhanced ultrasound. Contrast-enhanced ultrasound uses a microbubble-based contrast, similar to that used in echocardiography, which can outline gliomas, differentiate between tumor/edematous brain, provide grading information, show dynamic arterial/venous phases of the lesion, and be integrated to navigation systems as described previously.[29,30] A recent review from our group highlights the current state of the art.[31]

INTRAOPERATIVE MRI

iMRI in neurosurgery started at Brigham and Women's Hospital in Boston, Massachusetts in 1994 (**Fig. 2**).[2,32,33] Between 1995 and 2007, more than 1000 craniotomies using iMRI were completed.[4] General Electric working closely with Brigham and Women's Hospital in the early 1990s to develop an open-configuration iMRI consisting of two vertically oriented superconducting magnets with separate communicating cryo-coolers in a "double-donut" conformation.[3,4] The Signa System 0.5-T field machine (General Electric, Boston, MA) allowed for the patient's head to be placed in the vertical gap between the coils, as close as possible to the magnet isocenter,[3] minimizing spatial distortion and signal loss[34] while allowing for access to the patient by the surgeon and assistants. The system had the option of docking the operating table into the magnet sideways or lengthwise, depending on what configuration would maximize patient access.[3] The patient was fixed, and the MRI was also fixed; one did not need to move either to acquire iMRI. The main disadvantages of this early system were low field strength, which limited image resolution,

and the need for all surgical instruments and personnel to be MRI compatible.[3]

In later iMRI systems, the MRI was fixed, but the patient had to be rotated into the MRI machine, which was placed at a 160° angle to the OR table.[35,36] Other open-configuration iMRIs included the Siemens systems, including one with a table that could rotate into and out of a 1.5-T closed-bore magnet, and the Medtronic PoleStar system (Medtronic, Minneapolis, MN).[3] The advantage of these systems was that minimal modifications to OR suites had to be made, unlike the original iMRI. The major disadvantage was again the low field strength.[32]

A significant development in iMRIs was the modification of diagnostic closed-configuration MRI scanners for intraoperative use. One system (IMRIS, Deerfield Imaging, Minnetonka, MN) is a rail-mounted system that moves the MRI instrument to the patient allowing for minimal patient movement.[37,38] Launched commercially in 2005 and first launched in Europe in 2010,[35] more than 60 such systems have been installed worldwide to date.[32] A major advantage of iMRI with machines in or adjacent to ORs are that the patient does not need to be moved; therefore, intravenous lines, catheters, and endotracheal tubes are at less risk of dislodging.[35]

To reduce scanning time, which prolongs overall surgical time, iMRI sequences are tailored to particular types of tumors or lesions.[2] There is no universal iMRI protocol; rather, image sequences are obtained and reformatted into imaging planes, and if further resection is required, merged with stereotactic surgical navigation systems.[34] The standard sequences obtained during iMRI for glioma resections may include T1 (gadolinium enhanced or nonenhanced) T2, and fluid attenuated inversion recovery, and diffusion images.[39]

Glioblastoma and Extent of Resection

Maximal safe surgical resection of glioblastoma (GBM) is a key part of treatment. There are numerous studies showing a survival benefit with gross total resection of enhancing tumor.[40–42] iMRI can play a significant role in aiding the surgeon during the resection of GBMs including identifying incomplete resections (**Fig. 3**) and updating the neuronavigation dataset. In a prospective randomized control study, Senft and colleagues[43] showed that iMRI had more complete resections of the enhancing tumor than control subjects (96%) and a longer progression-free survival (226 days vs 98 days). Another study identified 47% of patients who underwent additional resection because of residual disease identified on the

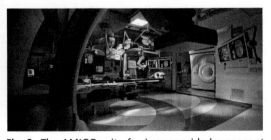

Fig. 2. The AMIGO suite for image-guided surgery at Brigham and Women's Hospital.

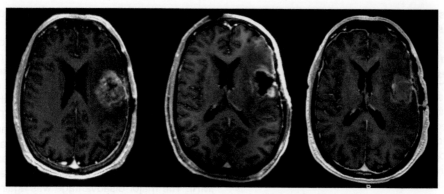

Fig. 3. Preoperative contrast-enhanced T1-weighted MRI of a recurrent GBM (*left*), intraoperative contrast-enhanced T1-weighted MRI showing residual tumor under the lip of the resection edge (*middle*), and postoperative T1-weighted contrasted MRI showing gross total resection of enhancing tumor (*right*).

intraoperative scan.[44] Napolitano and colleagues[45] also showed in a nonrandomized study that patients who underwent iMRI had a 17% improved quality of resection with 9% more gross total resection without additional morbidity. iMRI may have an increasingly important role in the future because there is increasing emphasis on maximizing the extent of resection for particular molecular subtypes of GBMs.[46,47]

Intraoperative MRI–Guided Biopsies

iMRI-guided frameless stereotactic brain biopsy can confirm intraoperatively that the biopsy needle has reached its target location and converts a blind procedure into a visualized procedure with high histologic yield.[48,49] A prospective analysis (June 2009 to April 2011) showed that frameless stereotactic iMRI-guided tumor biopsy increased diagnostic effectiveness and safety and decreased cost.[50] Several systems for iMRI-guided biopsies currently exist. Neurogate (Daum GmbH, Fuerth, Germany) is an magnetic resonance–compatible device for stereotactic biopsy of lesions.[51] A study of 28 patients between 1997 and 2000 with intracranial metastatic tumors or gliomas who underwent biopsy with Neurogate established stereotaxy in the open MRI as safe and accurate for intracranial biopsies.[51] Other available MRI-compatible biopsy systems include the Magnetic VisiOn (Magnetic VisiOn GmbH, Rueti, Switzerland), the Heidelberger Interventions-Trajektor (Pilling Weck Chirurgische Produkte GmbH, Karlstein, Germany), and the Navigus trajectory guide (Image-Guided Neurologics, Inc, Melbourne, FL).[51]

The Clearpoint Smartframe system (MRI Interventions, Irvine, CA) is an MRI-compatible stereotactic tripod system originally developed for MRI-guided placement of deep brain stimulating electrode, which can also be used for intracranial biopsies. The system consists of three circular fiducials and a cannula filled with gadolinium contrast.[52] It is typically mounted on the scalp through screws that pierce skin and penetrate the outer cranium table, or the frame is mounted directly on the skull.[53] It provides submillimeter accuracy for stereotaxy.[52] Another option is Hall and Truwit's "prospective stereotaxis" system, which uses iMRI to target the lesion, monitor needle advancement, and track progress in real time at one to three images per second, and the needle can be advanced manually or via remote control.[39,54,55]

LASER INTERSTITIAL THERMAL THERAPY

The advent of magnetic resonance thermometry allowed the controlled delivery of laser energy to the brain with near real-time monitoring of heating. Thermal therapy emerged from an observation in 1891 that an inoperable sarcoma went into remission after a patient had a febrile strep infection.[56,57] Treatment of cancer by thermal methods was bypassed in favor of radiation and chemotherapy until its resurgence in 1967, when Cavaliere and colleagues[58] proposed that cancer cells may be preferentially vulnerable to heat.[57,58] LITT was first used to ablate treatment-resistant focal metastatic intracranial tumors, and was then approved by the Food and Drug Administration for use of soft tissue ablation in neurosurgery (**Fig. 4**).[59,60] Its use was later expanded to glioma surgery.

In a first clinical study of LITT in gliomas, median survival of 16 patients with supratentorial GBM who underwent LITT after first relapse increased from 9.4 to 11.2 months (vs a natural history of survival <5 months or after temozolomide chemotherapy 5.4–7.1 months).[61] LITT has been used to ablate newly diagnosed and recurrent GBMs.

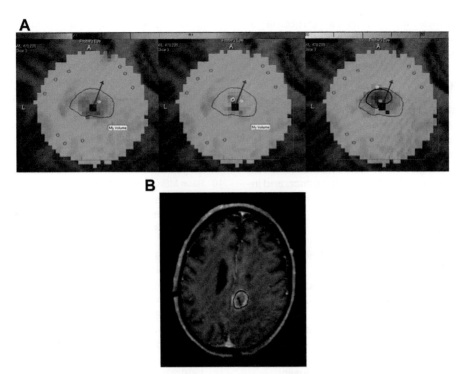

Fig. 4. (*A*) Magnetic resonance thermometry allows the operator to assess relative temperature maps in real-time. The three panels are the same slice taken at different time points in the ablation. (*Left*) The tumor (*pink outline*) preablation with a cooler center (*bluish hue*) as cooled CO_2 is sent around the catheter tip. (*Middle*) The same slice midablation with a relative warming up of the center of the catheter (*greenish hue*) and the beginnings of the thermal damage estimate beginning to appear (*yellow*). (*Right*) Further warming (*reddish hue*) and larger thermal damage estimate. (*B*) LITT ablation procedure performed in iMRI using magnetic resonance thermometry sequences to derive thermal damage estimates.

In a study of eight patients with newly diagnosed and 13 patients with recurrent GBMs, LITT extended median survival from 2 to 8 months in newly diagnosed GBM; medial survival of patients with recurrent GBMs who underwent LITT was 7 months, suggesting LITT may be an effective salvage therapy.[62] LITT can also be used in cases of radiographic progression, especially when patients have few other salvage treatment options.[63]

MRI-guided LITT is a major advancement because it allows for monitoring of ablation in real time with MRI.[64] Without MRI guidance, LITT harbored an unacceptably high risk of thermal damage to the surrounding healthy brain.[64] The Visualase System by Medtronic is an MRI-guided laser ablation system used in the United States since 2007. It gained CE approval in March 2018.[65,66] The Neuroblate System by Monteris (Plymouth, MN) is currently the only robotic LITT system.[67] MRI-guided LITT may be a safer alternative to patients in whom GBM is not accessible by surgery or in patients who are not surgical candidates because of medical comorbidities or other risks.[68]

INTRAOPERATIVE COMPUTED TOMOGRAPHY

Intraoperative computed tomography (iCT) for glioma surgery was first described in the 1980s.[69] The initial limitations were image quality and hardware artifact.[70] Current systems available include a multidetector CT, which provides high-resolution images of the soft tissue, or the cone-beam CT, which provides better bony resolution with decreased cost and radiation exposure.[71] Although the imaging quality when compared with iMRI of intra-axial malignant tumors is poor, there is a significant advantage in terms of acquisition time, cost, maintenance, workflow, and avoidance of room logistics, such as magnetic shielding.

Because iCT offers the ability to image with the patient's head fixed in pins, it is used to update neuronavigation, accommodate for brain shift, and obtain vascular imaging.[72] This has also paved the way for automated registration techniques using a low-dose CT scan to reduce mean target registration errors to less than 1 mm.[73] One study showed the workflow interruption to obtaining an intraoperative scan is around

10 to 15 minutes with one of their seven glioma patients needing further resection after the intraoperative scan.[70]

SUMMARY

Intraoperative imaging is a useful adjunct to achieving a maximally safe resection during high-grade glioma surgery. There are a variety of modalities available including iMRI, iUS, and iCT, all of which aim to give the surgeon more information, address brain shift, identify residual tumor, and increase the extent of surgical resection.

CLINICS CARE POINTS

- iMRI can demonstrate and aid compenstion for brain shift of up to 1 cm.
- iMRI requires significant site and personnel resources and can add up to 2 hours to craniotomy.
- intraoperative US can aid in detecting brain shift.
- iMRI can increase rate of gross total GBM resection and improve resection quality.
- iMRI has utility for brain biopsies.
- iMRI-guided LITT shows utility in new and recurrent GBMs.

DISCLOSURE

The authors have nothing to disclose.

REFERENCES

1. Bernadette H, Walsh Robert P. Intraoperative MRI for neurosurgical and general surgical interventions. Curr Opin Anaesthesiol 2014;27(4):448–52.
2. Daniel Thomas G, Swearingen B, Curry W, et al. 3 Tesla intraoperative MRI for brain tumor surgery. J Magn Reson Imaging 2014;39(6):1357–65.
3. Mislow John MK, Golby Alexandra J, Black Peter M. Origins of intraoperative MRI. Magn Reson Imaging Clin N Am 2010;18(1):1–10.
4. Black P, Jolesz Ferenc A, Khalid M. From vision to reality: the origins of intraoperative MR imaging. Acta Neurochir Suppl 2011;109:3–7.
5. Jenkinson Michael D, Barone Damiano G, Hart MG, et al. Intraoperative imaging technology to maximise extent of resection for glioma. Cochrane Database Syst Rev 2017. https://doi.org/10.1002/14651858. cd012788.
6. Ballantine HT Jr, Bolt RH, Hueter TF, et al. On the detection of intracranial pathology by ultrasound. Science 1950;112(2914):525–8.
7. Serra C, Stauffer A, Actor B, et al. Intraoperative high frequency ultrasound in intracerebral high-grade tumors. Ultraschall Med 2012;33(7): E306–12.
8. Aliasgar M, Shetty P. Objective assessment of utility of intraoperative ultrasound in resection of central nervous system tumors: a cost-effective tool for intraoperative navigation in neurosurgery. J Neurosci Rural Pract 2011;2(1):4–11.
9. Syed M, Rachael M, Qiu Z, et al. Intraoperative ultrasound-guided resection of gliomas: a meta-analysis and review of the literature. World Neurosurg 2016;92:255–63.
10. Ravn MBK, Asgeir Store J, Ingerid R, et al. The diagnostic properties of intraoperative ultrasound in glioma surgery and factors associated with gross total tumor resection. World Neurosurg 2018;115: e129–36.
11. Solheim O, Selbekk T, Asgeir Store J, et al. Ultrasound-guided operations in unselected high-grade gliomas: overall results, impact of image quality and patient selection. Acta Neurochir 2010; 152(11):1873–86.
12. Riccabona M, Nelson TR, Weitzer C, et al. Potential of three-dimensional ultrasound in neonatal and paediatric neurosonography. Eur Radiol 2003; 13(9):2082–93.
13. Gronningsaeter A, Kleven A, Ommedal S, et al. SonoWand, an ultrasound-based neuronavigation system. Neurosurgery 2000;47(6):1373–9 [discussion: 1379–80].
14. Hata N, Dohi T, Iseki H, et al. Development of a frameless and armless stereotactic neuronavigation system with ultrasonographic registration. Neurosurgery 1997;41(3):608–13 [discussion: 613–4].
15. Mercier L, Del Maestro Rolando F, Petrecca K, et al. New prototype neuronavigation system based on preoperative imaging and intraoperative freehand ultrasound: system description and validation. Int J Comput Assist Radiol Surg 2011;6(4):507–22.
16. Prada F, Massimiliano DB, Mattei L, et al. Fusion imaging for intra-operative ultrasound-based navigation in neurosurgery. J Ultrasound 2014;17(3): 243–51.
17. Erik Magnus B, Gulati S, Solheim O, et al. Functional magnetic resonance imaging and diffusion tensor tractography incorporated into an intraoperative 3-dimensional ultrasound-based neuronavigation system: impact on therapeutic strategies, extent of resection, and clinical outcome. Neurosurgery 2010;67(2):251–64.
18. Pierrick C, Hellier P, Xavier M, et al. 3D rigid registration of intraoperative ultrasound and preoperative MR brain images based on hyperechogenic structures. Int J Biomed Imaging 2012;2012: 531319.
19. Machado I, Matthew T, Luo J, et al. Non-rigid registration of 3D ultrasound for neurosurgery using

automatic feature detection and matching. Int J Comput Assist Radiol Surg 2018;13(10):1525–38.

20. Frisken S, Luo M, Machado I, et al. Preliminary results comparing thin plate splines with finite element methods for modeling brain deformation during neurosurgery using intraoperative ultrasound. Proc SPIE Int Soc Opt Eng 2019;10951. https://doi.org/10.1117/12.2512799.

21. Machado I, Matthew T, George E, et al. Deformable MRI-ultrasound registration using correlation-based attribute matching for brain shift correction: accuracy and generality in multi-site data. Neuroimage 2019;202:116094.

22. Mercier L, Vladimir F, Claire H, et al. Comparing two approaches to rigid registration of three-dimensional ultrasound and magnetic resonance images for neurosurgery. Int J Comput Assist Radiol Surg 2012;7(1):125–36.

23. Reinertsen I, Lindseth F, Unsgaard G, et al. Clinical validation of vessel-based registration for correction of brain-shift. Med Image Anal 2007;11(6):673–84.

24. Tronnier VM, Bonsanto MM, Staubert A, et al. Comparison of intraoperative MR imaging and 3D-navigated ultrasonography in the detection and resection control of lesions. Neurosurg Focus 2001;10(2):E3.

25. van Velthoven V. Intraoperative ultrasound imaging: comparison of pathomorphological findings in US versus CT, MRI and intraoperative findings. Acta Neurochir Suppl 2003;85:95–9.

26. Selbekk T, Asgeir Store J, Solheim Ole, et al. Ultrasound imaging in neurosurgery: approaches to minimize surgically induced image artefacts for improved resection control. Acta Neurochir 2013; 155(6):973–80.

27. Geirmund U, Millgård SL, Sébastien M, et al. A new acoustic coupling fluid with ability to reduce ultrasound imaging artefacts in brain tumour surgery-a phase I study. Acta Neurochir 2019;161(7): 1475–86.

28. Sidhu Paul S, Vito C, Dietrich Christoph F, et al. The EFSUMB guidelines and recommendations for the clinical practice of contrast-enhanced ultrasound (CEUS) in non-hepatic applications: update 2017 (long version). Ultraschall Med 2018;39(2):e2–44.

29. Prada F, Perin A, Alberto M, et al. Intraoperative contrast-enhanced ultrasound for brain tumor surgery. Neurosurgery 2014;74(5):542–52 [discussion: 552].

30. Del BM, Perin A, Casali C, et al. Advanced ultrasound imaging in glioma surgery: beyond grayscale B-mode. Front Oncol 2018;8:576.

31. Sastry R, Bi WL, Pieper S, et al. Applications of ultrasound in the resection of brain tumors. J Neuroimaging 2017;27(1):5–15.

32. Jones Pamela S. Swearingen Brooke. Intraoperative MRI for pituitary adenomas. Neurosurg Clin N Am 2019;30(4):413–20.

33. Schwartz RB, Hsu L, Wong TZ, et al. Intraoperative MR imaging guidance for intracranial neurosurgery: experience with the first 200 cases. Radiology 1999; 211(2):477–88.

34. Choudhri Asim F, Siddiqui A, Paul K Jr, et al. Intraoperative MRI in pediatric brain tumors. Pediatr Radiol 2015;45(Suppl 3):S397–405.

35. Feigl Guenther C, Heckl S, Marcel K, et al. Review of first clinical experiences with a 1.5 Tesla ceiling-mounted moveable intraoperative MRI system in Europe. Bosn J Basic Med Sci 2019;19(1):24–30.

36. Nimsky C, Ganslandt O, von Keller B, et al. Preliminary experience in glioma surgery with intraoperative high-field MRI. Acta Neurochir Suppl 2003;88: 21–9.

37. Sutherland GR, Louw DF. Intraoperative MRI: a moving magnet. CMAJ 1999;161(10):1293.

38. Sutherland GR, Kaibara T, Louw D, et al. A mobile high-field magnetic resonance system for neurosurgery. J Neurosurg 1999;91(5):804–13.

39. Arya N, Lutz D, Stark Andreas M, et al. Intraoperative MRI with 1.5 Tesla in neurosurgery. Neurosurg Clin N Am 2009;20(2):163–71.

40. Michel L, Abi-Said D, Fourney Daryl R, et al. A multivariate analysis of 416 patients with glioblastoma multiforme: prognosis, extent of resection, and survival. J Neurosurg 2001;95(2):190–8.

41. Nader S, Mei-Yin P, McDermott MW, et al. An extent of resection threshold for newly diagnosed glioblastomas. J Neurosurg 2011;115(1):3–8.

42. Grabowski Matthew M, Recinos Pablo F, Nowacki Amy S, et al. Residual tumor volume versus extent of resection: predictors of survival after surgery for glioblastoma. J Neurosurg 2014; 121(5):1115–23.

43. Senft C, Bink A, Franz K, et al. Intraoperative MRI guidance and extent of resection in glioma surgery: a randomised, controlled trial. Lancet Oncol 2011; 12(11):997–1003.

44. Mustafa Aziz H, Weinberg Jeffrey S, Suki D, et al. Impact of intraoperative high-field magnetic resonance imaging guidance on glioma surgery: a prospective volumetric analysis. Neurosurgery 2009; 64(6):1073–81 [discussion: 1081].

45. Napolitano M, Vaz G, Lawson TM, et al. Glioblastoma surgery with and without intraoperative MRI at 3.0T. Neurochirurgie 2014;60(4):143–50.

46. Molinaro Annette M, Hervey-Jumper S, Morshed Ramin A, et al. Association of maximal extent of resection of contrast-enhanced and non–contrast-enhanced tumor with survival within molecular subgroups of patients with newly diagnosed glioblastoma. JAMA Oncol 2020;495. https://doi.org/10.1001/jamaoncol.2019.6143.

47. Jason B, Suki D, Hess KR, et al. IDH1 mutant malignant astrocytomas are more amenable to surgical resection and have a survival benefit associated

with maximal surgical resection. Neuro Oncol 2014; 16(1):81–91.

48. Moriarty TM, Quinones-Hinojosa A, Larson PS, et al. Frameless stereotactic neurosurgery using intraoperative magnetic resonance imaging: stereotactic brain biopsy. Neurosurgery 2000;47(5):1138–45 [discussion: 1145–6].

49. Bernays René L, Kollias Spyros S, Khan N, et al. Histological yield, complications, and technological considerations in 114 consecutive frameless stereotactic biopsy procedures aided by open intraoperative magnetic resonance imaging. J Neurosurg 2002; 354–62. https://doi.org/10.3171/jns.2002.97.2.0354.

50. Marcin C, Tabakow P, Włodzimierz J, et al. Intraoperative magnetic resonance-guided frameless stereotactic biopsies: initial clinical experience. Neurol Neurochir Pol 2012;46(2):157–60.

51. Hans Ekkehart V, Winkler D, Strauss G, et al. NEUROGATE: a new MR-compatible device for realizing minimally invasive treatment of intracerebral tumors. Comput Aided Surg 2004;45–50. https://doi.org/10. 1080/10929080400006358.

52. Larson Paul S, Starr Philip A, Bates G, et al. An optimized system for interventional magnetic resonance imaging-guided stereotactic surgery: preliminary evaluation of targeting accuracy. Neurosurgery 2012;70(1 Suppl Operative):95–103 [discussion: 103].

53. Jiri B Jr, Alattar A, Margret J, et al. Biopsy and ablation of H3K27 glioma using skull-mounted smartframe device: technical case report. World Neurosurg 2019;127:436–41.

54. Hall WA, Martin AJ, Liu H, et al. Brain biopsy using high-field strength interventional magnetic resonance imaging. Neurosurgery 1999;44(4):807–13 [discussion: 813–4].

55. Hall Walter A, Martin A, Liu H, et al. Improving diagnostic yield in brain biopsy: coupling spectroscopic targeting with real-time needle placement. J Magn Reson Imaging 2001;13(1):12–5.

56. Hornback NB. Historical aspects of hyperthermia in cancer therapy. Radiol Clin North Am 1989;27(3): 481–8.

57. Lee TW, Murad Greg JA, Hoh Brian L, et al. Fighting fire with fire: the revival of thermotherapy for gliomas. Anticancer Res 2014;34(2):565–74.

58. Cavaliere R, Ciocatto EC, Giovanella BC, et al. Selective heat sensitivity of cancer cells. Biochemical and clinical studies. Cancer 1967;20(9):1351–81.

59. Curry Daniel J, Gowda A, McNichols Roger J, et al. MR-guided stereotactic laser ablation of epileptogenic foci in children. Epilepsy Behav 2012;24(4):408–14.

60. Alexandre C, McNichols Roger J, Jason SR, et al. Real-time magnetic resonance-guided laser thermal therapy for focal metastatic brain tumors. Neurosurgery 2008;63(1 Suppl 1):ONS21–8 [discussion: ONS28–9].

61. Hans-Joachim S, Frank E, von Tempelhoff W, et al. MR-guided laser-induced interstitial thermotherapy of recurrent glioblastoma multiforme: preliminary results in 16 patients. Eur J Radiol 2006;59(2):208–15.

62. Thomas Jonathan G, Rao G, Kew Y, et al. Laser interstitial thermal therapy for newly diagnosed and recurrent glioblastoma. Neurosurg Focus 2016; 41(4):E12.

63. Manmeet A, Barnett Gene H, Deng Di, et al. Laser ablation after stereotactic radiosurgery: a multicenter prospective study in patients with metastatic brain tumors and radiation necrosis. J Neurosurg 2018;130(3):804–11.

64. Medvid R, Ruiz A, Komotar RJ, et al. Current applications of MRI-guided laser interstitial thermal therapy in the treatment of brain neoplasms and epilepsy: a radiologic and neurosurgical overview. AJNR Am J Neuroradiol 2015;1998–2006. https:// doi.org/10.3174/ajnr.a4362.

65. LaRiviere Michael J, Gross Robert E. Stereotactic laser ablation for medically intractable epilepsy: the next generation of minimally invasive epilepsy surgery. Front Surg 2016. https://doi.org/10.3389/ fsurg.2016.00064.

66. Patel P, Patel Nitesh V, Danish Shabbar F. Intracranial MR-guided laser-induced thermal therapy: single-center experience with the Visualase thermal therapy system. J Neurosurg 2016;125(4):853–60.

67. Sloan Andrew E, Ahluwalia Manmeet S, Valerio-Pascua J, et al. Results of the NeuroBlate System first-in-humans phase I clinical trial for recurrent glioblastoma. J Neurosurg 2013;118(6):1202–19.

68. Usama S, Kumar Vinodh A, Madewell John E, et al. Neurosurgical applications of MRI guided laser interstitial thermal therapy (LITT). Cancer Imaging 2019;19(1):65.

69. Shalit MN, Israeli Y, Matz S, et al. Experience with intraoperative CT scanning in brain tumors. Surg Neurol 1982;17(5):376–82.

70. Christian S, Nicole T, Thorsteinsdottir J, et al. Intraoperative computed tomography in cranial neurosurgery. Neurosurg Clin N Am 2017;28(4):595–602.

71. Conley David B, Tan B, Bendok Bernard R, et al. Comparison of intraoperative portable CT scanners in skull base and endoscopic sinus surgery: single center case series. Skull Base 2011;21(4):261–70.

72. Giuseppe B, Massimiliano M, Peschillo S, et al. Intraoperative computed tomography, navigated ultrasound, 5-amino-levulinic acid fluorescence and neuromonitoring in brain tumor surgery: overtreatment or useful tool combination? J Neurosurg Sci 2019. https://doi.org/10.23736/S0390-5616.19. 04735-0.

73. Carl B, Miriam B, Benjamin S, et al. Reliable navigation registration in cranial and spine surgery based on intraoperative computed tomography. Neurosurg Focus 2019;47(6):E11.

Use of Intraoperative Fluorophores

Alexander J. Schupper, MD[a], Constantinos Hadjipanayis, MD, PhD[a,b],*

KEYWORDS

- Fluorescence-guided surgery • Fluorophores • Glioblastoma • GBM • 5-ALA • Fluorescein sodium
- ICG • Targeted fluorophores

KEY POINTS

- Maximal safe resection remains the standard of care for treatment of high grade glioma.
- Fluorescence-guided surgery provides an intraoperative adjunct for surgeons to maximally resect glioma tumors.
- Various fluorophores allow better detection of tumors, guiding surgeons to improve resection.

 Video content accompanies this article at http://www.neurosurgery.theclinics.com.

INTRODUCTION

Surgical resection of glioblastoma tumors has remained a mainstay of treatment in neurosurgical oncology. Our current surgical paradigm for glioblastoma, the most common high-grade glioma (HGG), focuses on complete resection of the contrast enhancing tumor (CRET) when safely possible. Multiple studies have confirmed that CRET results in better outcomes for patients with glioblastoma, especially when combined with adjuvant therapies such as chemoradiation.[1–6]

However, most glioblastoma tumor resections do not result in maximal resection of tumors owing to eloquent location of tumors, large tumor size, and difficulty visualizing the tumor at its infiltrative margin.[7] A common challenge during glioma resection is intraoperative identification of tumor tissue and delineation from surrounding brain tissue because HGGs typically infiltrate into the surrounding brain parenchyma.[7] To help the neurosurgeon maximally resect a tumor while preserving surrounding brain tissue, fluorescence-guided surgery (FGS) has been introduced into the field of neurosurgery.

In 1948, Dr G. E. Moore was the first to describe the use of fluorescein sodium for localization of brain tumors.[8] The intravascular and nonspecific accumulation of sodium fluorescein in brain tumors permitted visualization of yellow fluorescence by the naked eye and heralded the beginnings of FGS. Not until 1998 was the first clinical trial completed by Dr Walter Stummer studying the use of 5-aminolevulinic acid (5-ALA) for FGS of HGG tumors. In his original work, he was the first to describe how 5-ALA was metabolized to its fluorophore, protoporphyrin IX (PpIX), inside glioma cells.[9] Tumor tissue could be visualized with use of a modified operative microscope that could excite PpIX in tumor cells to visualize the violet-red fluorescence. Over the past 2 decades, the use of FGS has become a new paradigm in neurosurgical oncology.[10] Other fluorophores have been evaluated for the use of FGS in HGG surgery that are both nontargeted and targeted. These agents include endogenous fluorophores, molecular fluorophores, nanoparticles, and targeted antibodies.[9] In addition to the study of fluorescent agents for FGS of HGGs, technologies have also developed to permit

a Department of Neurosurgery, Icahn School of Medicine at Mount Sinai, Mount Sinai Health System, New York, NY, USA; b Department of Neurosurgery, Mount Sinai Beth Israel, New York, NY, USA
* Corresponding author. Mount Sinai Union Square, 10 Union Square East 5th Floor, Suite 5E, New York, NY 10003.
E-mail address: Constantinos.Hadjipanayis@mountsinai.org

Neurosurg Clin N Am 32 (2021) 55–64
https://doi.org/10.1016/j.nec.2020.08.001
1042-3680/21/© 2020 Elsevier Inc. All rights reserved.

improved visualization and detection of fluorescence in glioma cells.[11] This article describes the currently used fluorescent agents in glioblastoma surgery as well as the technologies investigated to improve visualization of fluorophores and resection of glioblastoma.

PRINCIPLES OF FLUORESCENT-GUIDED SURGERY

To understand the concept of FGS, it is important to understand the concept of fluorophore light absorption and light emission. In most cases, the emitted light of a fluorophore has a longer wavelength than the absorbed light. Light, or electromagnetic radiation, can be visible or invisible to the eye. Visible light is usually defined by wavelengths in the range of 400 to 700 nm which is between the invisible ultraviolet (10–400 nm) and infrared (>700 nm) light spectrums. Visible light is primarily composed of 3 different colors (blue, green, and red). Blue is a shorter wavelength of visible light (420–440 nm), green is a medium wavelength (534–545 nm), and red is a longer wavelength peaking near 564 to 580 nm. When fluorophores absorb light, the fluorophore enters an excited state of energy and, upon decay back to its resting state, it releases some of its energy as light, which can be detected as fluorescence. The most common fluorophore studied in cell and molecular biology is green fluorescent protein.[12] The gene that expresses green fluorescent protein is frequently used as a reporter of expression. This protein was isolated from the jellyfish *Aequorea victoria*. Green fluorescent protein exhibits bright green fluorescence when exposed to light in the blue to ultraviolet range. Different fluorophores emit light resulting in detection of fluorescence at different light wavelengths.

Glioblastoma Fluorescent-Guided Surgery

Overall, 5-aminolevulinc acid (5-ALA),[13,14] fluorescein sodium,[15] and indocyanine green (ICG),[16] have been the most widely studied fluorescent agents used clinically in patients for glioblastoma FGS. However, it is important to note that other fluorophores have been studied in glioma preclinical studies and include hypericin,[17] 5-aminofluorescein labeled to human serum albumin,[18] endogenous fluorophores,[19] various molecular targets,[20] nanoparticles,[21] and epidermal growth factor receptor (EGFR) antibodies.[22] This list is not exhaustive, but demonstrates the wide variety of potential targets for fluorescence of glioma cells.

5-Aminolevulinc Acid

To date, 5-ALA is the most common fluorescent agent studied for glioblastoma FGS. As a normal metabolite in the heme biosynthesis pathway, 5-ALA accumulates in glioma cells after oral administration at least 3 hours before surgery. After uptake by glioma cells, 5-ALA is metabolized in the mitochondrial heme biosynthesis pathway to its fluorophore metabolite, PpIX. PpIX accumulates in glioma cells and permits fluorescence detection owing to lower levels of the enzyme ferrochelatase, which catalyzes the production of heme from PpIX with the addition of iron. PpIX emits violet-red fluorescence (635 nm) in tumor cells after excitation by blue light (410 nm). A modified surgical microscope can switch between conventional white light and blue light for 5-ALA FGS.[9,23,24] By providing a light filter on the microscope, sufficient discrimination between background light and fluorescent tumor permits FGS because the surrounding brain tissue seems to be blue in color. Surrounding ambient light may interfere with proper visualization of PpIX and requires the operative lights to be turned off. Tumor peak fluorescence time is 6 to 8 hours after ingestion and can last for more than 12 hours.[24–26] First approved for use by the European Medicines Agency (EMA) in 2007, 5-ALA (as Gliolan), it was also recently was approved by the US Food and Drug Administration as Gleolan.[27] The approval of 5-ALA was based on a number of clinical trials and used in thousands of patients with glioma for FGS confirming safety. Minor adverse effects include transient liver enzyme elevations, nausea, and temporary skin photosensitivity within in 24 hours of administration.[14,28,29]

A number of studies have also confirmed that 5-ALA FGS permits greater resection of glioblastoma tumors that may impact patient outcomes.[10] The most notable study was a landmark randomized phase III study completed in 2006 comparing 5-ALA FGS to conventional microsurgery of HGGs. The multicenter study, led by Walter Stummer, included more than 300 patients with HGGs. Those patients that underwent 5-ALA FGS had significantly higher rates of CRET and progression-free survival at 6 months compared with those who did not undergo FGS.[14] After this study, there has been a wave of investigation into 5-ALA for HGG surgery. Since the initial Stummer trial reported CRET rates of 65%, other studies combining intraoperative navigation and cortical/subcortical mapping of eloquent tumors have improved the rates of CRET to more than 80% with the use of 5-ALA FGS (**Fig. 1**, Video 1).[30–32]

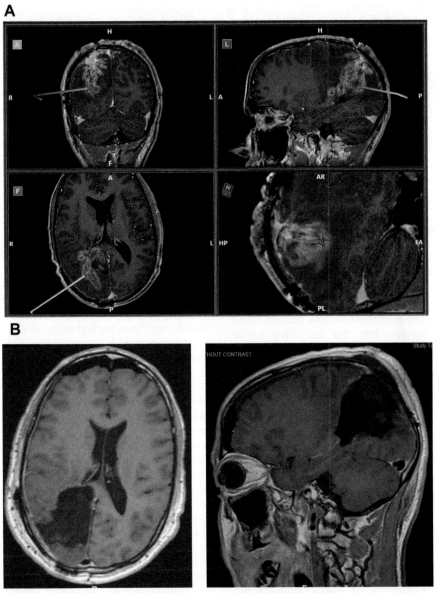

Fig. 1. (*A*) Preoperative MRI demonstrating large R parieto-occipital recurrent glioblastoma multiforme. (*B*) Postoperative MRI revealing complete resection of CRET on axial (*left*) and sagittal (*right*) sequences.

PpIX and 5-ALA fluorescence is highly diagnostic of HGG tumor tissue. A number of studies have confirmed the high sensitivity and specificity for differentiating glioblastoma tumor tissue from surrounding brain tissue at 83% to 87% and 89% to 100%, respectively.[33–36] Additionally, the positive predictive value of tissue fluorescence and presence of malignant tumor tissue has been shown to be close to 100% in both primary and recurrent gliomas.[37,38] The specificity and negative predictive value, however, are not found to be as high in most studies.[39–44] Owing to the infiltrative biology of HGGs, tumor cells are known to infiltrate centimeters away from the tumor bulk where fluorescence may be difficult to detect owing to the decreased presence of tumor cells with surrounding cells of the brain.[45]

The 5-ALA produces both a violet-red fluorescence in high-density tumor areas and a less vivid pink fluorescence toward the tumor infiltrative margin, where both surrounding brain tissue and tumor cells exist (**Fig. 2**).[38,46] With greater rates of CRET, 5-ALA FGS has been studied on its effect on patient outcomes including progression-free

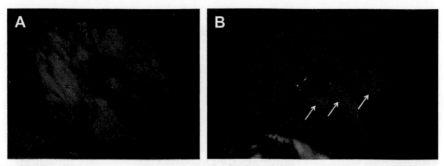

Fig. 2. (*A*) Bulk tumor fluorescence visualized during 5-ALA FGS (shown by *asterisk*). (*B*) Vague or weak fluorescence visualized at infiltrative tumor margin (shown by *arrows*).

survival and overall survival. Aldave and colleagues[47] found that, in 52 patients with glioblastoma who underwent complete resection of tumor fluorescence with 5-ALA, there was a significant overall survival benefit in comparison to patients with residual contrast enhancement (27 vs 17 months).

The 5-ALA FGS of HGG tumors permits more aggressive surgery into the infiltrative tumor margin that can improve patient outcomes. More aggressive surgery, however, may increase patient morbidity, especially for tumors located in or adjacent to eloquent regions of the brain. The 5-ALA FGS was found to be associated with a greater temporary impairment of neurologic function in the randomized phase III 5-ALA study.[14,48] A deterioration in the NIH-SS score by 1 point or more was observed in 26.2% of patients in the 5-ALA arm 48 hours after surgery, compared with 14.5% in the control group undergoing conventional microsurgery.

Recurrent High-Grade Glioma Fluorescent-Guided Surgery

Although the majority of 5-ALA glioblastoma studies have been performed on newly diagnosed glioblastoma, multiple studies have suggested a similar benefit in recurrent patients with glioblastoma who undergo 5-ALA FGS.[39–41,49,50] The sensitivity of 5-ALA fluorescence detection, however, may be slightly decreased in recurrent glioblastoma, because differentiating tumor from brain tissue may be more difficult owing to the presence of treatment effect in tumors and the surrounding brain tissue. In patients with recurrent glioblastoma, they almost always have undergone radiation and chemotherapy treatments that can result in radiation necrosis and gliosis.[41] False-positive tissue fluorescence has been reported in tumor areas with radiation necrosis and gliosis.[41]

FLUORESCEIN SODIUM FLUORESCENT-GUIDED SURGERY

Fluorescein sodium is one of the oldest studied fluorophores that has been primarily used for retinal examinations in ophthalmology.[51] In 1948, George E. Moore[52] described the properties of fluorescein in distinguishing healthy versus malignant tissue, and Murray[53] was the first to report the use of fluorescein in human brain tumor tissue. Fluorescein sodium is administered systemically at the time of anesthesia and its fluorescence can be detected in tumors in a limited time frame (approximately 3 hours). Fluorescein sodium excitation lies between 460 and 500 nm of visible light, with emission between 540 and 690 nm as a yellow-green fluorescence.[42] Modified operative microscopes with a special light filter can be used to visualize the yellow-green fluorescence; however, fluorescence can be visualized in the presence of surrounding ambient visible light. Fluorescein sodium is an intravascular fluorophore that accumulates in glioblastoma tumors owing to breakdown of the blood–brain barrier. The extracellular fluorophore is not taken up by tumor cells but accumulates by an enhanced permeability retention effect. Fluorescein sodium has several advantages over 5-ALA in that it is readily available, less expensive, and can be identified in the presence of ambient light.[43,44] However, a major criticism with fluorescein sodium is that it is less tumor-specific than 5-ALA because it is extracellular, time limited, and fluorescence accumulates in perilesional edema and surgical tissue injury.[45]

Glioblastoma Fluorescein Sodium Fluorescent-Guided Surgery

Several studies have reported the efficacy of fluorescein sodium in improving the resection of glioblastoma tumors,[54–57] with high CRET rates and good correlation between intraoperative fluorescence and contrast enhancement on neuronavigation MRI.[58] Unlike 5-ALA, there are no randomized controlled studies with fluorescein sodium FGS to determine if extent of tumor resection confers a progression-free survival or overall survival benefit, and therefore limited evidence is present for improved patient outcomes with fluorescein sodium FGS. In 2018, Acerbi and colleagues[15] conducted a phase II study (FLUGLIO) of fluorescein sodium for HGG surgery, and found that fluorescein was safe and effective, with a sensitivity and specificity of tumor cell detection of 80%. In a small prospective study, Chen and colleagues[59] found a progression-free survival benefit in the fluorescein sodium group; however, this effect has not been shown in a larger, randomized study.

There is no clear consensus on the dosage and timing of administration. However, timing seems to be critical, because extravasation and distribution of this agent follows a certain time course. After a half-life of 264 minutes, fluorescein will be extravasated and might stain peritumoral edema or surrounding brain, jeopardizing resection of nontumorous tissue.[60] Recently, simultaneous use of 5-ALA and fluorescein has been tested, and shown to improve background discrimination and have a potential role in future FGS investigations.[61]

INDOCYANINE GREEN

Similar to fluorescein, ICG has wide clinical applications in medicine; it has been used to assess hepatic function and ophthalmic angiography.[10] ICG has also had prior applications in neurosurgery, and is commonly used in cerebrovascular neurosurgery to assess aneurysm occlusion and vessel integrity (ICG video angiography).[62] Unlike 5-ALA and fluorescein sodium, the peak excitation of ICG is 805 nm and emission is 835 nm, placing it in the near-infrared (NIR) region of the light spectrum invisible to the naked eye.[63] The application of ICG in glioblastoma surgery is known as second window ICG, which allows passive accumulation of ICG in tumor tissue.[64] This occurs from higher doses of ICG being administered 24 hours before surgery, which accumulates in glioma tissue the following day owing to the enhanced permeability retention effect.[65] Fluorescence is detected by an NIR camera, which has been integrated into visualization devices that can permit an overlay of the NIR image on the conventional view with standard light. This technique may allow for the delineation of the tumor margins and, although the mechanism is not well understood, it is believed to accumulate from the disruption of the blood–brain barrier.[66] As the only US Food and Drug Administration-approved NIR fluorophore for ophthalmologic applications,[67] ICG is safely tolerated and has a low incidence of adverse events.[62]

In a small study using second window ICG for localization of HGGs, the majority of tumors were visualized with the NIR camera, and fluorescence correlated well with the degree of preoperative contrast enhancement, suggesting a potential benefit of NIR imaging for detection of residual tumor.[64,65]

Unlike the fluorophores that fluoresce in the visible light spectrum, such as 5-ALA and fluorescein sodium, ICG excites and emits in the NIR spectrum.[68] This longer wavelength allows visualization of fluorescence in deeper tissue regions owing to a high signal to noise ratio, which may improve surgical precision, with improved ability to visualize residual tumor beyond normal tissue.[68] Cho and colleagues[64] found 100% visualization of tumor before durotomy in tumors that reached the cortex, and adequate accuracy in overall detection. Two additional clinical trials have reported the use of ICG in glioma surgery, however, the rate of CRET with this fluorophore has not been well-established.[69,70] Despite several advantages of ICG in the NIR spectrum, similar to fluorescein, ICG can accumulate in areas of peritumoral edema and blood–brain barrier breakdown, which may lead to hindered specificity and false-positive staining.[64,65]

TARGETED FLUOROPHORES
BLZ-100 Fluorescent-Guided Surgery

BLZ-100 (tozuleristide, Blaze Bioscience Inc, Seattle, WA), commonly known as "tumor paint," is a conjugate of NIR with the tumor-specific peptide chlorotoxin.[66] Extracted from scorpion venom, chlorotoxin binds to the cell surface of low- and high-grade glial tumors[67,68] and can be visualized with a NIR camera.[69,70] In 2019, a phase I study showed safety for us of BLZ-100 in patients with primary and recurrent glioblastoma,[66] and there is current investigation in both the adult and pediatric populations to assess extent of resection and progression-free survival using BLZ-100 in malignant glioma surgery. As previously mentioned with ICG, there are benefits to using a fluorophore in the NIR spectrum, and BLZ-100 adds the advantage of a tumor-specific peptide to the benefits of ICG.

Tumor-Targeted Alkyl Phosphocholine Analogs

Alkylphosphocholine analogs are small synthetic phospholipid ether molecules, which have been shown to target a wide range of tumors types with a broad tumor targeting potential.[67] Following tumor cell uptake, alkylphosphocholine analogs have prolonged intracellular retention, thought to be due to lipid raft expression.[67] There have yet to be any clinical trials; however, preclinical studies have shown glioblastoma selectivity with 2 alkylphosphocholine analogs (CLR1501 and CLR1502, Cellectar Biosciences, Madison, WI) have been studied in a preclinical setting and found to label glioblastoma cells with a high cell selectivity.[71]

Targeting Epidermal Growth Factor Receptor

EGFR has been shown to be expressed on the cell surface of glioblastoma, which displays mutant forms of the EGF receptor.[10] Tagged with fluorescent dyes, anti-EGFR antibodies are able to distinguish glioblastoma multiforme-specific mutated EGFR from EGFR negative tumor with 100% sensitivity and specificity.[22] Only preclinical studies have been conducted to date; however, they have shown a potential role for future use in FGS surgery.[22,72]

Cetuximab-IRDye800

Cetuximab, an EGFR inhibitor, when conjugated with fluorescent dye (IRDye 800), has been shown in animal models to be effective in the NIR spectrum for glioma surgery.[73] Recently, a first-in-human study found that cetuximab-IRDye800 was not only safe and effective for use in patients undergoing intraoperative visualization of glioblastoma, but that the conjugate had an optimal signal to background ratio, with adequate tumor visualization. However, only 3 patients were included in this study, and further investigation is needed.[74]

VISUALIZATION TECHNOLOGIES

In conjunction with improved targeting of tumor tissue in glioblastoma FGS, greater visualization and detection of target tissue is required for improved results in the operating room. Over the past decade, technologies have been developed to improve the detection of tumor fluorescence, providing surgeons with better visualization of tumor infiltration than ever before. Newer detection devices can permit quantification of brain versus tumor tissue has become incredibly accurate. Here, we review the current standard practice, and some of these novel techniques currently under investigation.

Wide-Field Surgical Microscopy

As the historical and conventional method of visualization during brain tumor surgery, wide-field surgical microscopy has continued to improve over the past 2 decades and remains the standard for visualizing tumor fluorescence during FGS with modified light filters. Initially described in glioma resection in the late 1990s by Stummer and co-workers,[24] today all modern operative microscopes have the capability of visualizing the more common fluorophores in the visible and NIR spectrums. Despite its time-tested reliability, conventional microscopy is limited by its focal distance, creating vulnerability for blind spots of fluorescence in areas where the tumor may be covered by healthy tissue or blood products.[75]

Wide-Field Fluorescence Endoscopy

To improve visualization of deep or subcortical tumors in FGS surgery, endoscopic methods have been explored. Endoscopy may improve the ability to visualize fluorescence around blind spots that would be missed by conventional microscopy, which has previously been shown in 5-ALA FGS for intraventricular HGG.[76] Other technical studies have also shown improved HGG visualization with endoscopy for 5-ALA FGS.[77,78]

Quantitative Spectroscopy

There is little debate regarding the ability to visualize fluorescence at the center of a tumor mass; however, less distinguishable is the margin between healthy brain tissue and tumor. As described elsewhere in this article, fluorophores may exhibit a spectrum of colors between the signal of tumor fluorescence and normal tissue, rendering it challenging to discernably determine the margin. Resecting a safe margin is essential for progression-free and overall survival, with patients receiving a subtotal resection having a higher risk of mortality.[1] To combat this dilemma, quantitative spectroscopy has been used. At the margin, the tumor cell density can be calculated, guiding surgeons to accurately determine the resected margin outside of the defined margin on imaging. Handheld probes have been developed that can be placed on the target tissue to quantify tumor-cell density in real time.[79–81] As described by Wei and colleagues,[81] this tool can be useful at the end of a glioma resection, where a probe can be placed over critical locations to determine if additional resection is required. The limit to this technology is the amount of surface area that can be analyzed at once. Because only several millimeters can be quantified at a time, this limitation creates practical challenges in cases of large tumors with large associated resection cavities.[81] To improve detection ability, algorithms are being evaluated to allow faster detection of larger areas.[79,80]

Probe-Based Confocal Microscopy

In addition to changing the size and versatility of the microscope, the mechanics of microscopic visualization have been studied as well. Wide-field microscopy conventionally uses single axis confocal microscopy; however, to allow a small numerical aperture, longer working distance, and greater signal to noise background ratio, dual-axis confocal microscopy has been studied. By changing the configuration, it allows for improved contrast detection.[82] Handheld probes have previously been shown to both detect PpIX expression and quantification in 5-ALA resection of gliomas,[83] and by combining dual-axis confocal microscopy with a handheld probe, this strategy allows for a high rate of scanning with minimal motion artifact while analyzing the resection cavity.[84] The resolution has been shown to be strong enough that it correlates with histologically processed tissue sections. This technology has also been used with fluorescein, showing effective detection of gliomas.[85,86] Despite the current limitations of processing speeds and restricted area of visualization, by allowing for in vivo histologic tumor characteristics, this technology has provided surgeons with the ability to diagnosis tissue at the margin during surgery for the first time.

SUMMARY

As the technology of visualization devices has expanded over the past 2 decades, the use of intraoperative fluorophores has expanded. Although FGS has been studied among different brain tumors, glioblastoma and HGGs have been largely implicated for their high sensitivity and specificity for tumor fluorescence and provided surgeons with a useful adjunct in the operating room. The use of fluorophores in surgery for glioblastoma has made a significant contribution to the field, and as intraoperative visualization and detection devices continue to improve, this role will continue to expand in guiding surgeons toward maximal safe resection.

CLINICS CARE POINTS

- Intraoperative use of fluorescence provides surgeons with improved visualization of glioblastoma tissue.
- Many fluorophores have been studied, and 5-ALA, fluorescein, and ICG are the most commonly used in practice today.

- Innovation of visualization devices have allowed for improve detection and quantification of fluorescence in tumor tissue, especially at the infiltrative margin.

DISCLOSURE

C. Hadjipanayis is a consultant for NXDC and Synaptive Medical Inc. He receives royalties from NXDC. He has also received speaker fees by Carl Zeiss and Leica. A.J. Schupper has nothing to disclose.

SUPPLEMENTARY DATA

Supplementary data related to this article can be found online at https://doi.org/10.1016/j.nec.2020.08.001.

REFERENCES

1. Stupp R, Mason WP, van den Bent MJ, et al. Radiotherapy plus concomitant and adjuvant temozolomide for glioblastoma. N Engl J Med 2005;352(10): 987–96.
2. Brown TJ, Brennan MC, Li M, et al. Association of the extent of resection with survival in glioblastoma: a systematic review and meta-analysis. JAMA Oncol 2016;2(11):1460–9.
3. Lacroix M, Abi-Said D, Fourney DR, et al. A multivariate analysis of 416 patients with glioblastoma multiforme: prognosis, extent of resection, and survival. J Neurosurg 2001;95(2):190–8.
4. Marko NF, Weil RJ, Schroeder JL, et al. Extent of resection of glioblastoma revisited: personalized survival modeling facilitates more accurate survival prediction and supports a maximum-safe-resection approach to surgery. J Clin Oncol 2014;32(8): 774–82.
5. Sanai N, Berger MS. Glioma extent of resection and its impact on patient outcome. Neurosurgery 2008; 62(4):753–64 [discussion: 264–6].
6. Stummer W, Reulen HJ, Meinel T, et al. Extent of resection and survival in glioblastoma multiforme: identification of and adjustment for bias. Neurosurgery 2008;62(3):564–76 [discussion: 564–76].
7. Orringer D, Lau D, Khatri S, et al. Extent of resection in patients with glioblastoma: limiting factors, perception of resectability, and effect on survival. J Neurosurg 2012;117(5):851–9.
8. Moore GE, Peyton WT. The clinical use of fluorescein in neurosurgery; the localization of brain tumors. J Neurosurg 1948;5:392–8.
9. Stummer W, Stocker S, Novotny A, et al. In vitro and in vivo porphyrin accumulation by C6 glioma cells after exposure to 5-aminolevulinic acid. J Photochem Photobiol B 1998;45(2–3):160-169.

10. Senders JT, Muskens IS, Schnoor R, et al. Agents for fluorescence-guided glioma surgery: a systematic review of preclinical and clinical results. Acta Neurochir (Wien) 2017;159(1):151–67.

11. Hadjipanayis C, Stummer W. Fluorescence-guided neurosurgery. 1st edition. New York, NY: Thieme; 2018.

12. Jung D, Min K, Jung J, et al. Chemical biology-based approaches on fluorescent labeling of proteins in live cells. Mol Biosyst 2013;9(5):862–72.

13. Stummer W, Novotny A, Stepp H, et al. Fluorescence-guided resection of glioblastoma multiforme by using 5-aminolevulinic acid-induced porphyrins: a prospective study in 52 consecutive patients. J Neurosurg 2000;93(6):1003–13.

14. Stummer W, Pichlmeier U, Meinel T, et al. Fluorescence-guided surgery with 5-aminolevulinic acid for resection of malignant glioma: a randomised controlled multicentre phase III trial. Lancet Oncol 2006;7(5):392–401.

15. Acerbi F, Broggi M, Schebesch KM, et al. Fluorescein-guided surgery for resection of high-grade gliomas: a multicentric prospective phase II study (FLUOGLIO). Clin Cancer Res 2018; 24(1):52–61.

16. Zeh R, Sheikh S, Xia L, et al. The second window ICG technique demonstrates a broad plateau period for near infrared fluorescence tumor contrast in glioblastoma. PLoS One 2017;12(7):e0182034.

17. Ritz R, Daniels R, Noell S, et al. Hypericin for visualization of high grade gliomas: first clinical experience. Eur J Surg Oncol 2012;38(4):352–60.

18. Kremer P, Fardanesh M, Ding R, et al. Intraoperative fluorescence staining of malignant brain tumors using 5-aminofluorescein-labeled albumin. Neurosurgery 2009;64(3 Suppl):ons53–60 [discussion: ons60–1].

19. Jackson H, Muhammad O, Daneshvar H, et al. Quantum dots are phagocytized by macrophages and colocalize with experimental gliomas. Neurosurgery 2007;60(3):524–9 [discussion: 529–30].

20. Burden-Gulley SM, Zhou Z, Craig SE, et al. Molecular Magnetic Resonance Imaging of Tumors with a PTPmicro Targeted Contrast Agent. Transl Oncol 2013;6(3):329–37.

21. Cutter JL, Cohen NT, Wang J, et al. Topical application of activity-based probes for visualization of brain tumor tissue. PLoS One 2012;7(3):e33060.

22. Davis SC, Samkoe KS, O'Hara JA, et al. MRI-coupled fluorescence tomography quantifies EGFR activity in brain tumors. Acad Radiol 2010;17(3): 271–6.

23. Colditz MJ, Leyen K, Jeffree RL. Aminolevulinic acid (ALA)-protoporphyrin IX fluorescence guided tumour resection. Part 2: theoretical, biochemical and practical aspects. J Clin Neurosci 2012; 19(12):1611–6.

24. Stummer W, Stepp H, Moller G, et al. Technical principles for protoporphyrin-IX-fluorescence guided microsurgical resection of malignant glioma tissue. Acta Neurochir (Wien) 1998;140(10):995–1000.

25. Kaneko S, Suero Molina E, Ewelt C, et al. Fluorescence-based measurement of real-time kinetics of Protoporphyrin IX after 5-Aminolevulinic Acid administration in Human in situ Malignant Gliomas. Neurosurgery 2019;85(4):E739–46.

26. Suero Molina E, Wölfer J, Ewelt C. Dual-labeling with 5-aminolevulinic acid and fluorescein for fluorescence-guided resection of high-grade gliomas: technical note. J Neurosurg 2018;128(2): 399–405.

27. Hadjipanayis CG, Stummer W. 5-ALA and FDA approval for glioma surgery. J Neurooncol 2019; 141(3):479–86.

28. Chung SR, Choi YJ, Suh CH, et al. Diffusion-weighted magnetic resonance imaging for predicting response to chemoradiation therapy for head and neck squamous cell carcinoma: a systematic review. Korean J Radiol 2019;20(4):649–61.

29. Teixidor P, Arraez MA, Villalba G, et al. Safety and efficacy of 5-aminolevulinic acid for high grade glioma in usual clinical practice: a prospective cohort study. PLoS One 2016;11(2):e0149244.

30. Coburger J, Hagel V, Wirtz CR, et al. Surgery for glioblastoma: impact of the combined use of 5-aminolevulinic acid and intraoperative MRI on extent of resection and survival. PLoS One 2015;10(6): e0131872.

31. Della Puppa A, De Pellegrin S, d'Avella E, et al. 5-aminolevulinic acid (5-ALA) fluorescence guided surgery of high-grade gliomas in eloquent areas assisted by functional mapping. Our experience and review of the literature. Acta Neurochir (Wien) 2013;155(6):965–72 [discussion: 972].

32. Schucht P, Beck J, Abu-Isa J, et al. Gross total resection rates in contemporary glioblastoma surgery: results of an institutional protocol combining 5-aminolevulinic acid intraoperative fluorescence imaging and brain mapping. Neurosurgery 2012; 71(5):927–35 [discussion: 935–6].

33. Eljamel S. 5-ALA fluorescence image guided resection of glioblastoma multiforme: a meta-analysis of the literature. Int J Mol Sci 2015;16(5):10443–56.

34. Stummer W, Stocker S, Wagner S, et al. Intraoperative detection of malignant gliomas by 5-aminolevulinic acid-induced porphyrin fluorescence. Neurosurgery 1998;42(3):518–25 [discussion: 525–6].

35. Su X, Huang QF, Chen HL, et al. Fluorescence-guided resection of high-grade gliomas: a systematic review and meta-analysis. Photodiagnosis Photodyn Ther 2014;11(4):451–8.

36. Zhao S, Wu J, Wang C, et al. Intraoperative fluorescence-guided resection of high-grade malignant gliomas using 5-aminolevulinic acid-induced

porphyrins: a systematic review and meta-analysis of prospective studies. PLoS One 2013;8(5):e63682.

47. Diez Valle R, Tejada Solis S, Idoate Gastearena MA, et al. Surgery guided by 5-aminolevulinic fluorescence in glioblastoma: volumetric analysis of extent of resection in single-center experience. J Neurooncol 2011; 102(1):105–13.

48. Lau D, Hervey-Jumper SL, Chang S, et al. A prospective Phase II clinical trial of 5-aminolevulinic acid to assess the correlation of intraoperative fluorescence intensity and degree of histologic cellularity during resection of high-grade gliomas. J Neurosurg 2016;124(5):1300–9.

49. Suchorska B, Weller M, Tabatabai G, et al. Complete resection of contrast-enhancing tumor volume is associated with improved survival in recurrent glioblastoma-results from the DIRECTOR trial. Neuro Oncol 2016;18(4):549–56.

40. Hickmann AK, Nadji-Ohl M, Hopf NJ. Feasibility of fluorescence-guided resection of recurrent gliomas using five-aminolevulinic acid: retrospective analysis of surgical and neurological outcome in 58 patients. J Neurooncol 2015;122(1):151–60.

41. Kamp MA, Felsberg J, Sadat H, et al. 5-ALA-induced fluorescence behavior of reactive tissue changes following glioblastoma treatment with radiation and chemotherapy. Acta Neurochir (Wien) 2015;157(2):207–13 [discussion: 213–4].

42. Hohne J, Hohenberger C, Proescholdt M, et al. Fluorescein sodium-guided resection of cerebral metastases-an update. Acta Neurochir (Wien) 2017;159(2):363–7.

43. Manoharan R, Parkinson J. Sodium fluorescein in brain tumor surgery: assessing relative fluorescence intensity at tumor margins. Asian J Neurosurg 2020; 15(1):88-93.

44. Neira JA, Ung TH, Sims JS, et al. Aggressive resection at the infiltrative margins of glioblastoma facilitated by intraoperative fluorescein guidance. J Neurosurg 2017;127(1):111–22.

45. Stummer W. Fluorescein in brain metastasis and glioma surgery. Acta Neurochir (Wien) 2015;157:2199–200.

46. Schipmann S, Schwake M, Suero Molina E, et al. Markers for Identifying and Targeting Glioblastoma Cells during Surgery. J Neurol Surg A Cent Eur Neurosurg 2019;80(6):475–87.

47. Aldave G, Tejada S, Pay E, et al. Prognostic value of residual fluorescent tissue in glioblastoma patients after gross total resection in 5-aminolevulinic Acid-guided surgery. Neurosurgery 2013;72(6):915–20 [discussion: 920–1].

48. Stummer W, Tonn JC, Mehdorn HM, et al. Counterbalancing risks and gains from extended resections in malignant glioma surgery: a supplemental analysis from the randomized 5-aminolevulinic acid glioma resection study. Clinical article. J Neurosurg 2011;114(3):613–23.

49. Perrini P, Gambacciani C, Weiss A, et al. Survival outcomes following repeat surgery for recurrent glioblastoma: a single-center retrospective analysis. J Neurooncol 2017;131(3):585–91.

50. Ringel F, Pape H, Sabel M, et al. Clinical benefit from resection of recurrent glioblastomas: results of a multicenter study including 503 patients with recurrent glioblastomas undergoing surgical resection. Neuro Oncol 2016;18(1):96–104.

51. Rabb MF, Burton TC, Schatz H, et al. Fluorescein angiography of the fundus: a schematic approach to interpretation. Surv Ophthalmol 1978;22(6): 387–403.

52. Moore GE. Fluorescein as an Agent in the Differentiation of Normal and Malignant Tissues. Science 1947;106(2745):130–1.

53. Murray KJ. Improved surgical resection of human brain tumors: part I. A preliminary study. Surg Neurol 1982;17:316–9.

54. Okuda T, Yoshioka H, Kato A. Fluorescence-guided surgery for glioblastoma multiforme using high-dose fluorescein sodium with excitation and barrier filters. J Clin Neurosci 2012;19(12):1719–22.

55. Schebesch KM, Brawanski A, Hohenberger C, et al. Fluorescein sodium-guided surgery of malignant brain tumors: history, current concepts, and future project. Turk Neurosurg 2016;26(2):185–94.

56. Schebesch KM, Proescholdt M, Hohne J, et al. Sodium fluorescein-guided resection under the YELLOW 560 nm surgical microscope filter in malignant brain tumor surgery–a feasibility study. Acta Neurochir (Wien) 2013;155(4): 693–9.

57. Kuroiwa T, Kajimoto Y, Ohta T. Development of a fluorescein operative microscope for use during malignant glioma surgery: a technical note and preliminary report. Surg Neurol 1998;50(1):41–8 [discussion: 48–9].

58. Diaz RJ, Dios RR, Hattab EM, et al. Study of the biodistribution of fluorescein in glioma-infiltrated mouse brain and histopathological correlation of intraoperative findings in high-grade gliomas resected under fluorescein fluorescence guidance. J Neurosurg 2015;122(6):1360–9.

59. Chen B, Wang H, Ge P, et al. Gross total resection of glioma with the intraoperative fluorescence-guidance of fluorescein sodium. Int J Med Sci 2012;9(8):708–14.

60. Stummer W, Gotz C, Hassan A, et al. Kinetics of Photofrin II in perifocal brain edema. Neurosurgery 1993;33(6):1075–81 [discussion: 1081–2].

61. Stummer W. Poor man's fluorescence? Acta Neurochir (Wien) 2015;157(8):1379–81.

62. Raabe A, Beck J, Gerlach R, et al. Near-infrared indocyanine green video angiography: a new method for intraoperative assessment of vascular flow. Neurosurgery 2003;52(1):132–9 [discussion: 139].

63. Cherrick GR, Stein SW, Leevy CM, et al. Indocyanine green: observations on its physical properties, plasma decay, and hepatic extraction. J Clin Invest 1960;39:592–600.

64. Cho SS, Salinas R, De Ravin E, et al. Near-Infrared Imaging with Second-Window Indocyanine Green in Newly Diagnosed High-Grade Gliomas Predicts Gadolinium Enhancement on Postoperative Magnetic Resonance Imaging. Mol Imaging Biol 2019. [Epub ahead of print].

65. Lee JY, Thawani JP, Pierce J, et al. Intraoperative Near-Infrared Optical Imaging Can Localize Gadolinium-Enhancing Gliomas During Surgery. Neurosurgery 2016;79(6):856–71.

66. Patil CG, Walker DG, Miller DM, et al. Phase 1 Safety, Pharmacokinetics, and Fluorescence Imaging Study of Tozuleristide (BLZ-100) in Adults With Newly Diagnosed or Recurrent Gliomas. Neurosurgery 2019;85(4):E641–9.

67. Weichert JP, Clark PA, Kandela IK, et al. Alkylphosphocholine analogs for broad-spectrum cancer imaging and therapy. Sci Transl Med 2014;6(240):240ra275.

68. Hilgard P, Klenner T, Stekar J, et al. Alkylphosphocholines: a new class of membrane-active anticancer agents. Cancer Chemother Pharmacol 1993;32(2):90–5.

69. Kuo JS, Zhang RR, Pinchuk AN, et al. Creation of a Dual-Labeled Cancer-Targeting Alkylphosphocholine Analog for Dual Modality Quantitative Positron Emission Tomography and Intraoperative Tumor Visualization. Neurosurgery 2016;63(CN_suppl_1):208.

70. Zhang RR, Swanson KI, Hall LT, et al. Diapeutic cancer-targeting alkylphosphocholine analogs may advance management of brain malignancies. CNS Oncol 2016;5(4):223–31.

71. Swanson KI, Clark PA, Zhang RR, et al. Fluorescent cancer-selective alkylphosphocholine analogs for intraoperative glioma detection. Neurosurgery 2015;76(2):115–23 [discussion: 123–4].

72. Sexton K, Tichauer K, Samkoe KS, et al. Fluorescent affibody peptide penetration in glioma margin is superior to full antibody. PLoS One 2013. https://doi.org/10.1371/journal.pone.0060390.

73. Warram JM, de Boer E, Korb M, et al. Fluorescence-guided resection of experimental malignant glioma using cetuximab-IRDye 800CW. Br J Neurosurg 2015;29(6):850–8.

74. Miller SE, Tummers WS, Teraphongphom N, et al. First-in-human intraoperative near-infrared fluorescence imaging of glioblastoma using cetuximab-IRDye800. J Neurooncol 2018;139(1):135–43.

75. Wei L, Roberts DW, Sanai N, et al. Visualization technologies for 5-ALA-based fluorescence-guided surgeries. J Neurooncol 2019;141(3):495–505.

76. Tamura Y, Kuroiwa T, Kajimoto Y, et al. Endoscopic identification and biopsy sampling of an intraventricular malignant glioma using a 5-aminolevulinic acid-induced protoporphyrin IX fluorescence imaging system. Technical note. J Neurosurg 2007;106(3):507–10.

77. Belykh E, Miller EJ, Hu D, et al. Scanning Fiber Endoscope Improves Detection of 5-Aminolevulinic Acid-Induced Protoporphyrin IX Fluorescence at the Boundary of Infiltrative Glioma. World Neurosurg 2018;113:e51–69.

78. Potaov A, Usachey D, Loshakov V, et al. First experience in 5-ALA fluorescence-guided and endoscopically assisted microsurgery of brain tumors. Med Laser Appl 2008;23(4):202–8.

79. Valdes PA, Leblond F, Kim A, et al. Quantitative fluorescence in intracranial tumor: implications for ALA-induced PpIX as an intraoperative biomarker. J Neurosurg 2011;115(1):11–7.

80. Bravo JJ, Olson JD, Davis SC, et al. Hyperspectral data processing improves PpIX contrast during fluorescence guided surgery of human brain tumors. Sci Rep 2017;7(1):9455.

81. Wei L, Fujita Y, Sanai N, et al. Toward Quantitative Neurosurgical Guidance With High-Resolution Microscopy of 5-Aminolevulinic Acid-Induced Protoporphyrin IX. Front Oncol 2019;9:592.

82. Wei L, Yin C, Liu JTC. Dual-axis confocal microscopy for point-of-care pathology. IEEE J Sel Top Quantum Electron 2019;25(1):7100910.

83. Sanai N, Eschbacher J, Hattendorf G, et al. Intraoperative confocal microscopy for brain tumors: a feasibility analysis in humans. Neurosurgery 2011;68(2 Suppl Operative):282–90 [discussion: 290].

84. Wei L, Chen Y, Yin C, et al. Optical-sectioning microscopy of protoporphyrin IX fluorescence in human gliomas: standardization and quantitative comparison with histology. J Biomed Opt 2017;22(4):46005.

85. Martirosyan NL, Eschbacher JM, Kalani MY, et al. Prospective evaluation of the utility of intraoperative confocal laser endomicroscopy in patients with brain neoplasms using fluorescein sodium: experience with 74 cases. Neurosurg Focus 2016;40(3):E11.

86. Belykh E, Miller EJ, Patel AA, et al. Diagnostic accuracy of a confocal laser endomicroscope for in vivo differentiation between normal injured and tumor tissue during fluorescein-guided glioma resection: laboratory investigation. World Neurosurg 2018;115:e337–48.

Functional Mapping for Glioma Surgery, Part 1
Preoperative Mapping Tools

Sebastian Ille, MD, Sandro M. Krieg, MD, MBA*

KEYWORDS

- Preoperative • nTMS • Mapping • Motor function • Language • Neuropsychology • fMRI • MEG

KEY POINTS

- Noninvasive functional localization of eloquent cortex or subcortical fiber tracts can enhance extent of resection and functional outcome.
- Functional magnetic resonance imaging and tractography are magnetic resonance imaging–based techniques.
- Navigated transcranial magnetic stimulation and magnetoencephalography are neurophysiologic modalities.
- The combination of cortical mapping methods with tractography is able to assign function to tractography adding specific information to the otherwise unspecific tractography.
- Intraoperative neuromonitoring (IOM) starts but does not end with noninvasive mapping techniques; they are complementary methods.

INTRODUCTION

Proximity of tumors to highly significant functional areas, or so-called eloquent areas, still is a risk factor for progressive tumor, shorter progression-free survival, and overall survival.[1,2] Yet, a full comprehension of topographic anatomy is insufficient to conclude eligibility for gross total resection because nowadays the considerable interindividual variations in functional anatomy, especially in brain tumor patients, is known.[3–7] Thus, techniques for noninvasive mapping are useful when it comes to estimating resectability, surgical approach, or even risk stratification of a surgical procedure.[8]

Among those techniques are true electrophysiologic methods, such as navigated transcranial magnetic stimulation (nTMS) and magnetoencephalography (MEG), and magnetic resonance imaging (MRI)-based methods using surrogate parameters of function, that is, functional MRI (fMRI) and tractography by diffusion tensor imaging (DTI). Due to the increased use of such noninvasive options and optimized patient communication by such data, resection of tumors previously tagged as unresectable is regarded more frequently as a valid option at a tolerable morbidity.[9,10] Thus, among other sophisticated techniques in the neuro-oncological armamentarium of neurosurgeons, like image guidance, fluorescent dyes, ultrasound, and intraoperative MRI, those noninvasive mapping modalities represent an important pillar in modern surgical neuro-oncology.

They not only are able to map critical functional areas, like motor, language, and other neuropsychological functions, prior to surgery but also are able to guide intraoperative direct electrical stimulation of the cortex (DCS) or direct subcortical stimulation (SCS) by providing additional highly valuable information on function and location within the cortex and white matter.[11]

Department of Neurosurgery, Technical University of Munich, Germany, School of Medicine, Klinikum rechts der Isar, Ismaninger Strasse 22, Munich 81675, Germany
* Corresponding author.
E-mail address: Sandro.Krieg@tum.de

Neurosurg Clin N Am 32 (2021) 65–74
https://doi.org/10.1016/j.nec.2020.08.004
1042-3680/21/© 2020 Elsevier Inc. All rights reserved.

Recently, especially for language and also for motor function, several studies showed the large neuro-oncological impact of brain plasticity.[3–7,10,12] In particular, tumors generally stated by anatomy as language eloquent are situated regularly in brain regions not involved at all in language processing.[9,10,13,14] Additionally, functional reorganization facilitates tumor resection during the course of the disease.[6,7,12,15,16]

Thus, modern surgical neuro-oncology requires any noninvasive setup in order to get an approximate idea on the current individual functional anatomy at the current time point of the respective disease prior to surgery. Because mapping and monitoring of motor and language function are the most frequently applied techniques, this article also focuses on these 2 functions. Other approaches and functions also are discussed.

FUNCTIONAL MAGNETIC RESONANCE IMAGING

fMRI is a technique using blood oxygenation level–dependent effect as surrogate marker of neuronal activation. In theory, neuronal activation induces hyperperfusion via neurovascular coupling and these perfusion-related changes in the blood oxygen level of venous blood then can be detected by MRI.[17] Yet, a differentiation of essential versus nonessential areas for function is not possible. fMRI can detect only brain areas that are involved in any given function but is unable to identify essential regions (**Fig. 1**).

For more than 15 years, fMRI has been used for presurgical evaluation of functional areas prior to brain tumor surgery due to the broad availability of magnetic resonance scanners worldwide.[18]

Especially the presence of oxygen-consuming tumors or arteriovenous malformations (AVMs), however, can lead to a neurovascular uncoupling and bias the fMRI results, thus producing false-negative fMRI results, making them basically unreliable for resection planning.[19,20] For language mapping, Giussani and colleagues[21] provided a meta-analysis comparing presurgical fMRI to DCS and demonstrated that specificity ranged between 0% and 97% and sensitivity between 59% and 100% compared with intraoperative DCS mapping, thus making the described fMRI protocols unsuitable for presurgical decision making. For motor function, the accuracy and predictive values of fMRI seem different and better suited to sufficiently predict the location of motor function compared with DCS.[22–24] Yet, other studies still proved a large deviance between fMRI and DCS.[25–27]

In recent years, resting-state fMRI was introduced as a promising method to reduce noise and bias due to impaired tumor-induced oxygenation.[28] Nonetheless, what first was promoted as another promising approach also now is reported to be more or less mediocre in its clinical value.[29,30]

MAGNETOENCEPHALOGRAPHY

MEG, in contrast, does not measure surrogate markers but directly detects very small magnetic fields created by bioelectric currents from neuronal activation at picotesla or femtotesla levels.[31] This requires an elaborate setup of magnetic shielding and supraconductive sensors that allows, on the other hand, measurement of spontaneous or evoked brain activity with a high temporal but low spatial resolution. Coregistration of MEG detectors with anatomic MRI makes MEG eligible for presurgical planning. In doing so, MEG repeatedly was used for auditory, motor, language, and visual cortex mapping prior to surgery for brain tumor and for epilepsy patients.

Studies comparing the accuracy of preoperative MEG with intraoperative DCS are available for motor and language function and reported consistent outlining of motor areas compared with intraoperative DCS.[32–36] Concerning language, 12 patients were investigated by Tarapore and colleagues;[37]

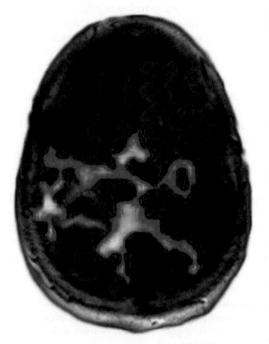

Fig. 1. fMRI shows activated brain regions by a finger-tapping task in a patient with a right-sided metastasis of the precentral gyrus.

MEG language sites outlined via verb generation and object naming tasks correlated with nTMS sites in 5 subjects and with DCS sites in 2 subjects. From the same group, Findlay and colleagues[27,37] investigated MEG for a global analysis of language lateralization, showing that it is capable to forecast postsurgical language function for eloquent glioma patients. Another study uses resection-related deficits, proving that the resection of motor functional tissue caused new surgery-related neurologic deficits in all cases if MEG-positive cortex was resected.[38]

Hence, the major limitation and reason of the scarce literature for the use in brain tumor patients of this powerful tool are its limited distribution due to the high apparative costs and required staff expertise.

NAVIGATED TRANSCRANIAL MAGNETIC STIMULATION

TMS was brought into clinical neurology in 1985.[39] The induced magnetic field penetrates the skull and induces an electric field inside the brain, which then stimulates neurons[40] (**Fig. 2**). TMS is painless and allows eliciting motor-evoked potentials (MEPs) similar to DCS. Yet, the implementation of very focal figure-of-8 coils and the combination with a neuronavigational device, enabling a proper calculation of strength and location of the induced electric field, allowed the application for neurosurgeons due to spatial resolution in the millimeter range.[41]

Since 2009, several studies proved the accuracy of nTMS compared with DCS motor mapping to be within the general inaccuracy of neuronavigation.[42] For language, repetitive, thus inhibitory, nTMS is used causing a so-called virtual lesion similar to the commonly used 50/60-Hz bipolar stimulation during awake surgery. A fundamental disparity to other noninvasive brain mapping modalities is its disruptive approach. If cortical areas elicit an assessable physiologic reaction, they are mandatory for the suppressed response. The other described methods detect areas participating in a given task without discriminating indispensable areas from only involved areas. Concerning neurosurgery, nTMS is CE-marked and Food and Drug Administration (FDA)-approved to identify motor-involved and language-involved cortical areas prior to surgery. Mapping other functions, such as face recognition, supplementary motor area, visuospatial attention, and arithmetical processing, have been described as well.[43–46]

Several current matched-pair analyses proved nTMS to show better functional and oncological outcome by cutting residual tumor from 42% to 22% and by reducing permanent deficits both for gliomas and metastases.[47–50]

Compared with other technologies, nTMS is inexpensive and proved accurate. Moreover, its methodological approach is similar to intraoperative techniques, which currently promotes its further international spread.

Concerning nTMS language mapping, several studies have investigated the predictive value compared with awake DCS mapping, resulting in a low positive but high negative predictive value.[51] This means that nTMS identifies regions that not

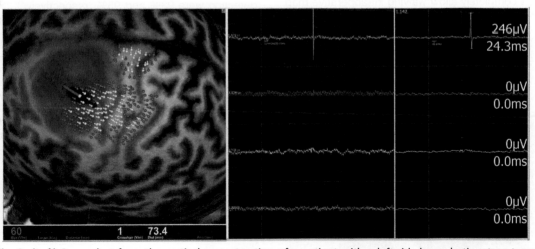

Fig. 2. (*Left*) Screenshot from the cortical reconstruction of a patient with a left-sided anaplastic astrocytoma showing the stimulated cortical area (*between blue and red arrows*) and MEP-positive cortex (*white points*). (*Right*) Electromyography (EMG) shows the immediate muscle potential due to stimulation of the respective cortical spot.

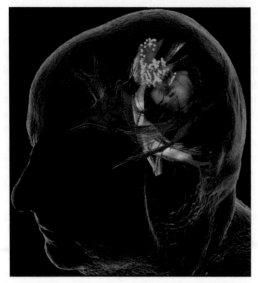

Fig. 3. This neuronavigational 3-dimensional screenshot shows cortical nTMS points for language (purple points) and motor function (green) as well as nTMS-based tractography of the CST (yellow) and language tracts, such as the arcuate fascicle (purple fibers) in a patient with a left parietal GBM (blue).

only are essential but also are involved in language function. For neurosurgical applications, the nTMS-negative areas can be resected or serving as entry zones for corticotomy in a reliable way[52] (**Fig. 3**). Moreover, nTMS language also was described as a tool for follow-up examinations prior to repeated awake surgery in order to identify any language shift and thus reveal cortical plasticity in brain tumor patients.[12,16,53,54]

In general, due to the comparable methodology and accuracy, nTMS as presurgical mapping does not completely allow waiving intraoperative mapping or monitoring but serves as an adjunct to estimate resectability, extent of resection, and surgical approaches prior to surgery and eases intraoperative DCS mapping.[11] Yet, only superficial but not deep cortical areas are accessible for nTMS.

Concerning safety, the authors have data from a large, prospective multicenter cohort of 733 neurosurgical patients across 3 institutions and 2 countries. No adverse events were observed.[55] Moreover, nTMS also is approved for pediatric patients as well as for epilepsy surgery.[56,57]

TRACTOGRAPHY

DTI is the methodology used most commonly for neurosurgical tractography. First described in 1994, it uses the direction of water diffusion parallel to white matter fibers as a surrogate marker to visualize the latter.[58–60] Due to FDA approval, DTI is widely distributed to calculate white matter tracts using DTI fiber tracking (FT) in neurosurgical patients for preoperative work-up. DTI FT is able to visualize fiber bundles originating from a defined cortical or subcortical region, which has to be outlined by the investigator, called regions of interest (ROIs). Thus, it does not harbor any information on the particular function of the reconstructed fibers.

The most common use of DTI FT is the visualization of the corticospinal tract (CST) close to subcortical tumors.[61–66] The accuracy of current preoperative or intraoperative DTI FT protocols repeatedly has been compared with intraoperative subcortical stimulation mapping, showing excellent intraoperative correlation of DTI FT and SCS if the intraoperative brain shift was taken into account.[61,67–69] Sensitivity and specificity of CST detection were 93% and 95%, respectively.[61–63] A prospective randomized trial investigated 238

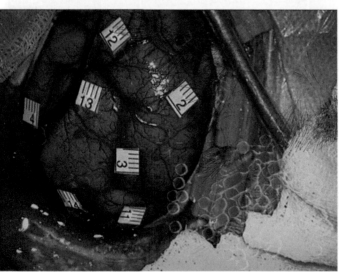

Fig. 4. This microscope screenshot shows the intraoperative cortical surface after finishing DCS mapping in a left parietal GBM patient. The heads-up display provides an overlay showing cortical nTMS points for language (purple), motor (green), and calculation function (blue). One-digit numbers represent DCS positive language areas; 2-digit numbers represent DCS positive calculation areas.

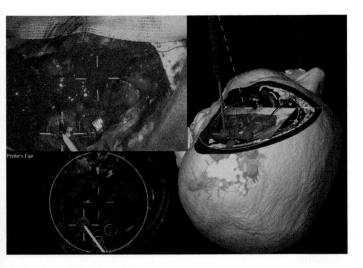

Fig. 5. The figure is a combination using a navigated microscope showing the overlay between preoperative language mapping (pink) and sterile number tags of DCS mapping in a large insular GBM. Blue dashed line and blue circular line, microscope orientation and focus; green line and pointer, reconstruction of the intraoperative navigational pointer.

patients using preoperative DTI FT for CST reconstruction demonstrated improved neurologic outcome and larger extent of resection compared with the control group.[70]

In a more sophisticated approach, cortical functional mapping by fMRI, MEG, or nTMS can serve as an adjunct to provide functional instead of anatomic ROI data[8,71–74] (see **Fig. 3**). Without function-based ROIs, the reconstruction of subcortical tracts by diffusion tensor vectors is only a pure anatomic surrogate without being or representing true electrophysiologic or functional data.

In contrast to fMRI and MEG, this approach of function-based DTI FT already was assessed and investigated extensively for nTMS as a cortical mapping modality. In 1 study comparing fMRI and nTMS as ROI, nTMS was shown superior due to the neurovascular decoupling in the vicinity of tumors, discussed previously.[74] This is not surprising because for motor function nTMS identifies areas eliciting MEPs, and its use as ROI then visualizes all fibers originating from this particular area called the CST. For language, cortical areas whose inhibition elicited some type of naming error serve as ROI, leading to a considerably stable reconstruction of the subcortical language network.[73]

For neurosurgical applications, tractography provides helpful information for consulting of patients, planning surgical approaches, and guiding intraoperative subcortical stimulation.[62,75] For function-based DTI FT, several studies also reported excellent and stable data for use as a preoperative risk stratification tool.[8,76] Several studies investigated function-based compared with anatomy-based DTI FT and reported a higher level of standardization of the function-based approach.[77,78]

For intraoperative use, brain shift represents a major limitation, which can range between −8 mm and 15 mm and is not predictable in terms of preferred direction.[79] DTI FT, therefore, is another valuable adjunct not only for preoperative planning but also for intraoperative guidance. Its intraoperative use, however, should be applied with caution and combined with intraoperative electrical stimulation mapping.[67,79,80]

DISCUSSION

The modalities, discussed previously, currently show a large variation in use between countries and also between departments. This seems to be a sign that not only functional mapping of tumors within eloquent brain regions but also the neuro-oncological approach is changing. Deficit rates are going down while overall survival and surgical indications for gross total resection are increasing.[48,81] Therefore, not only are adopting and investigating potentially new adjuncts to the armamentarium compelled but also gaining expertise in applying them properly needed. Especially, taking tumor-induced neuroplasticity into account for decision making and surgical considerations seems to be a compelling approach for most surgical neuro-oncologists.[53,54,82–84]

Thus, after all, there are now 4 different applications of presurgical mapping modalities:

1. Decision of resection versus biopsy[85]
2. Indication planning of awake surgery versus asleep surgery versus biopsy versus wait and scan
3. Providing seed regions for function-based DTI FT (see **Fig. 3**)

4. Providing data for the intraoperative use to guide DCS mapping[11] (**Figs. 4** and **5**).

Worth mentioning, presurgical mapping data can guide and therefore shorten intraoperative DCS mapping, but it is not supposed to replace DCS mapping or monitoring (see **Fig. 5**). For surgeons and departments experienced in monitoring and mapping, noninvasive mapping provides highly valuable information but does not represent a competing modality. On the contrary, intraoperative neuromonitoring starts rather than ends with presurgical mapping.

Intraoperatively, presurgical mapping data are prone to brain shift and, therefore, spatial distortion. Techniques, such as intraoperative elastic fusion of presurgical mapping data on intraoperative MRI data, can be other tools to overcome this limitation. Recent studies report preliminary but convincing results.[86,87]

No matter which noninvasive techniques are used, it is crucial to assure a full integration into the electronic infrastructure because surgical decision making is based on such data. Moreover, full integration into the respective cancer center's clinical workflow is helpful to allow participation of other specialties like radiation oncologists. Concerning radiation oncology, some studies in the past investigated noninvasive functional data for radiosurgery and radiation therapy planning and reported reduced dosage to eloquent cortex without affecting the treatment dose.[88–92]

SUMMARY

Noninvasive mapping can provide valuable information, which nowadays can be reliable enough to alter indications or approach planning. Nonetheless, it has to be acquired and experience and trust gained over some time. Only then can accurate and standardized noninvasive mapping data provide beneficial data for surgery and patient consultation.

CLINICS CARE POINTS

- Noninvasive mapping can improve surgical results.[48]
- fMRI, MEG, nTMS, and tractography can serve as functional mapping prior to brain tumor surgery.
- Such data allow for preoperative risk assessment and patient counseling.[8]
- Noninvasive mapping can guide intraoperative DCS mapping.[11]

DISCLOSURE

S.M. Krieg is consultant for Nexstim Plc (Helsinki, Finland), Brainlab AG (Munich, Germany), and Spineart Deutschland GmbH (Frankfurt, Germany) and received honoraria from Medtronic (Meerbusch, Germany) and Carl Zeiss Meditec (Oberkochen, Germany). S. Ille is consultant for Brainlab AG (Munich, Germany). Both authors, however, declare that they have no conflict of interest regarding the materials used or the results presented in this article. Both authors declare no other relationships or activities that could appear to have influenced the submitted work.

REFERENCES

1. Jakola AS, Unsgard G, Myrmel KS, et al. Low grade gliomas in eloquent locations - implications for surgical strategy, survival and long term quality of life. PLoS One 2012;7(12):e51450.
2. Chang EF, Clark A, Smith JS, et al. Functional mapping-guided resection of low-grade gliomas in eloquent areas of the brain: improvement of long-term survival. Clinical article. J Neurosurg 2011; 114(3):566–73.
3. Conway N, Wildschuetz N, Moser T, et al. Cortical plasticity of motor-eloquent areas measured by navigated transcranial magnetic stimulation in patients with glioma. J Neurosurg 2017;127(5): 981–91.
4. Bulubas L, Sollmann N, Tanigawa N, et al. Reorganization of motor representations in patients with brain lesions: a navigated transcranial magnetic stimulation study. Brain Topogr 2018;31(2):288–99.
5. Bulubas L, Sardesh N, Traut T, et al. Motor cortical network plasticity in patients with recurrent brain tumors. Front Hum Neurosci 2020;14:118.
6. Southwell DG, Hervey-Jumper SL, Perry DW, et al. Intraoperative mapping during repeat awake craniotomy reveals the functional plasticity of adult cortex. J Neurosurg 2016;124(5):1460–9.
7. Traut T, Sardesh N, Bulubas L, et al. MEG imaging of recurrent gliomas reveals functional plasticity of hemispheric language specialization. Hum Brain Mapp 2019;40(4):1082–92.
8. Sollmann N, Zhang H, Fratini A, et al. Risk assessment by presurgical tractography using navigated TMS maps in patients with highly motor- or language-eloquent brain tumors. Cancers (Basel) 2020;12(5):1264.
9. Krieg SM, Schnurbus L, Shiban E, et al. Surgery of highly eloquent gliomas primarily assessed as nonresectable: risks and benefits in a cohort study. BMC Cancer 2013;13:51.
10. Southwell DG, Birk HS, Han SJ, et al. Resection of gliomas deemed inoperable by neurosurgeons

based on preoperative imaging studies. J Neurosurg 2018;129(3):567–75.

11. Ille S, Gempt J, Meyer B, et al. nTMS guidance of awake surgery for highly eloquent gliomas. Neurosurg Focus 2018;45(VideoSuppl2):V9.

12. Ille S, Engel L, Albers L, et al. Functional reorganization of cortical language function in glioma patients-a preliminary study. Front Oncol 2019;9:446.

13. Southwell DG, Riva M, Jordan K, et al. Language outcomes after resection of dominant inferior parietal lobule gliomas. J Neurosurg 2017;127(4):781–9.

14. Tate MC, Herbet G, Moritz-Gasser S, et al. Probabilistic map of critical functional regions of the human cerebral cortex: Broca's area revisited. Brain 2014; 137(Pt 10):2773–82.

15. Picart T, Herbet G, Moritz-Gasser S, et al. Iterative surgical resections of diffuse glioma with awake mapping: how to deal with cortical plasticity and connectomal constraints? Neurosurgery 2019; 85(1):105–16.

16. Krieg SM, Sollmann N, Hauck T, et al. Repeated mapping of cortical language sites by preoperative navigated transcranial magnetic stimulation compared to repeated intraoperative DCS mapping in awake craniotomy. BMC Neurosci 2014;15:20.

17. Ogawa S, Tank DW, Menon R, et al. Intrinsic signal changes accompanying sensory stimulation: functional brain mapping with magnetic resonance imaging. Proc Natl Acad Sci U S A 1992;89(13): 5951–5.

18. Liegeois F, Cross JH, Gadian DG, et al. Role of fMRI in the decision-making process: epilepsy surgery for children. J Magn Reson Imaging 2006;23(6): 933–40.

19. Fujiwara N, Sakatani K, Katayama Y, et al. Evoked-cerebral blood oxygenation changes in false-negative activations in BOLD contrast functional MRI of patients with brain tumors. Neuroimage 2004;21(4):1464–71.

20. Ulmer JL, Hacein-Bey L, Mathews VP, et al. Lesion-induced pseudo-dominance at functional magnetic resonance imaging: implications for preoperative assessments. Neurosurgery 2004;55(3):569–79 [discussion: 580–1].

21. Giussani C, Roux FE, Ojemann J, et al. Is preoperative functional magnetic resonance imaging reliable for language areas mapping in brain tumor surgery? Review of language functional magnetic resonance imaging and direct cortical stimulation correlation studies. Neurosurgery 2010;66(1):113–20.

22. Roux FE, Boulanouar K, Ranjeva JP, et al. Usefulness of motor functional MRI correlated to cortical mapping in Rolandic low-grade astrocytomas. Acta Neurochir (Wien) 1999;141(1):71–9.

23. Krings T, Schreckenberger M, Rohde V, et al. Functional MRI and 18F FDG-positron emission tomography for presurgical planning: comparison with electrical cortical stimulation. Acta Neurochir (Wien) 2002;144(9):889–99 [discussion: 899].

24. Jack CR Jr, Thompson RM, Butts RK, et al. Sensory motor cortex: correlation of presurgical mapping with functional MR imaging and invasive cortical mapping. Radiology 1994;190(1):85–92.

25. Krieg SM, Shiban E, Buchmann N, et al. Presurgical navigated transcranial magnetic brain stimulation for recurrent gliomas in motor eloquent areas. Clin Neurophysiol 2013;124(3):522–7.

26. Krieg SM, Shiban E, Buchmann N, et al. Utility of presurgical navigated transcranial magnetic brain stimulation for the resection of tumors in eloquent motor areas. J Neurosurg 2012;116(5): 994–1001.

27. Findlay AM, Ambrose JB, Cahn-Weiner DA, et al. Dynamics of hemispheric dominance for language assessed by magnetoencephalographic imaging. Ann Neurol 2012;71:668–86.

28. Zhang D, Johnston JM, Fox MD, et al. Preoperative sensorimotor mapping in brain tumor patients using spontaneous fluctuations in neuronal activity imaged with functional magnetic resonance imaging: initial experience. Neurosurgery 2009;65(6 Suppl): 226–36.

29. Voets NL, Plaha P, Parker Jones O, et al. Presurgical localization of the primary sensorimotor cortex in gliomas : when is resting state FMRI beneficial and sufficient? Clin Neuroradiol 2020. https://doi.org/10.1007/s00062-020-00879-1.

30. Azad TD, Duffau H. Limitations of functional neuroimaging for patient selection and surgical planning in glioma surgery. Neurosurg Focus 2020;48(2):E12.

31. Makela JP, Forss N, Jaaskelainen J, et al. Magnetoencephalography in neurosurgery. Neurosurgery 2007;61(1 Suppl):147–64 [discussion: 164–5].

32. Tarapore PE, Tate MC, Findlay AM, et al. Preoperative multimodal motor mapping: a comparison of magnetoencephalography imaging, navigated transcranial magnetic stimulation, and direct cortical stimulation. J Neurosurg 2012;117(2):354–62.

33. Kirsch HE, Zhu Z, Honma S, et al. Predicting the location of mouth motor cortex in patients with brain tumors by using somatosensory evoked field measurements. J Neurosurg 2007;107(3):481–7.

34. Nagarajan S, Kirsch H, Lin P, et al. Preoperative localization of hand motor cortex by adaptive spatial filtering of magnetoencephalography data. J Neurosurg 2008;109(2):228–37.

35. Korvenoja A, Kirveskari E, Aronen HJ, et al. Sensorimotor cortex localization: comparison of magnetoencephalography, functional MR imaging, and intraoperative cortical mapping. Radiology 2006; 241(1):213–22.

36. Schiffbauer H, Berger MS, Ferrari P, et al. Preoperative magnetic source imaging for brain tumor surgery: a quantitative comparison with intraoperative

sensory and motor mapping. J Neurosurg 2002; 97(6):1333–42.

37. Tarapore PE, Martino J, Guggisberg AG, et al. Magnetoencephalographic imaging of resting-state functional connectivity predicts postsurgical neurological outcome in brain gliomas. Neurosurgery 2012;71(5):1012–22.

38. Schiffbauer H, Ferrari P, Rowley HA, et al. Functional activity within brain tumors: a magnetic source imaging study. Neurosurgery 2001;49(6):1313–20 [discussion: 1320–1].

39. Barker AT, Jalinous R, Freeston IL. Non-invasive magnetic stimulation of human motor cortex. Lancet 1985;1(8437):1106–7.

40. Hess CW, Mills KR, Murray NM. Responses in small hand muscles from magnetic stimulation of the human brain. J Physiol 1987;388:397–419.

41. Brasil-Neto JP, Cohen LG, Panizza M, et al. Optimal focal transcranial magnetic activation of the human motor cortex: effects of coil orientation, shape of the induced current pulse, and stimulus intensity. J Clin Neurophysiol 1992;9(1):132–6.

42. Takahashi S, Vajkoczy P, Picht T. Navigated transcranial magnetic stimulation for mapping the motor cortex in patients with rolandic brain tumors. Neurosurg Focus 2013;34(4):E3.

43. Maurer S, Tanigawa N, Sollmann N, et al. Non-invasive mapping of calculation function by repetitive navigated transcranial magnetic stimulation. Brain Struct Funct 2016;221(8):3927–47.

44. Maurer S, Giglhuber K, Sollmann N, et al. Non-invasive mapping of face processing by navigated transcranial magnetic stimulation. Front Hum Neurosci 2017;11:4.

45. Giglhuber K, Maurer S, Zimmer C, et al. Mapping visuospatial attention: the greyscales task in combination with repetitive navigated transcranial magnetic stimulation. BMC Neurosci 2018;19(1):40.

46. Schramm S, Sollmann N, Ille S, et al. Application of navigated transcranial magnetic stimulation to map the supplementary motor area in healthy subjects. J Clin Neurophysiol 2020;37(2):140–9.

47. Krieg SM, Picht T, Sollmann N, et al. Resection of motor eloquent metastases aided by preoperative nTMS-based motor maps-comparison of two observational cohorts. Front Oncol 2016;6:261.

48. Krieg SM, Sabih J, Bulubasova L, et al. Preoperative motor mapping by navigated transcranial magnetic brain stimulation improves outcome for motor eloquent lesions. Neuro Oncol 2014;16(9):1274–82.

49. Krieg SM, Sollmann N, Obermueller T, et al. Changing the clinical course of glioma patients by preoperative motor mapping with navigated transcranial magnetic brain stimulation. BMC Cancer 2015;15:231.

50. Picht T, Frey D, Thieme S, et al. Presurgical navigated TMS motor cortex mapping improves outcome in glioblastoma surgery: a controlled observational study. J Neurooncol 2016;126(3):535–43.

51. Krieg SM, Tarapore PE, Picht T, et al. Optimal timing of pulse onset for language mapping with navigated repetitive transcranial magnetic stimulation. Neuroimage 2014;100C:219–36.

52. Ille S, Sollmann N, Butenschoen VM, et al. Resection of highly language-eloquent brain lesions based purely on rTMS language mapping without awake surgery. Acta Neurochir (Wien) 2016;158(12):2265–75.

53. Krieg SM, Sollmann N, Hauck T, et al. Functional language shift to the right hemisphere in patients with language-eloquent brain tumors. PLoS One 2013;8(9):e75403.

54. Rosler J, Niraula B, Strack V, et al. Language mapping in healthy volunteers and brain tumor patients with a novel navigated TMS system: evidence of tumor-induced plasticity. Clin Neurophysiol 2014;125(3):526–36.

55. Tarapore PE, Picht T, Bulubas L, et al. Safety and tolerability of navigated TMS for preoperative mapping in neurosurgical patients. Clin Neurophysiol 2016;127(3):1895–900.

56. Hameed MQ, Dhamne SC, Gersner R, et al. Transcranial magnetic and direct current stimulation in children. Curr Neurol Neurosci Rep 2017;17(2):11.

57. Lehtinen H, Makela JP, Makela T, et al. Language mapping with navigated transcranial magnetic stimulation in pediatric and adult patients undergoing epilepsy surgery: comparison with extraoperative direct cortical stimulation. Epilepsia Open 2018;3(2):224–35.

58. Moseley ME, Cohen Y, Kucharczyk J, et al. Diffusion-weighted MR imaging of anisotropic water diffusion in cat central nervous system. Radiology 1990;176(2):439–45.

59. Moseley ME, Kucharczyk J, Asgari HS, et al. Anisotropy in diffusion-weighted MRI. Magn Reson Med 1991;19(2):321–6.

60. Sakuma H, Nomura Y, Takeda K, et al. Adult and neonatal human brain: diffusional anisotropy and myelination with diffusion-weighted MR imaging. Radiology 1991;180(1):229–33.

61. Ohue S, Kohno S, Inoue A, et al. Accuracy of diffusion tensor magnetic resonance imaging-based tractography for surgery of gliomas near the pyramidal tract: a significant correlation between subcortical electrical stimulation and postoperative tractography. Neurosurgery 2012;70(2):283–93 [discussion: 294].

62. Bello L, Gambini A, Castellano A, et al. Motor and language DTI fiber tracking combined with intraoperative subcortical mapping for surgical removal of gliomas. NeuroImage 2008;39(1):369–82.

63. Berman JI, Berger MS, Chung SW, et al. Accuracy of diffusion tensor magnetic resonance imaging tractography assessed using intraoperative subcortical stimulation mapping and magnetic source imaging. J Neurosurg 2007;107(3):488–94.

64. Nimsky C, Ganslandt O, Hastreiter P, et al. Preoperative and intraoperative diffusion tensor imaging-based fiber tracking in glioma surgery. Neurosurgery 2005;56(1):130–7 [discussion: 138].

65. Stadlbauer A, Nimsky C, Gruber S, et al. Changes in fiber integrity, diffusivity, and metabolism of the pyramidal tract adjacent to gliomas: a quantitative diffusion tensor fiber tracking and MR spectroscopic imaging study. AJNR Am J Neuroradiol 2007;28(3): 462–9.

66. Bauer MH, Barbieri S, Klein J, et al. Boundary estimation of fiber bundles derived from diffusion tensor images. Int J Comput Assist Radiol Surg 2011;6(1):1–11.

67. Zhu FP, Wu JS, Song YY, et al. Clinical application of motor pathway mapping using diffusion tensor imaging tractography and intraoperative direct subcortical stimulation in cerebral glioma surgery: a prospective cohort study. Neurosurgery 2012; 71(6):1170–83 [discussion 1183–4].

68. Ostry S, Belsan T, Otahal J, et al. Is intraoperative diffusion tensor imaging at 3.0T comparable to subcortical corticospinal tract mapping? Neurosurgery 2013;73(5):797–807 [discussion: 806–7].

69. Zolal A, Hejcl A, Vachata P, et al. The use of diffusion tensor images of the corticospinal tract in intrinsic brain tumor surgery: a comparison with direct subcortical stimulation. Neurosurgery 2012;71(2): 331–40 [discussion: 340].

70. Wu JS, Zhou LF, Tang WJ, et al. Clinical evaluation and follow-up outcome of diffusion tensor imaging-based functional neuronavigation: a prospective, controlled study in patients with gliomas involving pyramidal tracts. Neurosurgery 2007;61(5):935–48 [discussion: 948–9].

71. Gaetz W, Scantlebury N, Widjaja E, et al. Mapping of the cortical spinal tracts using magnetoencephalography and diffusion tensor tractography in pediatric brain tumor patients. Childs Nerv Syst 2010;26(11): 1639–45.

72. Sollmann N, Kelm A, Ille S, et al. Setup presentation and clinical outcome analysis of treating highly language-eloquent gliomas via preoperative navigated transcranial magnetic stimulation and tractography. Neurosurg Focus 2018;44(6):E2.

73. Sollmann N, Zhang H, Schramm S, et al. Function-specific tractography of language pathways based on nTMS mapping in patients with supratentorial lesions. Clin Neuroradiol 2020;30(1):123–35.

74. Weiss Lucas C, Tursunova I, Neuschmelting V, et al. Functional MRI vs. navigated TMS to optimize M1 seed volume delineation for DTI tractography. A prospective study in patients with brain tumours

adjacent to the corticospinal tract. Neuroimage Clin 2017;13:297–309.

75. Carrabba G, Fava E, Giussani C, et al. Cortical and subcortical motor mapping in rolandic and perirolandic glioma surgery: impact on postoperative morbidity and extent of resection. J Neurosurg Sci 2007;51(2):45–51.

76. Rosenstock T, Grittner U, Acker G, et al. Risk stratification in motor area-related glioma surgery based on navigated transcranial magnetic stimulation data. J Neurosurg 2017;126(4):1227–37.

77. Krieg SM, Buchmann NH, Gempt J, et al. Diffusion tensor imaging fiber tracking using navigated brain stimulation—a feasibility study. Acta Neurochir (Wien) 2012;154(3):555–63.

78. Frey D, Strack V, Wiener E, et al. A new approach for corticospinal tract reconstruction based on navigated transcranial stimulation and standardized fractional anisotropy values. Neuroimage 2012; 62(3):1600–9.

79. Nimsky C, Ganslandt O, Hastreiter P, et al. Preoperative and intraoperative diffusion tensor imaging-based fiber tracking in glioma surgery. Neurosurgery 2007;61(1 Suppl):178–85 [discussion: 186].

80. Ozawa N, Muragaki Y, Nakamura R, et al. Shift of the pyramidal tract during resection of the intraaxial brain tumors estimated by intraoperative diffusion-weighted imaging. Neurol Med Chir (Tokyo) 2009; 49(2):51–6.

81. Sollmann N, Ille S, Hauck T, et al. The impact of preoperative language mapping by repetitive navigated transcranial magnetic stimulation on the clinical course of brain tumor patients. BMC Cancer 2015; 15:261.

82. Kawashima A, Krieg SM, Faust K, et al. Plastic reshaping of cortical language areas evaluated by navigated transcranial magnetic stimulation in a surgical case of glioblastoma multiforme. Clin Neurol Neurosurg 2013;115(10):2226–9.

83. Robles SG, Gatignol P, Lehericy S, et al. Long-term brain plasticity allowing a multistage surgical approach to World Health Organization Grade II gliomas in eloquent areas. J Neurosurg 2008;109(4): 615–24.

84. Ius T, Angelini E, Thiebaut de Schotten M, et al. Evidence for potentials and limitations of brain plasticity using an atlas of functional resectability of WHO grade II gliomas: towards a "minimal common brain". Neuroimage 2011;56(3):992–1000.

85. Picht T, Schulz J, Hanna M, et al. Assessment of the influence of navigated transcranial magnetic stimulation on surgical planning for tumors in or near the motor cortex. Neurosurgery 2012;70(5):1248–56 [discussion: 1256–7].

86. Ille S, Schroeder A, Wagner A, et al. Deterministic clinical tractography is highly accurate in the vicinity

of eloquent gliomas: a study by IONM and elastic fusion based on intraoperative MRI data. Virtual American Association of Neurological Surgeons Annual Meeting; April 24, 2020, 2020.

87. Gerhardt J, Sollmann N, Hiepe P, et al. Retrospective distortion correction of diffusion tensor imaging data by semi-elastic image fusion - Evaluation by means of anatomical landmarks. Clin Neurol Neurosurg 2019;183:105387.

88. Conti A, Pontoriero A, Ricciardi GK, et al. Integration of functional neuroimaging in CyberKnife radiosurgery: feasibility and dosimetric results. Neurosurg Focus 2013;34(4):E5.

89. Tokarev AS, Rak VA, Sinkin MV, et al. Appliance of navigated transcranial magnetic stimulation in radiosurgery for brain metastases. J Clin Neurophysiol 2020;37(1):50–5.

90. Diehl CD, Schwendner MJ, Sollmann N, et al. Application of presurgical navigated transcranial magnetic stimulation motor mapping for adjuvant radiotherapy planning in patients with high-grade gliomas. Radiother Oncol 2019;138:30–7.

91. Schwendner MJ, Sollmann N, Diehl CD, et al. The role of navigated transcranial magnetic stimulation motor mapping in adjuvant radiotherapy planning in patients with supratentorial brain metastases. Front Oncol 2018;8:424.

92. Picht T, Schilt S, Frey D, et al. Integration of navigated brain stimulation data into radiosurgical planning: potential benefits and dangers. Acta Neurochir (Wien) 2014;156(6):1125–33.

Functional Mapping for Glioma Surgery, Part 2
Intraoperative Mapping Tools

Ramin A. Morshed, MD[a,b], Jacob S. Young, MD[a,b], Anthony T. Lee, MD PhD[a,b], Shawn L. Hervey-Jumper, MD[a,b],*

KEYWORDS

- Intraoperative mapping • Awake craniotomy • Language mapping • Direct cortical stimulation

KEY POINTS

- Intraoperative motor mapping can involve direct bipolar or monopolar stimulation and motor-evoked potential monitoring via a transcranial or direct cortical strip electrode approach.
- Intraoperative language testing may assess several language domains including naming, repetition, reading, writing, and syntax.
- Intraoperative cognitive mapping is less frequently used but has been increasingly recognized as important for maintaining quality of life.
- Appropriate patient selection and preoperative optimization of risk factors including seizures and anxiety are important.

INTRODUCTION

Surgical resection is a mainstay of treatment for patients who are diagnosed with a presumed glioma, even when involving areas of the brain with presumed functional significance (ie, eloquent cortex). Care must be taken to preserve neurologic function while striving for maximal extent of resection, as permanent postoperative neurologic impairments, particularly involving language and motor function, are associated with worse overall survival and lower quality of life.[1–4] Intraoperative functional mapping of lesional and perilesional tissue is a well-established technique for avoiding permanent neurologic deficits.[5,6] It involves the administration of short pulses of electrical stimulation to identify specific functions and is either activating (eg, eliciting a motor response) or disruptive (eg, speech arrest).

This article describes techniques used for motor and language mapping, as well as less traditional intraoperative testing paradigms for cognition mapping. Finally, the article discusses complications associated with mapping and insights into their management.

SENSORIMOTOR MAPPING

Accurate motor mapping is imperative to successfully resect tumors within or near the sensorimotor cortex.[7,8] Classically, intraoperative sensory-motor function was identified with neurophysiological monitoring that used motor-evoked potentials (MEPs) and motor stimulation in asleep patients to visualize motor contraction (ie, stimulation producing a positive response) (**Table 1**).[9] MEPs can be generated via transcranial stimulation, direct cortical, or subcortical

Funding: Robert Wood Johnson Foundation 74259 (S.L. Hervey-Jumper), NINDS K08 110919-01 (S.L. Hervey-Jumper), Loglio Collective (S.L. Hervey-Jumper), National Center for Advancing Translational Sciences of the NIH (R.A. Morshed), Neurosurgery Research and Education Foundation (R.A. Morshed).

[a] Department of Neurological Surgery, University of California San Francisco, San Francisco, CA, USA; [b] Helen Diller Family Comprehensive Cancer Center, University of California San Francisco, San Francisco, CA, USA
* Corresponding author. Department of Neurological Surgery, University of California at San Francisco, 505 Parnassus Avenue, Room M-779, San Francisco, CA 94143-0112.
E-mail address: shawn.hervey-jumper@ucsf.edu

Neurosurg Clin N Am 32 (2021) 75–81
https://doi.org/10.1016/j.nec.2020.09.001
1042-3680/21/© 2020 Elsevier Inc. All rights reserved.

Table 1
Advantages and disadvantages of different stimulation techniques

Modality	Advantages	Disadvantages
Motor Evoked Potentials (MEP)	• Direct cortical MEP allows for continuous stimulation and verification of tract continuity • Transcranial MEPs allow both hemispheres to be tested simultaneously and compared against each other	• Signal can be affected by anesthetic, muscle relaxant, neuromuscular blockade, patient temperature, brain shift, and hypotension • Cortical strip placement can lead to vein injury • Transcranial MEP often painful for awake patients
Bipolar stimulation	• Key component of cortical and subcortical mapping of language and motor cortex • More focused area of stimulation leads to accurate identification of eloquent tissue	• Positive response subcortically usually means that subcortical fibers usually already within 5 mm • Increased seizure frequency when compared to monopolar stimulation in some studies
Monopolar Stimulation	• Key component of cortical and subcortical mapping of language and motor cortex • Stimulation intensity correlates with distance to tracts (1 mA ≈ 1 mm)	• More diffuse area of stimulation that can lead to spatially inaccurate eloquent cortex identification • Theoretic increased risk of tissue damage when compared to bipolar stimulation

stimulation, with the magnitude and latency of the responses impacted by factors such as the depth of anesthesia, recent muscle relaxant, and neuromuscular blockade.[10]

After identifying the motor cortex and central sulcus with phase reversal, continuous direct cortical MEP monitoring allows for a real-time confirmation of a functional pyramidal tract.[11] Transcranial monitoring on the other hand has the advantage of allowing both hemispheres to be tested simultaneously and compared against each other, and it does not require the placement of a cortical strip electrode that has the potential to injure the cortex or a bridging vein, although its sensitivity relative to direct cortical MEPs is debated.[12] Numerous studies have found that MEP recordings can be successfully obtained in nearly all patients, and the irreversible loss of greater than 50% amplitude in the MEPs is a strong predictor of a permanent postoperative paresis.[13–16] However, there are still a small percentage of false-positive changes in MEP, possibly because of brain shift during tumor resection, hypotension, or changes to the anesthetic regimen.

Utilization of direct cortical and subcortical electrical stimulation to map the eloquent cortex and axonal pathways of the sensorimotor system has become a standard of care.[17] There are 2 major methods for stimulating cortical and subcortical fibers: (1) monopolar stimulation, which delivers short trains of high frequency (250–500 Hz) square wave monophasic pulses and requires electromyography (EMG) to visualize firing; and (2) bipolar stimulation, which uses low frequency (60 Hz) to deliver long biphasic pulses.[18,19] The amplitude intensity of stimulation must be adjusted for the type of anesthetic used, with higher amplitudes required for asleep patients. Monopolar stimulation is useful for identifying the motor tracts at a safe distance and estimating their proximity with a reasonably linear relationship of 1 mA of current for every 1 mm of distance between the probe and the white matter tract (generally consistent up to 25 mA).[18,20] Bipolar stimulation is more targeted, and detection of a motor response subcortically with the bipolar probe indicates a close proximity to the motor system (usually within 5 mm) and an increased risk for a permanent postoperative deficit. Recent work suggests that combinatorial techniques involving transcranial MEPs with concurrent monopolar and bipolar stimulation of the subcortical pathways can improve detection of the corticospinal tract and largely avoid severe postoperative deficits.[1,21]

Unlike language mapping, awake mapping of the motor system is not necessary to achieve excellent outcomes, even for tumors within the primary motor cortex itself.[22,23] Fundamentally, major differences in mapping technique exist between awake and asleep approaches; awake patients can voluntarily move muscle groups to confirm the presence or absence of a deficit if there is a change in the mapping signals. Multiple studies have shown that, infrequently, false -positive changes in MEP can occur, with discrepancies existing between the postoperative clinical examination and the intraoperative MEP findings.[16,24] However, some studies have suggested there is an increased risk of seizures during awake motor mapping, although this is likely dependent on the stimulation parameters used.[25,26] Moreover, the ability to map MEPs may be limited in an awake patient, as transcranial MEPs are often painful for the patient. Finally, when resections involve regions such as the supplementary motor area that are critical for movement planning and initiation, awake patients may become slow and/or apraxic despite intact corticospinal tract signaling and inevitable functional recovery, potentially pushing surgeons to stop tumor resection prematurely.[27,28]

LANGUAGE MAPPING

Intraoperative language mapping is a well-established technique for avoiding permanent language deficits.[29] Stimulation is thought to result in focal disruption of networks involved in speech and language processing as demonstrated by correct and incorrect patient responses to various testing paradigms. Intraoperatively, electrical cortical stimulation (ECS) can be performed using low-frequency (60 Hz, 1.0 msec biphasic square wave) bipolar stimulation. Intraoperative electrocorticography is performed using a 16-channel electrode and holder assembly (Grass Model CE1, Natus Medical Inc., Pleasanton, California) and interpreted by an epileptologist. Stimulation begins at 2 mA and then increases until positive sites are identified, after-discharge potentials occur, or a maximum current of 5 mA is reached (although other groups have used higher currents).[30] Current is applied for 3 to 4 seconds, with 4 to 10 seconds between tasks. If a site causes an error, then it is tested at least 2 more times, and in general any site with greater than 50% error rate is marked and persevered.

Intraoperative language testing can involve assessment of several components of language and include picture naming, counting, repetition, reading, writing, sentence completion, and assessing language syntax. The most common intraoperative language mapping task employed is picture naming, which is used for its speed, simplicity, and ability to detect gross language disruption. Errors during picture naming have been aggregated into 6 categories: semantic paraphasias (king -> queen), circumlocutions (pen -> thing used to write), phonological paraphasias (deletions or substitutions of syllables), neologisms (made-up words), performance errors (slurred or stuttered responses), and no response errors.[31] Counting is another commonly used task to identify speech arrest sites. The patient is asked to slowly count to either 5 or 10 while stimulation is applied to different cortical and subcortical sites. If the patient can continue to move his or her arm and tongue but counting is interrupted, this is consistent with speech arrest. Alternatively, if arm movement or tongue movement are also impaired, the response is more consistent with either motor arrest or anarthria, respectively.

Word repetition is not as frequently employed as picture naming and counting in the operating room but is still a useful adjunct for assessing language. Patients with conduction aphasia generally have fluent natural speech and preserved perception capabilities, but an inability to repeat words verbatim. To test word repetition, patients are first familiarized with a list of words usually between 2 to 4 syllables long and containing simple and difficult words (ie, words with consonant clusters and pseudo-words) that are derived from scrambled real words (eg, delight → ledite). Patients are then instructed to repeat individual words while ECS is applied to the cortex.

Reading tasks involve having the patient read short, unrelated sentences that have not been previously rehearsed. While the patient is reading, stimulation is applied to assess for interference in function. Writing tasks involve hand writing dictated text by using the dominant hand. Patients should be able to see what they are writing, and a writing pad is often held up to them at a visible distance by other operating room staff. While writing, direct cortical stimulation is applied, and writing deficits may include letter omissions, writing arrest, or illegible script.[32] To date, language syntax is the least commonly tested language domain with intraoperative mapping. Given the need to test more than a single word to investigate syntax, the tasks are more complex, take more time, and are harder to perform in the operating room setting.

NONLANGUAGE COGNITIVE MAPPING

Although language mapping remains the predominant eloquent function mapped in awake patients, many other cognitive domains, such as memory, attention, motivation, and emotion are affected in patients with intrinsic brain tumors.[33] Moreover, deficits in these domains undeniably impact quality of life, and efforts should be made to preserve these higher-order cognitive functions when possible in patients. Although a few patients have an improvement in their cognitive function after tumor resection, cognitive decline is common after surgery, with attention and processing speed being the most impacted.[34]

Complex executive functions like selective attention, working memory, inhibitory control, and mental flexibility, are challenging to measure and test intraoperatively. An intraoperative version of the Stroop task, which measures the patient's ability to resist interference, has been developed to assess some of these executive functions. Puglisi and colleagues[35,36] found positive stimulation sites in the right inferior frontal gyrus and frontostriatal white matter pathways, and showed that preserving positive sites identified with this task reduced early and late deficits in post-operative executive function.

A calculation task has been utilized during resections of the dominant angular gyrus and nondominant parietal lobe in an attempt to preserve this cognitive ability, and the positive subcortical sites have been identified and preserved intraoperatively with good patient outcomes.[37,38] Also, a working memory task, called the double task, has been used in Perisylvian resections near the superior longitudinal fasciculus.[39] During this task, the patient completes a movement while simultaneously performing a picture naming task. Should patients develop an ideational apraxia, they can perform the movements spontaneously but not upon request. Finally, ECS has been used to try to identify regions critical for memory storage and retrieval during resection of lesions in the left anterior temporal lobe, frontal lobe, and fornix.[40,41] The selection of which executive functions to map should be tailored to individual patients' goals. Additionally, given there are numerous cognitive domains, future work is needed to address which tasks are best suited to preserve cognitive function possible within the time constraints of a surgical resection.

MANAGEMENT OF INTRAOPERATIVE COMPLICATIONS ASSOCIATED WITH MAPPING

There are several issues that can arise when performing intraoperative mapping including stimulation-induced seizures, loss of airway, and patient non-compliance. As with any surgical procedure, patient selection and preoperative optimization of risk factors are critical to avoid intraoperative complications. A full assessment of a patient's medical comorbidities, neurologic deficits, seizure frequency, body habitus, and level of anxiety should be taken into consideration when formulating the operative plan.

Stimulation-induced intraoperative seizures are the biggest contributor to awake craniotomy failure.[5,42,43] Historically, intraoperative stimulation-induced seizures were controlled with intravenous lorazepam, but this often-necessitated cessation of intraoperative testing due to patient sedation. More recent methods for seizure abortion include first irrigating with iced Lactated Ringer's solution applied locally to the cortical surface followed by intravenous Propofol if seizures do not abate. Intraoperative electrocorticography may help as a preventative measure as it allows not only for the identification of after-discharge potentials, but also for identifying an appropriate stimulation current for intraoperative testing. Patients should always be continued on their prior antiepileptics leading up to a craniotomy or should receive an intraoperative agent before starting the craniotomy. Using these interventions, awake mapping failure rates can be as low as 0.5%.[5]

Airway compromise is another concern when performing awake procedures. Patients who are over-sedated or are obese can develop hypercapnia which can precipitate cerebral edema or hypoxia. Tools such as nasal trumpets and laryngeal mask airways (LMA) have significantly enhanced airway options for these patients. Selection of an appropriate anesthetic regimen is also important for maintaining a balance between patient sedation and wakefulness to allow for intraoperative mapping. The two major techniques for performing awake craniotomy are the "asleep-awake-asleep" approach utilizing a combination of propofol-remifentanil and the "conscious sedation" technique. In a randomized control trial comparing dexmedetomidine to propofol-remifentanyl, the dexmedetomidine group was associated with fewer respiratory adverse events and there was no difference in the degree of sedation or the ability of patients to perform mapping tasks.[44] In general, our group begins with propofol-remifentanil and adds dexmedetomidine (with or without continuing propofol) if required.[5]

Managing patient expectations and experience during intraoperative mapping is also critical for a successful operation, especially for patients who already suffer from anxiety at baseline. Patients must be well informed about the procedure, steps involved, neurologic symptoms they may xperience during mapping, and management of ntraoperative pain and sedation. With sudden novements, patients are at risk of scalp lacerations due to pin slippage, contamination of the peration field, and other bodily injury. Patient's vith a high degree of anxiety should be optimized preoperatively on anxiolytics; however, some patient's may not be awake mapping candidates due to anxiety or confusion and may need to be done under general anesthesia. Working with an experienced anesthesia team can help alleviate sudden erratic behavior due to changes in the level of sedation intraoperatively. Additionally, repeated communication between the surgeon and patient s essential for behavior management throughout he case.

SUMMARY AND FUTURE DIRECTIONS

As the neurosurgical armamentarium expands, future advances in intraoperative mapping will need to consider the optimal combination of functional mapping techniques to complement ECS. As the understanding of basic human neuroscience advances, particularly in aspects of cognition, emotion, and higher-order communication, more agnostic techniques such as functional MRI will be essential to guide intraoperative validation with ECS. Advances in intraoperative imaging will provide real-time feedback to help account for brain shifts that occur following craniotomy and tumor debulking. Even ECS is not immune to further technological advances, as evidence by the recently published train-of-five bipolar technique for mapping motor cortex.[45]

CLINICS CARE POINTS

- For motor mapping, MEPs are generated with transcranial stimulation or a subdural strip electrode placed over the primary motor cortex. This can be performed in addition to direct bipolar and/or monopolar stimulation.
- Subcortical mapping techniques are important for both motor and language mapping
- Intraoperative language testing can involve assessment of picture naming, counting, repetition, reading, writing, and assessing language syntax.
- As with any surgical procedure, patient selection and preoperative optimization of risk factors are critical to avoid intraoperative complications.

DISCLOSURE

The authors have nothing to disclose.

REFERENCES

1. Han Seunggu J, Morshed Ramin A, Troncon I, et al. Subcortical stimulation mapping of descending motor pathways for perirolandic gliomas: Assessment of morbidity and functional outcome in 702 cases. J Neurosurg 2019;131(1):201–8.
2. Keles GE, Lundin DA, Lamborn KR, et al. Intraoperative subcortical stimulation mapping for hemispherical perirolandic gliomas located within or adjacent to the descending motor pathways: evaluation of morbidity and assessment of functional outcome in 294 patients. J Neurosurg 2004; 100(3):369–75.
3. Rahman M, Abbatematteo J, De Leo Edward K, et al. The effects of new or worsened postoperative neurological deficits on survival of patients with glioblastoma. J Neurosurg 2017. https://doi.org/10.3171/2016.7.JNS16396.
4. Duffau H, Capelle L, Denvil D, et al. Usefulness of intraoperative electrical subcortical mapping during surgery for low-grade gliomas located within eloquent brain regions: Functional results in a consecutive series of 103 patients. J Neurosurg 2003. https://doi.org/10.3171/jns.2003.98.4.0764.
5. Hervey-Jumper Shawn L, Li J, Lau D, et al. Awake craniotomy to maximize glioma resection: methods and technical nuances over a 27-year period. J Neurosurg 2015;123(2):325–39.
6. Sanai N, Mirzadeh Z, Berger Mitchel S. Functional outcome after language mapping for glioma resection. N Engl J Med 2008;358(1):18–27.
7. Ius T, Angelini E, Thiebaut de Schotten M, et al. Evidence for potentials and limitations of brain plasticity using an atlas of functional resectability of WHO grade II gliomas: Towards a "minimal common brain. Neuroimage 2011. https://doi.org/10.1016/j.neuroimage.2011.03.022.
8. McGirt Matthew J, Mukherjee D, Chaichana Kaisorn L, et al. Association of surgically acquired motor and language deficits on overall survival after resection of glioblastoma multiforme. Neurosurgery 2009. https://doi.org/10.1227/01.NEU.0000349763.42238.
9. Saito T, Tamura M, Chernov Mikhail F, et al. Neurophysiological Monitoring and Awake Craniotomy for Resection of Intracranial Gliomas. Prog Neurol Surg 2017. https://doi.org/10.1159/000464387.
10. Yingling Charles D, Ojemann S, Dodson B, et al. Identification of motor pathways during tumor surgery facilitated by multichannel electromyographic recording. J Neurosurg 1999. https://doi.org/10.3171/jns.1999.91.6.0922.
11. Sala F, Lanteri P. Brain surgery in motor areas: The invaluable assistance of intraoperative neurophysiological monitoring. J Neurosurg Sci 2003;47(2):79–88.

12. Li F, Deshaies Eric M, Allott G, et al. Direct cortical stimulation but not transcranial electrical stimulation motor evoked potentials detect brain ischemia during brain tumor resection. Neurodiagn J 2011. https://doi.org/10.1080/1086508X.2011.11079819.

13. Neuloh G, Pechstein U, Cedzich C, et al. Motor Evoked Potential Monitoring with Supratentorial Surgery. Neurosurgery 2004. https://doi.org/10.1227/01.NEU.0000119326.15032.00.

14. Zhou Henry H, Kelly Patrick J. Transcranial electrical motor evoked potential monitoring for brain tumor resection. Neurosurgery 2001. https://doi.org/10.1227/00006123-200105000-00021.

15. Fujiki M, Furukawa Y, Kamida T, et al. Intraoperative corticomuscular motor evoked potentials for evaluation of motor function: A comparison with corticospinal D and I waves. J Neurosurg 2006. https://doi.org/10.3171/jns.2006.104.1.85.

16. Krieg Sandro M, Shiban E, Droese D, et al. Predictive value and safety of intraoperative neurophysiological monitoring with motor evoked potentials in glioma surgery. Neurosurgery 2012. https://doi.org/10.1227/NEU.0b013e31823f5ade.

17. De Witt Hamer Philip C, Robles SG, Zwinderman Aeilko H, et al. Impact of intraoperative stimulation brain mapping on glioma surgery outcome: a meta-analysis. J Clin Oncol 2012;30(20):2559–65.

18. Bello L, Riva M, Fava E, et al. Tailoring neurophysiological strategies with clinical context enhances resection and safety and expands indications in gliomas involving motor pathways. Neuro Oncol 2014. https://doi.org/10.1093/neuonc/not327.

19. Szelényi A, Senft C, Jardan M, et al. Intra-operative subcortical electrical stimulation: A comparison of two methods. Clin Neurophysiol 2011. https://doi.org/10.1016/j.clinph.2010.12.055.

20. Plans G, Fernández-Conejero I, Rifà-Ros X, et al. Evaluation of the high-Frequency monopolar stimulation technique for mapping and monitoring the corticospinal tract in patients with supratentorial gliomas. a proposal for intraoperative management based on neurophysiological data analysis in a series of. Clin Neurosurg 2017. https://doi.org/10.1093/neuros/nyw087.

21. Gogos Andrew J, Young Jacob S, Morshed Ramin A, et al. Triple motor mapping: transcranial, bipolar, and monopolar mapping for supratentorial glioma resection adjacent to motor pathways. J Neurosurg 2020;1–10. https://doi.org/10.3171/2020.3.JNS193434.

22. Magill ST, Han SJ, Li J, et al. Resection of primary motor cortex tumors: feasibility and surgical outcomes. J Neurosurg 2018;129(4):961–72.

23. Suarez-Meade P, Marenco-Hillembrand L, Prevatt C, et al. Awake vs. asleep motor mapping for glioma resection: a systematic review and meta-analysis. Acta Neurochir (Wien) 2020. https://doi.org/10.1007/s00701-020-04357-y.

24. Szelényi A, Hattingen E, Weidauer S, et al. Intraoperative motor evoked potential alteration in intracranial tumor surgery and its relation to signal alteration in postoperative magnetic resonance imaging. Neurosurgery 2010. https://doi.org/10.1227/01.NEU.0000371973.46234.46.

25. Nossek E, Matot I, Shahar T, et al. Intraoperative seizures during awake craniotomy: incidence and consequences: analysis of 477 patients. Neurosurgery 2013;73(1):135–40 [discussion: 140].

26. Gonen T, Grossman R, Sitt R, et al. Tumor location and IDH1 mutation may predict intraoperative seizures during awake craniotomy. J Neurosurg 2014;121(5):1133–8.

27. Young Jacob S, Morshed Ramin A, Mansoori Z, et al. Disruption of Frontal Aslant Tract Is Not Associated with Long-Term Postoperative Language Deficits. World Neurosurg 2020. https://doi.org/10.1016/j.wneu.2019.09.128.

28. Fernández Coello A, Moritz-Gasser S, Martino J, et al. Selection of intraoperative tasks for awake mapping based on relationships between tumor location and functional networks. J Neurosurg 2013;119(6):1380–94.

29. Wang DD, Deng H, Hervey-Jumper Shawn L, et al. Seizure Outcome After Surgical Resection of Insular Glioma. Neurosurgery 2018;83(4):709–18.

30. Roux FE, Durand JB, Djidjeli I, et al. Variability of intraoperative electrostimulation parameters in conscious individuals: Language cortex. J Neurosurg 2017;126(5):1641–52.

31. Corina DP, Loudermilk BC, Detwiler L, et al. Analysis of naming errors during cortical stimulation mapping: Implications for models of language representation. Brain Lang 2010. https://doi.org/10.1016/j.bandl.2010.04.001.

32. Lubrano V, Roux FE. Démonet Jean-François. Writing-specific sites in frontal areas: a cortical stimulation study. J Neurosurg 2004;101(5):787–98.

33. Klein M, Duffau H, De Witt Hamer Philip C. Cognition and resective surgery for diffuse infiltrative glioma: an overview. J Neurooncol 2012;108(2):309–18.

34. Hendriks Eef J, Habets Esther JJ, Taphoorn Martin JB, et al. Linking late cognitive outcome with glioma surgery location using resection cavity maps. Hum Brain Mapp 2018;39(5):2064–74.

35. Puglisi G, Howells H, Sciortino T, et al. Frontal pathways in cognitive control: direct evidence from intraoperative stimulation and diffusion tractography. Brain 2019;142(8):2451–65.

36. Puglisi G, Sciortino T, Rossi M, et al. Preserving executive functions in nondominant frontal lobe glioma surgery: An intraoperative tool. J Neurosurg 2019.

37. Della Puppa A, De Pellegrin S, Lazzarini A, et al. Subcortical mapping of calculation processing in

the right parietal lobe. J Neurosurg 2015. https://doi.org/10.3171/2014.10.JNS14261.

38. Duffau H, Denvil D, Lopes M, et al. Intraoperative mapping of the cortical areas involved in multiplication and subtraction: An electrostimulation study in a patient with a left parietal glioma. J Neurol Neurosurg Psychiatry 2002. https://doi.org/10.1136/jnnp.73.6.733.

39. Pramstaller PP, Marsden CD. The basal ganglia and apraxia. Brain 1996. https://doi.org/10.1093/brain/119.1.319.

40. Perrine K, Devinsky O, Uysal S, et al. Left temporal neocortex mediation of verbal memory: Evidence from functional mapping with cortical stimulation. Neurology 1994. https://doi.org/10.1212/wnl.44.10.1845.

41. Brandling-Bennett EM, Bookheimer SY, Horsfall JL, et al. A paradigm for awake intraoperative memory mapping during forniceal stimulation. Neurocase 2012. https://doi.org/10.1080/13554794.2010.547509.

42. Pereira LCV, Oliveira Karina M, L'Abbate Gisele L, et al. Outcome of fully awake craniotomy for lesions near the eloquent cortex: analysis of a prospective surgical series of 79 supratentorial primary brain tumors with long follow-up. Acta Neurochir (Wien) 2009;151(10):1215–30.

43. Nossek E, Matot I, Shahar T, et al. Failed awake craniotomy: a retrospective analysis in 424 patients undergoing craniotomy for brain tumor. J Neurosurg 2013;118(2):243–9.

44. Goettel N, Bharadwaj S, Venkatraghavan L, et al. Dexmedetomidine vs propofol-remifentanil conscious sedation for awake craniotomy: A prospective randomized controlled trial. Br J Anaesth 2016. https://doi.org/10.1093/bja/aew024.

45. Bander Evan D, Shelkov E, Modik O, et al. Use of the train-of-five bipolar technique to provide reliable, spatially accurate motor cortex identification in asleep patients. Neurosurg Focus 2020;48(2):E4.

Surgical Adjuncts for Glioblastoma

Sara Hartnett, MD[a], Derek Kroll, DO[b], Michael A. Vogelbaum, MD, PhD[b],*

KEYWORDS

• Glioblastoma • Surgery • Blood–brain barrier • Drug delivery • Therapeutic development

KEY POINTS

• Surgery and systemic medical therapies alone are not curative for glioblastoma.
• The blood–brain barrier and blood–tumor barrier limit the effectiveness of systemically administered therapies.
• The use of adjuncts that can be delivered during surgery for glioblastoma can provide more effective therapeutic access to tumor infiltrated brain tissue.
• These adjuncts can consist of specialized formulations for slow release of drugs, or of engineered biological therapies.

INTRODUCTION

Gliomas are the most common primary brain tumors in adults with approximately 20,000 new cases diagnosed each year in the United States.[1] The World Health Organization grades gliomas from I to IV, based on histopathologic analysis. High-grade gliomas include grades III and IV, whereas the term glioblastoma (GBM) is reserved for grade IV disease.[2] GBMs are classically associated with a poor prognosis, of which the median length of survival is approximately 16 to 20 months.[3,4] The unfavorable characteristics of GBM include the highly infiltrative nature, chemoresistance, propensity for recurrence, and poor long-term survival. With recurrent disease, maximal treatment provides an additional median survival of only 6 to 8 months.[5]

The current standard therapy for GBM includes maximal safe surgical resection as a means of cytoreduction. The positive impact of cytoreductive therapies is a concept that has slowly gained more widespread acceptance.[6] Treatment of GBM with chemotherapy and radiation therapy without any surgical cytoreductive therapies is associated with poorer outcomes.[6] Although surgery alone can never be considered a curative therapy for GBM, owing to its intrinsically infiltrative nature, resection of the enhancing mass, in the setting of maximal medical therapy, is associated with longer survival and there is an association between the completeness of resection and duration of survival. There is also evidence supporting further benefit of extending the resection beyond the enhancing mass, but this benefit seems to be limited to a very small subset of GBMs.[7]

Unfortunately, even in the setting of a complete resection of the enhancing tumor, adjuvant medical therapies also are not curative. The current standard of care use of fractionated radiation therapy and temozolomide during and after radiation was shown to extend overall and 2-year survival,[3] which was subsequently shown to be further extended via use of a tumor treating fields technology.[4] Despite these advances, the median survival of the most favorable patients with GBM still remains less than 2 years and 5-year survival is still measured in single digit percentages.

The single most important challenge to improving the efficacy of systemically applied therapies for GBM is that of overcoming the

a Department of Neurosurgery, USF Morsani School of Medicine, Tampa, FL, USA; b Department of NeuroOncology, Moffitt Cancer Center, Tampa, FL, USA
* Corresponding author. 12902 Magnolia Drive, Tampa, FL 33612,
E-mail address: Michael.Vogelbaum@moffitt.org
Twitter: @DrVogelbaum (M.A.V.)

Neurosurg Clin N Am 32 (2021) 83–91
https://doi.org/10.1016/j.nec.2020.08.005
1042-3680/21/© 2020 Elsevier Inc. All rights reserved.

blood–brain barrier (BBB) and blood–tumor barrier. These barriers prevent most chemotherapies and targeted therapies from reaching tumor cells in the brain at clinically effective concentrations.[8] Even the few chemotherapies known to have activity against GBM are limited to brain concentrations of less than 50% of their systemic concentration.[9] The strategy of increasing systemic dosing level (and hence systemic concentration) is typically not an option because these drugs produce systemic side effects, sometimes irreversible, and are already being used at their systemically defined maximum tolerable doses. It is a common misconception to state that a systemic drug is "brain penetrant" when preclinical evaluations are performed in orthotopic xenograft models, which represent the enhancing component of tumor only (with its partially impaired blood–tumor barrier). These models do not effectively model drug penetration into nonenhancing tumor, which is what is left after a complete resection of enhancing tumor is performed in the clinical setting, and the small molecule targeted therapies in particular are substrates for the drug-excluding pumps that actively maintain the BBB. Early attempts to increase the concentration of drug delivered to target tumor cells was via intra-arterial administration of chemotherapy. Yamada and colleagues[10] demonstrated an increased concentration of chloroethylnitrosurea within brain tumor tissue when given via intra-arterial infusion compared with the traditional intravenous route. Additionally, a study by Savaraj and colleagues[11] revealed a 4-fold increase in concentration of etoposide when administered intra-arterially versus intravenously. Similarly, a 2-fold increased concentration of drug within brain tumors was observed when cisplatin was administered intra-arterially compared with intravenously.[12] However, none of the aforementioned studies demonstrated significant improvement in overall survival in the intra-arterial versus intravenously administered groups. This method of systemic chemotherapy delivery is, unsurprisingly, also limited by an increased risk of systemic toxicities, as well as an inability to treat the contralateral cerebral hemisphere.[10–12]

Alternative strategies for overcoming the effects of the BBB and blood–tumor barrier have been explored. In general terms, these strategies can be lumped into the categories of drug modification, BBB disruption, and BBB bypass via direct brain delivery. This article focuses on the delivery of adjuvant therapies via direct brain delivery (surgical adjuncts). A summary of the approaches discussed can be seen in **Table 1**.

DISCUSSION
Intrathecal Delivery

Intraventricular or intrathecal delivery of chemotherapeutic agent has been used in the treatment of patients with malignancies of the central nervous system. Obtaining high levels of circulating drug within the cerebral spinal fluid space, however, does not produce clinically meaningful distribution within the brain parenchyma.[13] The current literature supports limiting the use of intraventricular or intrathecal delivery of chemotherapy to patients with leptomeningeal involvement of disease, most often seen in various types of metastatic carcinomas, as well as primary central nervous system lymphoma.[14,15] Studies that have focused on the use of this approach for GBM have not shown meaningful promise.

Intracavitary Delivery

Local delivery of chemotherapeutic agents inherently limits drug exposure to normal cells while bypassing the restrictive BBB and brain–tumor barriers, thus minimizing potential adverse systemic effects. To traverse the BBB and establish intratumoral access, a more invasive technique is warranted. This goal may be achieved by injection of the drug into the tumor cavity or by direct implantation of a drug-loaded system. Of the early surgically implantable systems, initial promising results focused on development of implantable drug-loaded polymers.

In the 1990s, several clinical trials were conducted to assess the safety and efficacy regarding the placement of implantable biodegradable polymers within the resection cavity. The implant consists of a drug-impregnated wafer designed to allow consistently adequate level of drug within the tumor. This strategy allows for immediate drug delivery with sustained distribution of agent over time. Carmustine (1,3-Bis(2-chloroethyl)-1-nitrosourea [BCNU]) is an alkylating agent administered intravenously in patients with GBM. Given the tolerability and efficacy in this patient population when given intravenously, carmustine was the chemotherapeutic agent selected for incorporation in the initial surgically implantable polymer system. Each wafer implant contains 7.7 mg of bioavailable agent (3.85% BCNU) designed for controlled release over the degradation period of the polymer.[16]

Brem and colleagues[16] conducted a randomized trial assessing the role of implanting carmustine wafers in patients with recurrent GBMs undergoing tumor resection. In 222 patients, median overall survival was increased in the BCNU-impregnated group compared with the placebo

Table 1
Approaches for surgically delivered adjuvant therapies

Approach	Advantages	Disadvantages	Examples
Intrathecal delivery	Well-established route of delivery FDA approved drugs available Efficacy established for PCNSL Can be performed intermittently or chronically	Poor equilibration with parenchyma No evidence suggesting efficacy in GBM	Intrathecal chemotherapy for carcinomatous meningitis or PCNSL[14,15]
Intracavitary delivery	Straightforward access at the time of surgical resection Can use a variety of substrate formulations to control timing of drug release Wide range of established agents can be incorporated into a variety of well-understood polymer substrates Proof of principle established with limited survival benefit associated with carmustine wafers	Relies on diffusion into tissue surrounding resection cavity Large concentration gradient between surface and surrounding tumor infiltrated brain	Carmustine wafers[16,17,19] Other intracavitary formulations[33–42]
Intraparenchymal delivery	Potential for delivery to a large volume of tumor infiltrated brain More uniform drug concentration profile Can target specific areas of tumor and tumor infiltrated brain Can be performed as a minimal access procedure Multiple types of drugs and biologics can be delivered	Delivery technology is still evolving; no permanently implanted devices currently on the market Difficult to directly image actual volume of distribution Currently no FDA-approved therapeutics for this approach	Viral gene therapies[45–55] Nonviral vectors[56–58] Convection enhanced delivery[65–73]

Abbreviations: FDA, US Food and Drug Administration; PCNSL, primary central nervous system lymphoma.

wafer group (31 weeks vs 23 weeks).[17] This finding resulted in the first implantable product approved by the US Food and Drug Administration (FDA) for the treatment of recurrent GBMs in 1997. Based on results demonstrating increased survival in patients with recurrent GBM, 2 double-blind trials were then designed to investigate potential benefit in newly diagnosed GBMs. Both trials demonstrated a similar increase in median overall survival in the BCNU wafer group compared with those who received placebo implantation. The study by Valtonen and colleagues[18] demonstrated a median overall survival of 58.1 weeks in the implanted wafer group compared with 39.9 weeks with placebo, although only 32 patients were included. A trial conducted by Westphal and colleagues[19] included 240 randomized patients and resulted in a median overall survival increase from 11.6 months to 13.9 months in the placebo versus BCNU wafer groups, respectively. Subsequently in 2003, carmustine wafers were FDA approved for treatment of newly diagnosed high-grade gliomas (World Health Organization grades III and IV) undergoing surgical resection.

Although it produces marginal improvement in median overall survival, the use of implantable BCNU wafers as a standard of care in GBM remains controversial. Much opposition stems from potential adverse events that may negatively impact quality of life in the late phases of the disease. Several large reviews have been conducted; the adverse events noted include but are not limited to edema, healing abnormalities, infection, seizure, and intracranial hypertension.[20–23] Additionally, there are limitations with drug delivery in carmustine wafers, including its rigid structure, minimum height of resection cavity required for proper wafer placement, number of wafers required for optimal BCNU dose, inadequate contact against tumor cavity interface, and dose fall off, as well as the inability of drug to reach the infiltrative aspects that are responsible for the high rate of local recurrence.[24–26]

In addition, the clinical trials that demonstrated the activity of carmustine wafers were performed before temozolomide became available. Its more robust clinical activity and similar mechanism of action raise questions as to whether carmustine wafers would provide similar or even additive benefit. Only about one-third of patients with GBM are responsive to alkylating agents.[27] Because the BCNU in the wafers and temozolomide are both DNA alkylating therapies, temozolomide, with its greater clinical activity, largely replaced the use of carmustine wafers. Yet, given the success of carmustine wafers as a proof of principle, efforts were made to include other chemotherapeutic agents in similar implantable systems. Polyanhydride-based polymer wafers have been impregnated with paclitaxel (PTX), doxorubicin, mitoxantrone, camptothecin, minocycline, and combined riluzole with memantine.[28–32] These drug-eluting wafers have been effectively implanted in intracranial animal models; however, their efficacy has not yet been established in human studies.

Another approach used for intracavitary delivery involves the use of hydrogels. Hydrogels are 3-dimensional networks of cross-linked hydrophilic polymers with a high affinity for body fluids at physiologic conditions and have been used in various areas medicine, including tissue engineering and contact lenses, as well as a vehicle for the delivery of therapeutics.[33–36] Advanced biochemical capabilities have allowed encapsulation of suitable bioactive agents within the gel matrix. The unique properties of hydrogels allow delivery in liquid form but solidifies in situ. As the hydrogel matrix dissolves over time, biologically active agent is released. Although beyond the scope of this section, it is important to note that each injectable hydrogel system is composed of one of several principle polymer components. For example, the polymer network may be based on polyphosphospazenes, polyacrylates, polyaxomers, chitosan, or other polysaccharides. This principle structural base composition has important clinical implications, such as degradation time, rate of drug release, and stimuli responsivity (ie, pH, thermosensitivity, photosensitivity, or multisensitivity).[33–35]

Polylactic-co-glycolic acid and polyethylene glycol

In contrast with the traditional hydrophilic drug-carrying hydrogels, polymeric networks of hydrophobic matrices were designed using polylactic-co-glycolic acid (PLGA). PLGA-based hydrogels have limited water absorption capabilities and are FDA approved for numerous parenteral drug delivery systems.[37] PLGA has been one of the most successful polymers used owing to its safety profile. Hydrolysis of PLGA results in formation of lactic and glycolic acid, which are endogenous byproducts metabolized by the citric acid (Krebs) cycle, minimizing potential toxicity.[38,39] Akbar and colleagues[40] developed a PLGA-based hydrogel with temozolomide and tested it in a surgical resection model for glioma in rats. A significant tumor load reduction (94%) was seen in the 30% temozolomide-loaded hydrogel group compared with the blank control group.[40] Mixtures of polyethylene glycol dimethacrylate and water have been loaded with temozolomide and PTX, in separate models. In the study by Fourniols and colleagues,[41] when this solution was loaded with temozolomide and combined with a photoinitiator, it was well-tolerated intracranially in mice in vivo. With respect to efficacy, tumor growth was significantly decreased in mice treated with the photopolymerized temozolomide hydrogel compared with the control group and greater apoptosis was observed at the center of the tumor.[41] Zhao and colleagues[42] used a similar polyethylene glycol dimethacrylate solution and photoinitiator that were loaded with PTX and tested in mice. As in the aforementioned study, tolerability was seen in vitro. Resection of the tumor was completed 13 days after initial implantation and the PTX-loaded hydrogel was injected into the tumor cavity at time of resection. This led to a more than 50% increase in the long-term survival mice (mean, 150 days) compared with the controls (mean, 52 days), implying a potential role in delay of GBM recurrence.[42]

Intraparenchymal Delivery

Surgically delivered gene therapy

Gene therapy is the transfer of recombinant nucleic acid (DNA) to cells of a patient to result in therapeutic effect using the cell's own machinery of transcription and translation to treat disease.[43] Viral vectors are the most studied and considered to be the most effective of all gene delivery methods for in vivo gene transfer. The viral genome is genetically modified to make it replication incompetent, nonpathogenic, and further modified to make space for the inserted gene (transgene).[44,45] Viruses are able to efficiently carry and transfer genetic material and are relatively easy to modify. In addition, viruses are able to induce cellular immune response and elicit a bystander cytotoxic effect.[46] Herpes simplex virus was one of the first delivery systems evaluated in clinical trials for glioma gene therapy. Retroviruses were chosen owing to their persistence in neuronal cells, their ability to hold a large number of genes, and the ease to produce recombinant vectors.[47,48] The initial trials studied cells containing retroviral herpes simplex virus-thymidine kinase with ganciclovir. The herpes simplex virus-thymidine kinase functioned as a suicide gene and converted the prodrug into its active form to inhibit DNA replication and cell division. The study showed intratumorally implanted retroviral vector-producing cells mediated herpes simplex virus-thymidine kinase transfection and antitumor activity in treated tumors.[45] Phase I clinical trials have studied another retroviral vector, Toca 511 which delivers suicide gene cytosine deaminase and mediates conversion of 5-fluorocytosine into the active antineoplastic drug 5-fluorouracil in transfected tumor cells.[49] A phase II/III clinical trial of this therapeutic completed enrollment, but did not reach its primary end point in terms of survival benefit (manuscript in preparation).

Adenoviral vectors have also been widely studied in clinical trials. The adenovirus serotype 5 has been most commonly used. GBM cells poorly express HAd5 receptors; therefore, the capsid of the virus is modified with additional carbohydrate binding domain to better allow it to infect GBM cells.[50] Phase I and II trials of adenovirus carrying the wild-type p53 gene (Ad-p53) have demonstrated safety and tolerability.[51,52] CD3+ T cells have been found in tumors analyzed after treatment, indicative of an immune activation. Transfected cells were only detected within 5 mm of the injection site, demonstrating the limited ability of the viral vector to further penetrate the tumor tissue.[51] Clinical studies have also evaluated adenoviral vector containing herpes simplex virus-thymidine kinase combined with valacyclovir. Using gene-mediated cytotoxic immunotherapy, thymidine kinase mediates the conversion of the prodrug into toxic nucleotide analogs, inducing tumor cell death and activation of antitumor immune cells.[53] AdV-tk injected into the tumor resection bed followed by the standard of care of radiation and temozolomide resulted in a small increase in 2- and 3-year survival over resection, radiation therapy, and temozolomide alone. A phase III trial of Ad-Tk delivered intratumorally during surgery did not demonstrate improved overall survival, but did show increased time to reintervention.[54]

Although viral vectors have been studied extensively, so far they have only resulted in marginal increases in overall survival and have yet to achieve clinical translation through FDA approval to treat patients with GBM. Viral vector effectiveness is largely limited by tumor penetration. A primary safety concern with viral vectors is the activation of natural immune defense systems which can lead to overactivation of inflammatory responses and potentially lead to multiorgan failure.[55] Other vectors, such as stem cells and nanoparticles, are being developed to overcome these challenges.

Nonviral vectors, although not yet approved by the FDA, have been explored for delivery of glioma gene therapy in preclinical studies. Liposomes, gold nanoparticles, and RNA nanoparticles have been evaluated clinically for GBM gene therapy. SGT-53, a transferrin receptor-targeted liposomal vector encapsulating wild-type p53 plasmid DNA, is able to cross the BBB and target GBM cells, resulting in a reduction of MGMT and apoptosis in GBM xenografts in mice.[56] NU-0129, a spherical nucleic acid gold nanoparticle containing small interfering RNAs targeting Bcl-2–like protein 12, which is involved in tumor progression and resistance to apoptosis is in early phase I clinical trials for patients with recurrent GBM.[57] RNA nanoparticles completely composed of RNA are being used in preclinical trials for delivery to inhibit oncogenic miR-21 in xenograft GBM models in mice.[58]

Convection-enhanced delivery

Convection-enhanced delivery (CED) involves the infusion of agents directly into brain tissue under continuous positive pressure at a low rate (microliters per minute).[59] With this approach, CED takes advantage of the principle of bulk fluid flow and it allows targeted delivery around the BBB. It also permits the real-time monitoring of infusion if a tracer is used.[60] Preclinical modeling and early clinical experience with CED has shown that mechanical tissue injury is avoided as long as the infusion rates are sufficiently low, although the extent of distribution also depends on the rate of delivery with a higher rate typically leading to a larger volume of distribution. Toxicity associated with CED is more likely to be attributable to the agent itself; flow rate–induced symptoms generally resolve once the rate is lowered.[61]

The volume of distribution that can be achieved by CED depends on factors such as the infusion rate, the duration of treatment, and the characteristics of the tissue itself. CED in enhancing brain tumor tissue produces a much more limited volume of distribution from that observed in nonenhancing, tumor infiltrated brain tissue owing to the higher efflux rate of the infusate in the setting of leaky blood vessels.[62–65] Novel catheters have been developed to try to optimize the volume of distribution by minimizing backflow around the catheter itself and allowing for extended delivery in some situations.[65,66]

A number of types of therapeutic agents have been investigated in clinical trials. For an agent to be considered for CED it needs to be safe to infuse in normal brain tissue when placed into solution, and the solutions need to have a low enough viscosity to be delivered via a cannula with a very small (submillimeter) outer diameter. Both small and large molecules have been investigated for CED delivery through a series of phase I and II trials, and 1 agent completed a phase III trial.[67–71] Ultimately, the phase III trial of an IL-13–linked cytotoxin delivered via CED failed to meet its goal of improving survival more than 50% over carmustine wafers.[71] A subsequent series of analyses pointed out the technological issues that were preventing CED from moving forward, and new trials have been launched with the use of updated technology and techniques.[72,73] Although there have been examples of success in small, largely single-center trials, CED remains an investigational approach because there are no drugs that are yet approved by the FDA for delivery directly to the brain via this approach.

SUMMARY

Surgical resection remains an important diagnostic and therapeutic approach for managing patients with GBM, but it will never be curative on its own. That said, with the limited ability of therapeutics to reach residual GBM disease via systemic routes of administration, there is the opportunity to take advantage of the surgeon's access to the other side of the BBB and administer therapeutics directly to the brain. Proof of principle of the value of this approach comes in the form of carmustine wafers, yet there remains the opportunity and need to provide more durable clinical impact than has been demonstrated with that particular therapeutic. Multiple novel formulations, biologics and delivery techniques remain under investigation and require support from the funding and clinical trial communities.

CLINICS CARE POINTS

- Therapeutic failure in GBM is in large part due to the restricted access of drugs and biologics to the CNS.
- The OR presents an opportunity to directly deliver therapeutics to residual GBM cells that cannot be removed surgically.
- Loco-regional delivery approaches remain under development, although past work has demonstrated proof-of-principle efficacy of this approach.
- Specialized formulations that can be safely delivered to the CNS present an opportunity for new drug development.

DISCLOSURES

M.A. Vogelbaum has indirect equity interests in Infuseon Therapeutics, Inc., and patent royalty interests in the Cleveland Multiport Catheter, which he invented. He has received honoraria from Tocagen, Inc., and Celgene. Infuseon and Celgene are funding clinical trials that he is conducting at Moffitt Cancer Center (funding to institution only). The other authors have nothing to disclose.

REFERENCES

1. Ostrom QT, Gittleman H, Liao P, et al. CBTRUS statistical report: primary brain and other central nervous system tumors diagnosed in the United States in 2010-2014. Neuro Oncol 2017;19(suppl_5):v1–88.
2. Louis DN, Perry A, Reifenberger G, et al. The 2016 world health organization classification of tumors of the central nervous system: a summary. Acta Neuropathol 2016;131(6):803–20.
3. Stupp R, Mason WP, van den Bent MJ, et al. Radiotherapy plus concomitant and adjuvant temozolomide for glioblastoma. N Engl J Med 2005;352(10):987–96.
4. Stupp R, Taillibert S, Kanner A, et al. Effect of tumor-treating fields plus maintenance temozolomide vs maintenance temozolomide alone on survival in patients with glioblastoma: a randomized clinical trial. JAMA 2017;318(23):2306–16.

5. Tan AC, Ashley DM, Lopez GY, et al. management of glioblastoma: state of the art and future directions. CA Cancer J Clin 2020;70(4):299–312.

6. Jackson C, Choi J, Khalafallah AM, et al. A systematic review and meta-analysis of supratotal versus gross total resection for glioblastoma. J Neurooncol 2020;148(3):419–31.

7. Beiko J, Suki D, Hess KR, et al. IDH1 mutant malignant astrocytomas are more amenable to surgical resection and have a survival benefit associated with maximal surgical resection. Neuro Oncol 2014;16(1):81–91.

8. Harder BG, Blomquist MR, Wang J, et al. Developments in blood-brain barrier penetrance and drug repurposing for improved treatment of glioblastoma. Front Oncol 2018;8:462.

9. Agarwal S, Manchanda P, Vogelbaum MA, et al. Function of the blood-brain barrier and restriction of drug delivery to invasive glioma cells: findings in an orthotopic rat xenograft model of glioma. Drug Metab Dispos 2013;41(1):33–9.

10. Yamada K, Ushio Y, Hayakawa T, et al. Distribution of radiolabeled 1-(4-amino-2-methyl-5-pyrimidinyl) methyl-3-(2-chloroethyl)-3-nitrosourea hydrochloride in rat brain tumor: intraarterial versus intravenous administration. Cancer Res 1987;47(8):2123–8.

11. Savaraj N, Lu K, Feun LG, et al. Comparison of CNS penetration, tissue distribution, and pharmacology of VP 16-213 by intracarotid and intravenous administration in dogs. Cancer Invest 1987;5(1):11–6.

12. Nakagawa H, Fujita T, Izumoto S, et al. cis-diamminedichloroplatinum (CDDP) therapy for brain metastasis of lung cancer. I. Distribution within the central nervous system after intravenous and intracarotid infusion. J Neurooncol 1993;16(1):61–7.

13. Burch PA, Grossman SA, Reinhard CS. Spinal cord penetration of intrathecally administered cytarabine and methotrexate: a quantitative autoradiographic study. J Natl Cancer Inst 1988;80(15):1211–6.

14. Le Rhun E, Preusser M, van den Bent M, et al. How we treat patients with leptomeningeal metastases. ESMO Open 2019;4(Suppl 2):e000507.

15. Korfel A, Schlegel U. Diagnosis and treatment of primary CNS lymphoma. Nat Rev Neurol 2013;9(6): 317–27.

16. Brem H, Mahaley MS Jr, Vick NA, et al. Interstitial chemotherapy with drug polymer implants for the treatment of recurrent gliomas. J Neurosurg 1991; 74(3):441–6.

17. Brem H, Piantadosi S, Burger PC, et al. Placebo-controlled trial of safety and efficacy of intraoperative controlled delivery by biodegradable polymers of chemotherapy for recurrent gliomas. The polymer-brain tumor treatment group. Lancet 1995; 345(8956):1008–12.

18. Valtonen S, Timonen U, Toivanen P, et al. Interstitial chemotherapy with carmustine-loaded polymers for high-grade gliomas: a randomized double-blind study. Neurosurgery 1997;41(1):44–8 [discussion: 48–9].

19. Westphal M, Hilt DC, Bortey E, et al. A phase 3 trial of local chemotherapy with biodegradable carmustine (BCNU) wafers (Gliadel wafers) in patients with primary malignant glioma. Neuro Oncol 2003; 5(2):79–88.

20. Chowdhary SA, Ryken T, Newton HB. Survival outcomes and safety of carmustine wafers in the treatment of high-grade gliomas: a meta-analysis. J Neurooncol 2015;122(2):367–82.

21. Hart MG, Grant R, Garside R, et al. Chemotherapy wafers for high grade glioma. Cochrane Database Syst Rev 2011;(3):CD007294.

22. Perry J, Chambers A, Spithoff K, et al. Gliadel wafers in the treatment of malignant glioma: a systematic review. Curr Oncol 2007;14(5):189–94.

23. Xing WK, Shao C, Qi ZY, et al. The role of Gliadel wafers in the treatment of newly diagnosed GBM: a meta-analysis. Drug Des Devel Ther 2015;9: 3341–8.

24. Ashby LS, Smith KA, Stea B. Gliadel wafer implantation combined with standard radiotherapy and concurrent followed by adjuvant temozolomide for treatment of newly diagnosed high-grade glioma: a systematic literature review. World J Surg Oncol 2016;14(1):225.

25. Bastiancich C, Danhier P, Preat V, et al. Anticancer drug-loaded hydrogels as drug delivery systems for the local treatment of glioblastoma. J Control Release 2016;243:29–42.

26. Bregy A, Shah AH, Diaz MV, et al. The role of Gliadel wafers in the treatment of high-grade gliomas. Expert Rev Anticancer Ther 2013;13(12):1453–61.

27. Silber JR, Bobola MS, Blank A, et al. O(6)-methylguanine-DNA methyltransferase in glioma therapy: promise and problems. Biochim Biophys Acta 2012;1826(1):71–82.

28. Walter KA, Cahan MA, Gur A, et al. Interstitial taxol delivered from a biodegradable polymer implant against experimental malignant glioma. Cancer Res 1994;54(8):2207–12.

29. DiMeco F, Li KW, Tyler BM, et al. Local delivery of mitoxantrone for the treatment of malignant brain tumors in rats. J Neurosurg 2002;97(5):1173–8.

30. Sawyer AJ, Saucier-Sawyer JK, Booth CJ, et al. Convection-enhanced delivery of camptothecin-loaded polymer nanoparticles for treatment of intracranial tumors. Drug Deliv Transl Res 2011;1(1):34–42.

31. Wait SD, Prabhu RS, Burri SH, et al. Polymeric drug delivery for the treatment of glioblastoma. Neuro Oncol 2015;17(Suppl 2):ii9–23.

32. Yohay K, Tyler B, Weaver KD, et al. Efficacy of local polymer-based and systemic delivery of the anti-glutamatergic agents riluzole and memantine in rat glioma models. J Neurosurg 2014;120(4):854–63.

33. Cirillo G, Spizzirri UG, Curcio M, et al. Injectable hydrogels for cancer therapy over the last decade. Pharmaceutics 2019;11(9):486.

34. Norouzi M, Nazari B, Miller DW. Injectable hydrogel-based drug delivery systems for local cancer therapy. Drug Discov Today 2016;21(11):1835–49.

35. Raucher D. Tumor targeting peptides: novel therapeutic strategies in glioblastoma. Curr Opin Pharmacol 2019;47:14–9.

36. Raucher D, Dragojevic S, Ryu J. Macromolecular drug carriers for targeted glioblastoma therapy: preclinical studies, challenges, and future perspectives. Front Oncol 2018;8:624.

37. Hines DJ, Kaplan DL. Poly(lactic-co-glycolic) acid-controlled-release systems: experimental and modeling insights. Crit Rev Ther Drug Carrier Syst 2013;30(3):257–76.

38. Arvold ND, Armstrong TS, Warren KE, et al. Corticosteroid use endpoints in neuro-oncology: response assessment in neuro-oncology working group. Neuro Oncol 2018;20(7):897–906.

39. Yang H, Leffler CT. Hybrid dendrimer hydrogel/poly(lactic-co-glycolic acid) nanoparticle platform: an advanced vehicle for topical delivery of antiglaucoma drugs and a likely solution to improving compliance and adherence in glaucoma management. J Ocul Pharmacol Ther 2013;29(2):166–72.

40. Akbar U, Jones T, Winestone J, et al. Delivery of temozolomide to the tumor bed via biodegradable gel matrices in a novel model of intracranial glioma with resection. J Neurooncol 2009;94(2):203–12.

41. Fourniols T, Randolph LD, Staub A, et al. Temozolomide-loaded photopolymerizable PEG-DMA-based hydrogel for the treatment of glioblastoma. J Control Release 2015;210:95–104.

42. Zhao M, Danhier F, Bastiancich C, et al. Post-resection treatment of glioblastoma with an injectable nanomedicine-loaded photopolymerizable hydrogel induces long-term survival. Int J Pharm 2018;548(1):522–9.

43. Blau HM, Springer ML. Gene therapy–a novel form of drug delivery. N Engl J Med 1995;333(18):1204–7.

44. Zlokovic BV, Apuzzo ML. Cellular and molecular neurosurgery: pathways from concept to reality–part II: vector systems and delivery methodologies for gene therapy of the central nervous system. Neurosurgery 1997;40(4):805–12 [discussion: 812–3].

45. Rainov NG, Ren H. Gene therapy for human malignant brain tumors. Cancer J 2003;9(3):180–8.

46. Kwiatkowska A, Nandhu MS, Behera P, et al. Strategies in gene therapy for glioblastoma. Cancers (Basel) 2013;5(4):1271–305.

47. Chiocca EA, Choi BB, Cai WZ, et al. Transfer and expression of the lacZ gene in rat brain neurons mediated by herpes simplex virus mutants. New Biol 1990;2(8):739–46.

48. Latchman DS. Herpes simplex virus-based vectors for the treatment of cancer and neurodegenerative disease. Curr Opin Mol Ther 2005;7(5):415–8.

49. Cloughesy TF, Landolfi J, Hogan DJ, et al. Phase 1 trial of vocimagene amiretrorepvec and 5-fluorocytosine for recurrent high-grade glioma. Sci Transl Med 2016;8(341):341ra375.

50. Kim JW, Glasgow JN, Nakayama M, et al. An adenovirus vector incorporating carbohydrate binding domains utilizes glycans for gene transfer. PLoS One 2013;8(2):e55533.

51. Lang FF, Bruner JM, Fuller GN, et al. Phase I trial of adenovirus-mediated p53 gene therapy for recurrent glioma: biological and clinical results. J Clin Oncol 2003;21(13):2508–18.

52. Vecil GG, Lang FF. Clinical trials of adenoviruses in brain tumors: a review of Ad-p53 and oncolytic adenoviruses. J Neurooncol 2003;65(3):237–46.

53. Chiocca EA, Aguilar LK, Bell SD, et al. Phase IB study of gene-mediated cytotoxic immunotherapy adjuvant to up-front surgery and intensive timing radiation for malignant glioma. J Clin Oncol 2011;29(27):3611–9.

54. Westphal M, Yla-Herttuala S, Martin J, et al. Adenovirus-mediated gene therapy with sitimagene ceradenovec followed by intravenous ganciclovir for patients with operable high-grade glioma (ASPECT): a randomised, open-label, phase 3 trial. Lancet Oncol 2013;14(9):823–33.

55. Thomas CE, Ehrhardt A, Kay MA. Progress and problems with the use of viral vectors for gene therapy. Nat Rev Genet 2003;4(5):346–58.

56. Kim SS, Rait A, Kim E, et al. A nanoparticle carrying the p53 gene targets tumors including cancer stem cells, sensitizes glioblastoma to chemotherapy and improves survival. ACS Nano 2014;8(6):5494–514.

57. Jensen SA, Day ES, Ko CH, et al. Spherical nucleic acid nanoparticle conjugates as an RNAi-based therapy for glioblastoma. Sci Transl Med 2013;5(209):209ra152.

58. Lee TJ, Yoo JY, Shu D, et al. RNA nanoparticle-based targeted therapy for glioblastoma through inhibition of oncogenic miR-21. Mol Ther 2017;25(7):1544–55.

59. Bobo RH, Laske DW, Akbasak A, et al. Convection-enhanced delivery of macromolecules in the brain. Proc Natl Acad Sci U S A 1994;91(6):2076–80.

60. Varenika V, Dickinson P, Bringas J, et al. Detection of infusate leakage in the brain using real-time imaging of convection-enhanced delivery. J Neurosurg 2008;109(5):874–80.

61. Vogelbaum MA. Convection enhanced delivery for treating brain tumors and selected neurological disorders: symposium review. J Neurooncol 2007;83(1):97–109.

62. Hall WA, Sherr GT. Convection-enhanced delivery: targeted toxin treatment of malignant glioma. Neurosurg Focus 2006;20(4):E10.

63. Vogelbaum MA. Convection enhanced delivery for the treatment of malignant gliomas: symposium review. J Neurooncol 2005;73(1):57–69.

64. Vogelbaum MA, Iannotti CA. Convection-enhanced delivery of therapeutic agents into the brain. Handb Clin Neurol 2012;104:355–62.

65. Vogelbaum MA, Brewer C, Barnett GH, et al. First-in-human evaluation of the Cleveland multiport catheter for convection-enhanced delivery of topotecan in recurrent high-grade glioma: results of pilot trial 1. J Neurosurg 2018;1–10. https://doi.org/10.3171/2017.10.JNS171845.

66. Krauze MT, Saito R, Noble C, et al. Reflux-free cannula for convection-enhanced high-speed delivery of therapeutic agents. J Neurosurg 2005;103(5):923–9.

67. Weaver M, Laske DW. Transferrin receptor ligand-targeted toxin conjugate (Tf-CRM107) for therapy of malignant gliomas. J Neurooncol 2003;65(1):3–13.

68. Weber FW, Floeth F, Asher A, et al. Local convection enhanced delivery of IL4-Pseudomonas exotoxin (NBI-3001) for treatment of patients with recurrent malignant glioma. Acta Neurochir Suppl 2003;88:93–103.

69. Weber F, Asher A, Bucholz R, et al. Safety, tolerability, and tumor response of IL4-Pseudomonas exotoxin (NBI-3001) in patients with recurrent malignant glioma. J Neurooncol 2003;64(1–2):125–37.

70. Kunwar S, Prados MD, Chang SM, et al. Direct intracerebral delivery of cintredekin besudotox (IL13-PE38QQR) in recurrent malignant glioma: a report by the cintredekin besudotox intraparenchymal study group. J Clin Oncol 2007;25(7):837–44.

71. Kunwar S, Chang S, Westphal M, et al. Phase III randomized trial of CED of IL13-PE38QQR vs Gliadel wafers for recurrent glioblastoma. Neuro Oncol 2010;12(8):871–81.

72. Sampson JH, Archer G, Pedain C, et al. Poor drug distribution as a possible explanation for the results of the PRECISE trial. J Neurosurg 2010;113(2):301–9.

73. Mueller S, Polley MY, Lee B, et al. Effect of imaging and catheter characteristics on clinical outcome for patients in the PRECISE study. J Neurooncol 2011;101(2):267–77.

Window of Opportunity Clinical Trials to Evaluate Novel Therapies for Brain Tumors

Visish M. Srinivasan, MD[a,b], Chibawanye Ene, MD PhD[a,c],
Brittany Parker Kerrigan, PhD[a,c], Frederick F. Lang, MD[a,c],*

KEYWORDS

- Oncology • Brain tumors • Biologic end points • Window of opportunity • Clinical trials
- Molecular markers • Biomarkers • Immunotherapy

KEY POINTS

- Window of opportunity clinical trials, also called biologic end point trials, are designed to provide molecular or cellular evidence from post-treatment human specimens that an experimental therapeutic is capable of entering tumor cells and inducing the desired molecular or cellular changes, which it was designed to produce.
- When combined with classic phase I or phase II trial end points, which define the maximal tolerated doses and a clinically effective dose, window of opportunity trials prove that these doses are also biologically effective doses.
- Window of opportunity trials are based on three requirements: acquisition of post-treatment tumor specimens, predetermined assays to detect alterations in defined molecular targets in these post-treatment tumor samples, and control untreated tissues against which the molecular changes in the post-treatment specimens can be compared.
- When standard phase I and II clinical trials are designed to include window of opportunity components, investigators gain valuable insights into why molecularly targeted agents do or do not show clinical benefit in GBM.

INTRODUCTION

Glioblastoma (GBM) is the most common primary brain tumor in adults.[1] Despite aggressive surgical resection followed by radiotherapy and temozolomide-based chemotherapy, the median overall survival (OS) remains only 15 months.[2] Unfortunately, over the last few decades, OS has improved by only a few months indicating that there is an urgent need for more effective therapies.

Following preclinical development, new anticancer therapeutics undergo a series of progressively complex and larger prospective clinical trials whose goals are to identify the maximal tolerated dose (MTD) of a new agent that can be given without serious side effects (phase I), to determine whether the agent works against particular tumors at this dose (phase II), and to compare the safety and efficacy of the new agent with the current standard of care (phase III).[3,4] Unfortunately, for most brain tumors, particularly GBM, many new therapies fail in large and expensive phase III clinical trials, despite perceived success in earlier phase I and phase II trials.[5–8] Of equal concern, many agents that seem to be efficacious

a Department of Neurosurgery, The University of Texas MD Anderson Cancer Center, 1515 Holcombe Boulevard, Unit 442, Houston, TX 77030, USA; b Department of Neurosurgery, Baylor College of Medicine, Houston, TX, USA; c The Brain Tumor Center, The University of Texas MD Anderson Cancer Center, Houston, TX, USA
* Corresponding author.
E-mail address: flang@mdanderson.org

Neurosurg Clin N Am 32 (2021) 93–104
https://doi.org/10.1016/j.nec.2020.09.002
1042-3680/21/© 2020 Elsevier Inc. All rights reserved.

in preclinical animal studies are dismissed as ineffective after phase II testing without knowledge of why the agent did not work against human GBMs.[9] As a result, there have been few new therapeutics for GBM approved by the Food and Drug Administration in the past 30 years.[5]

Multiple factors likely contribute to the overall low number of agents that successfully pass through the translational continuum and become new therapeutics for GBM, including the highly resistant phenotype of GBM, the uniqueness of the central nervous system microenvironment, the limitations to delivery imposed by the blood-brain barrier (BBB), and the lack of preclinical models that recapitulate the human disease and predict clinical success.[10–14] However, this poor outcome is also caused at least in part by the current methods used to evaluate new brain tumor therapeutics in patients (**Fig. 1**). Specifically, traditional phase I dose escalation trials typically identify the MTD based purely on assessments of systemic toxicity, such as nausea, vomiting, or diarrhea.[15] Likewise, phase II trials usually determine efficacy based on indirect measures, typically radiographic response, progression-free survival (PFS), and OS (see **Fig. 1**).[16] Indeed, traditional early stage trials of brain tumor therapeutics do not include direct assessments of tumor tissue, and therefore, do not determine whether the agent is capable of doing what it is intended to do in GBM tumors in human patients, which is arguably the most important end points of early stage drug development. As a result, agents that do not show radiographic response when used as monotherapy are dismissed, although they may in fact hit their target in the tumor cells and could be used in combination with other agents.[17] Alternatively, such agents as bevacizumab, which produce radiographic responses as measured by changes in contrast enhancement on MRI, may be deemed effective and move on to large phase III trials, although they have little ability to inhibit tumor growth.[6,18]

To address these shortfalls and expedite the discovery of new effective agents for GBM, more than 20 years ago, concurrent with the development of molecularly targeted therapeutic agents, and building on proposals in other solid tumors,[19] we[20] and others[21,22] proposed modifications to traditional early phase clinical trials for the treatment of GBM. The primary goal of these modifications was to demonstrate that the new agent was able to do what it was intended to do, namely, that it crossed the BBB and entered the brain tumor, hit its molecular target, and caused cell death and/or induced physiologically important changes in the tumor microenvironment (eg, enhance antiglioma T-cell populations[23]). To achieve this goal, it was proposed that the new therapeutic agent should be administered preoperatively to patients with surgically resectable tumors, the tumor be removed at surgery, and that the post-treatment tumor specimen be analyzed for drug penetrance and biologic activity, essentially recapitulating what is done during preclinical testing in the laboratory (see **Fig. 1**). These trials were originally designated as "biologic end point" trials because changes in the molecular biology of the tumor defined outcome.[20,21,24] However, soon these trials became known as "window of opportunity" trials because surgical resection provided an opportunity to obtain a post-treatment specimens that could give a window into the molecular effects of the agent on the tumor.[25] Over the past 20 years, window of opportunity trials have become increasingly accepted as an important component of the development of novel therapeutics of solid tumors, including brain tumors like GBM, and are considered by many as the gold standard of early stage clinical drug development.[22]

Execution of an effective window of opportunity trial for brain tumors is particularly complex because of the difficulties inherent in obtaining tumor tissue from the brain. Therefore, in this review, we define what constitutes window of opportunity trials. We discuss novel designs for incorporating biologic end points into early stage trials in the context of GBM, and through examples of successful window of opportunity trials, we illustrate the power of window of opportunity trials in the development of novel therapeutics for GBM.

DEFINING FEATURES OF A WINDOW OF OPPORTUNITY TRIAL

Window of opportunity trials are designed specifically to determine the extent to which a new therapeutic agent hits the molecular target against which it is designed and/or appropriately modulates the tumor microenvironment for therapeutic effect. When combined with traditional metrics of safety (eg, clinical toxicity) and efficacy (eg, radiographic response), data from window of opportunity trials provide critical molecular or cellular information about why agents succeed or fail during clinical trials. These results guide modifications early in the clinical trial continuum, including making go/no go decisions before expensive and time-consuming late-stage clinical trials. Window of opportunity trials incorporate several critical features that must be considered in the trial design, including tissue acquisition, molecular assays, and dose schedules (see **Fig. 1**).

Window of Opportunity Trial Concept

<u>Key Components</u>
1. Tissue acquisition
2. Molecular Assay
3. Dosing schedule

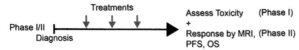

Result: Biologically Effective Dose

Traditional Clinical Trial

Fig. 1. Schema comparing window of opportunity trial concept with traditional clinical trials. In window of opportunity trials, following diagnosis, novel therapies are administered before tissue acquisition during surgery. Biologic assessment is performed on treated tissue and an untreated or control tissue to determine if the novel therapy modified its intended target within the tumor (biologic end point). This assists with determination of the biologically effective dose. Following surgery, the novel therapy can be continued to determine the maximum tolerated dose. In traditional clinical trials, novel therapies are administered following diagnosis. Maximum tolerated dose and clinical response are assessed without knowledge of the target modification within the tumor. PFS, progression-free survival.

Tissue Acquisition

The most important element of a window of opportunity trial is tissue acquisition after drug treatment. For brain tumors, tissue acquisition is a significant hurdle because of the potential complications associated with invasive brain procedures.[26] Tissue is obtained either through stereotactic biopsy or through open craniotomy and tumor resection. Stereotactic biopsy has the advantage that it is minimally invasive and affords the opportunity for serial biopsies before and after drug treatment, which is highly desirable because the pretreatment sample provides a baseline untreated (control) tissue (see later); however, the tissue samples are often small, limiting the number of assays that can be performed, and underevaluating the true heterogeneity of the tumor. Alternatively, open craniotomy and surgical resection often provides large amounts of tumor for analysis. Given the significant spatial heterogeneity of different clonal subpopulations within GBM,[27] optimal specimens for analyses are achieved using resection techniques where the tumor is

removed by circumferential dissection as previously described (**Fig. 2**).[28] This approach not only provides a large tumor sample for multiple analyses, but also preserves the tumor architecture, permitting assessments across the various tumor zones, including areas of solid tumor, infiltrating tumor cells and assessing the impact of the new therapy on different clones of tumor cells residing in different niches within the tumor, such as hypoxic areas, which may contribute to treatment resistance.[29]

Because of the complexities of including craniotomies in trial designs, many window of opportunity trials have optional arms for tissue acquisition. However, the most effective window of opportunity trials incorporate tumor acquisition specifically into clinical trial protocols. For phase I window of opportunity dose escalation trials, inclusion of two arms, a standard treatment arm and a biologic end point arm, is optimal in our experience (**Fig. 3**).[24,30] In the first arm (standard treatment arm), drug is given, and patients are simply followed for standard toxicity measures, providing traditional assessments of drug-induced toxicity.

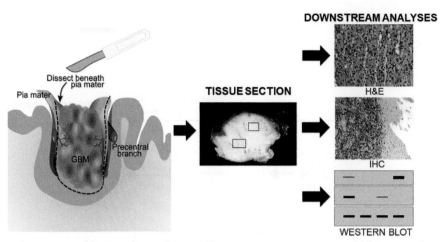

Fig. 2. Preserving tumor architecture for analysis. En bloc tumor resection using a subpial approach preserves tissue architecture for downstream biologic analysis including hematoxylin and eosin (H&E) stains, immunohistochemistry (IHC), and Western blot analysis.

In the second arm (biologic end point or window of opportunity arm), patients are treated with drug and then undergo craniotomy and tumor resection, thereby providing a post-treatment biologic specimen for analysis of drug-induced changes. We successfully used this strategy in a trial of an adenovirus-mediated p53 gene therapy (Ad-p53) and in another trial of Delta-24-RGD oncolytic virus.[24,30] In these trials, both arms were enrolled at each dose cohort, with arm 2 (biologic end point arm) enrolling after arm 1 (standard treatment arm) (**Fig. 4**; Strategy A). An alternative strategy, which is more cost efficient, is to enroll successive cohorts in arm 1 (standard arm) until the MTD is reached. Then, once the MTD is determined, patients are enrolled into arm 2 (biologic end point) (see **Fig. 4**; Strategy B). Whereas the former strategy defines the biologic outcome at each dose cohort, the latter strategy first defines the MTD and then assesses whether the MTD dose results

in target engagement/alteration. In our most recent window of opportunity trial,[31] we have followed this latter strategy because it allows for faster dose escalation, is less costly, and requires fewer patients.

Molecular Assays

The second critical component of a window of opportunity trial is a predefined molecular assay that assesses the desired molecular outcome. Determining the optimal assay is paramount to the success of any window of opportunity trial. One of the most basic assays that should be included in nearly all window of opportunity trials of drugs is a simple assay of drug levels in the tissue. This is particularly important in brain tumors where the BBB can prevent drug from reaching the tumor. Indeed, a major goal of window of opportunity trials is to simply demonstrate therapeutic levels of the drug in the tumor after the drug is delivered

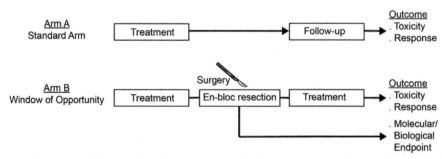

Fig. 3. Strategy for incorporating window of opportunity trial design into standard early phase clinical trials. The window of opportunity component is achieved by designing a separate arm as part of the standard trial. Specifically, Arm A represents the standard arm in which patients are treated with the novel therapeutic and standard clinical outcomes are measured. Patients with resectable tumors are enrolled into Arm B, which is design to provide post-treatment specimens for analysis.

Strategy **A**

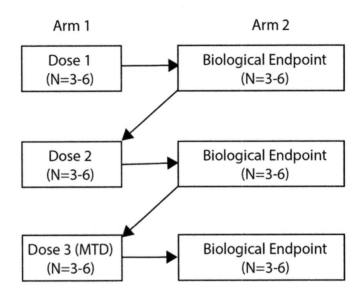

Strategy **B**

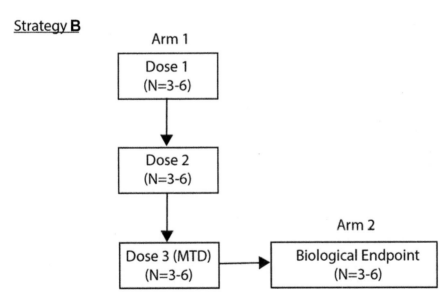

Fig. 4. Strategies for dose-escalation during window of opportunity trials. In strategy A, both arms are enrolled at each dose cohort, with arm 2 (biologic end point arm) enrolling after arm 1 (standard treatment arm). An alternative strategy (*B*), which is more cost efficient, is to enroll successive cohorts in arm 1 (standard arm) until the MTD is reached. Then, once the MTD is determined, patients are enrolled into arm 2 (biologic end point).

at the dose and schedule that will be moved forward into later stage trials. Because the BBB is difficult to assess in animal models,[32] the simple documentation that adequate concentrations of drug are present in a tumor is an important outcome of window of opportunity trials.

Equally important, is incorporating molecular assays that prove that the drug is interacting with

its target. Ideally, the target of the agent is known and an assay for assessing engagement with that target is available. For example, determinations of the effectiveness of tyrosine kinase inhibitors may require assays that document inhibition of phosphorylation of the target receptor.[17] Likewise, the effectiveness of an immunotherapeutic agent may be shown by assays that assess increases in antitumoral T cells.[23] Importantly, these assays must be applicable to clinical tissue specimens. Assays that assess target inhibition on tissue slices (eg, immunohistochemistry [IHC]) are preferred because they provide molecular information in the context of spatial distribution.[24,30,33] Nevertheless, most molecular assays that are developed in preclinical laboratory testing can be applied in window of opportunity trials, including Western blotting,[17] IHC,[24,30] in situ hybridization,[27] mass cytometry (CYTOF), and single-cell RNA sequencing.[34]

In this context, it is important that a major goal of preclinical animal studies of new targeted agents is the development of assays of target engagement that can be translated to clinical specimens. Indeed, most preclinical studies of new agents use animal models to prove efficacy by determining whether the agent improves animal survival.[35] However, an equally important application of preclinical animal models is developing critical assays that can be translated to clinical specimens. For example, in our work on Delta-24-RGD, an oncolytic virus, we developed a tissue-based assay using intracranial tumors from mice in which we documented the presence of active virus based on IHC using antibodies against viral proteins (hexon and E1A).[30,36] We showed in our animal models that intratumoral injections of Delta-24-RGD resulted in three concentric zones indicative of virus propagating through the tumor: (1) a central zone of necrosis (where the virus had killed cells), (2) a surrounding zone of cells that stained positively for hexon or E1B protein on IHC (where the virus was actively replicating in tumor cells), and (3) a third zone of tumor cells (where the virus had not reached yet) (**Fig. 5**).[36] This immunohistochemical assay and the zones of activity were translated to our clinical specimens and used to prove that Delta-24-RGD could infect and replicate in human tumors from patients with GBM.[30]

Assays that measure direct effects of a drug are preferable to assays that measure indirect effects or downstream effects. For example, if a drug is known to inhibit a particular molecular target, such as by blocking phosphorylation, the ideal assay would measure the phosphorylation status of the target (eg, by Western blotting).[17] Measurements of downstream effects, such as induction of apoptosis (as measured by cleaved caspase-3 activity) are less desirable.[37]

In this context, the heterogeneity of molecular events within any tumor mandates careful consideration of control tissue for comparison of molecular outcomes in any window of opportunity clinical trial. Although some molecular outcomes may not require a control (eg, level of a drug in a

tissue or identification of a therapeutic oncolytic virus in a tumor), baseline levels of most molecular targets vary greatly across tumors. For example, assaying inhibition of phosphorylation of a tyrosine kinase, such as epidermal growth factor receptor (EGFR), requires knowing the baseline level of phosphorylation before treatment.[17] Consequently, although inclusion of controls is not standard in traditional phase I or phase II clinical trials, defining the baseline levels of a molecular target is critical for the success of a window of opportunity clinical trial. Although comparing an untreated specimen with a treated specimen is ideal, acquiring an untreated specimen may be difficult in patients with brain tumors because a biopsy before and after treatment would be needed. Therefore, several novel avenues for acquiring control tissue have been proposed (see later) and many windows of opportunity have exploited these methods.

Dose Schedules

The last critical element of a window of opportunity trial is the dose and schedule of the experimental agent that is given to the patient. The defining feature of window of opportunity trials is that the delivered dose is a therapeutic dose that has the potential to be effective against the tumor. Using a therapeutic dose distinguishes window of opportunity trials from so called phase 0 trials. Unlike window of opportunity trials, phase 0 clinical trials are carried out early in drug development.[38] Here, investigators give a subtherapeutic dose of an investigational agent without diagnostic or therapeutic intent.[39] The primary goal of these studies is to assess the pharmacokinetics and pharmacodynamics of new agents that have never been tested in humans.[40,41] If these agents are found to meet the pharmacokinetic and pharmacodynamic thresholds, these candidate drugs then proceed to phase I dose escalation studies to assess safety and toxicity.[39] Whereas giving subtherapeutic doses of a drug and assaying blood levels of the agent may give valuable information about drug kinetics, phase 0 trials offer little value in terms of defining whether therapeutic levels of a drug enter a tissue or hit its target, particularly for brain tumors where subtherapeutic levels are not likely to cross the BBB. In window of opportunity trials, however, therapeutic doses of new agents are administered with a biologic end point as the goal.

In addition to the dose, a critical element of window of opportunity trials is deciding the length of treatment before tissue acquisition and the amount of time after treatment that the tissue will

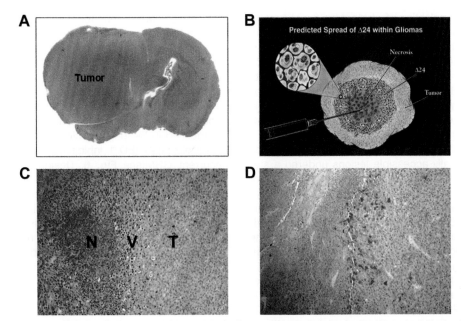

Fig. 5. Preclinical models for evaluating Delta-24 RGD before window of opportunity clinical trials. Preclinical animal models are important for developing assays that can be translated to clinical trials. For example, in the development of Delta-24-RGD, human gliomas were grown in preclinical mouse model as shown by H&E stains of mouse brains (*A*). To develop an assay that would prove viral replication and that could be translated to the clinic, we reasoned that there would be three zones of viral replication (*B*) when animals were sacrificed several days after intratumoral injection: a central zone of necrosis (N, where the virus had killed cells), a surrounding zone of cells that stained positively for hexon or E1B protein (V, where the virus was actively replicating in tumor cells), and a third zone of yet-to-be-infected tumor cells (T, where the virus had not reached yet). These zones were demonstrated in mouse tumors based on H&E (*C*) and after staining for E1A (*red staining* in *D*).

be acquired. Given that the goal of these trials is to determine the extent to which the drug hits its target or causes a desired molecular or cellular effect, consideration should be given to treating the patient for an extended period of time to maximize the potential molecular effects of the experimental agent. For example, lapatinib, an EGFR inhibitor, is typically dosed on a twice-daily schedule, and so in a recent window of opportunity trial this drug was given twice daily for 7 days before the tumor was resected.[17] This strategy ensured that the drug levels detected in the tumor were clinically relevant. In this context, a common approach is to treat for a long enough period of time so as to reach the steady state drug level (typical five half-lives of the agent) before tissue acquisition. Similarly, window of opportunity designs must carefully consider how much time should elapse between the last dose and tissue acquisition. Indeed, the molecular effects of the experimental agent may be delayed relative to drug delivery, particularly when the assayed effect is downstream of the molecular target. For example, in a currently ongoing trial assessing the ability of bone marrow stem cells to deliver Delta-24-RGD to brain tumors after intra-arterial injection, post-

treatment tissue is acquired 14 days after the injection based on preclinical studies showing it takes this much time for the cells to arrive in the tumor, release the virus, and then maximally infect the tumor cells.[31]

INCORPORATING WINDOW OF OPPORTUNITY TRIALS INTO EARLY PHASE TRIALS OF BRAIN TUMORS

Given the multiple considerations discussed previously, several strategies have been suggested for tailoring phase I and phase II trials to incorporate biologic end points and thereby meet the goals of window of opportunity trials for brain tumors. We have previously proposed several approaches that are worthy of review, and it is anticipated that new approaches will emerge to meet the needs of particular experimental agents.[20]

Phase I Trials

The goal of phase I clinical trials is to determine the MTD or the recommended phase II dose (RP2D) that can be given to a patient without causing undue toxicity. Incorporation of biologic end points in a window of opportunity phase I trial provides the further determination of whether the new agent influences the molecular end point being targeted, and therefore proves that the MTD or RP2D is also an effective biologic dose. Indeed, in some cases the effective biologic dose may prove to be lower than the MTD, although such examples are rare. We have previously suggested several strategies of carrying out effective phase I window of opportunity clinical trials.[20]

In the ideal design (**Fig. 6**, Design A), patients with surgically accessible lesions undergo a stereotactic biopsy to collect pretreatment tissue for baseline molecular analysis using the same assays that will be assessed after treatment After this baseline (control) tissue is obtained, the experimental therapeutic is administered based on the preplanned dose and schedule. At the completion of the drug treatment, a craniotomy and en bloc tumor resection is performed (alternatively another biopsy may be performed if tumor resection is not feasible). The post-treatment tumor specimen undergoes molecular analyses to determine tissue pharmacokinetic and drug-related molecular changes. After the patient recovers from the surgery, the agent is given (typically at the same dose given before surgery) to determine clinical toxicity according to standard phase I criteria. This two-stage design has the advantage that it allows comparisons to be made between untreated (control) and treated specimens from the same patient. However, the need for two procedures makes this design less desirable to many patients. A version of this strategy was used in our recent clinical trial of DNX-2401 oncolytic virus therapy for recurrent GBM,[24,30] in which post-treatment specimens were compared with untreated (control) tissue taken at the initial resection from the same patient (albeit not immediately before treatment).

To minimize the number of biopsies, several alternatives are possible. One strategy (see **Fig. 6**, Design B) is to randomize patients with surgically accessible lesions to a group that receives the therapy versus a group that does not receive the therapy or that receives a placebo. Patients in both groups undergo craniotomy and en bloc tumor resection. Molecular analyses are performed on all tumor specimens with the specimens from the untreated/placebo group serving as control specimens for the treated group. Following surgery, both groups receive the agent and are followed for clinical toxicity using standard phase I criteria. In this strategy the number of patients entered depends on the test-variability of the molecular analyses, which defines the number of patients needed to achieve statistical significance. This strategy has the advantage of requiring only one surgical intervention for each patient; however, it suffers from requiring the use of statistical methods to determine the variability in the baseline levels of the targeted molecule and to determine whether there is an overall impact of the therapy on the molecular target. Another alternative is to use banked specimens as the untreated control group for comparison with the treated group, exemplified in the phase II clinical trial assessing pembrolizumab (PD-1 inhibitor) in patients with recurrent GBM(see **Fig. 6**, Design C).[42,43] This strategy eliminates the need for randomizing patients to drug versus no-drug treatment and therefore requires less patients, but is limited by its reliance on noncontemporaneous historical control specimens that may have been handled and processes differently from the prospectively obtained post-treatment specimens.

Phase II Trials

Design strategies similar to those proposed for phase I trials can also be applied to phase II trials, again recognizing that these phase II trials must retain the goal of determining clinical efficacy while incorporating biologic end points. Similar to the ideal phase I strategy, in the ideal phase II approach, patients undergo a stereotactic biopsy before treatment, after which they are treated with the therapeutic agent using the dose defined in phase I. After treatment with the therapeutic agent, patients undergo surgical resection providing a post-treatment specimen that is compared with the pretreatment specimen to determine whether the agent hit its target or altered the tumor microenvironment to the degree established in the phase I setting. In this approach, the molecular end point can be used as a response criterion to define the efficacy of an agent, such that agents that repeatedly hit their target or induce the desired molecular effect are deemed efficacious.[30] This efficacy analysis is extended further by administering the experimental agent after surgical resection and by then following the patient to determine PFS or OS, based on MRI analyses of tumor recurrence. This is exemplified in the window of opportunity phase II trial assessing the efficacy of lapatinib (EGFR inhibitor) for recurrent GBM.[17] Here, patients with surgically resectable recurrent GBM were treated with lapatinib (750 mg orally twice daily) for 7 days before surgical removal of the tumor. The surgical specimen was analyzed for levels of lapatinib and for inhibition of EGFR phosphorylation. After recovery from surgery patients were treated with daily lapatinib until tumor recurrence to assess the impact of the drug on PFS. Because the tumor is largely

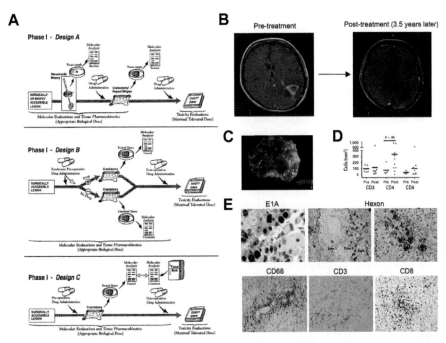

Fig. 6. Proposed designs for phase I clinical trials of agents for which molecular targets can be tested and window of opportunity trial assessing the oncolytic virus, Delta-24-RGD. Window of opportunity trials can take on several designs (*A*). Optimal design (Design A). A biopsy can be used to determine the baseline value of the target before treatment. Patients are then treated with drug, and the effects of the agent on the tumor are determined in a post-treatment surgical specimen. In design B, which avoids pretreatment biopsy, patients are randomized to receive drug or not. Post-treatment tumor reaction allows comparisons to be made between untreated specimen (control specimens) and treated specimens. In design C, control specimens are obtained from specimens in a tumor bank. Execution and outcome of a window of opportunity trial for Delta-24-RGD oncolytic virus is shown in *B–E*. (*B*) MRI with contrast of long-term survivor 3.5 years following Delta-24 treatment and surgery. (*C*) Photomicrographs of sections from en bloc resection specimens taken 14 days after virus injection. (*D*) Biologic response based on quantitative analyses of $CD3^+$, $CD4^+$, and $CD8^+$ cell infiltration in pretreatment (pre; n = 5) and post-treatment (post; n = 10) tumor specimens. The mean values are noted by *horizontal bars*; although $CD3^+$ changes were not evident, $CD4^+$ and $CD8^+$ cells increased after treatment, with increases in $CD4^+$ cells reaching statistical significance. (*E*) Immunohistochemical staining for viral E1A protein (*left*), which is a marker of viral infection, and for viral hexon protein (*right*), which is a marker of replication. E1A immunostaining (*left*) is primarily intranuclear, as would be expected for actively infecting virus. Immunohistochemical staining for $CD68^+$ macrophages, $CD3^+$, and $CD8^+$ T cells. ([*A*] *From* Lang FF, Gilbert MR, Puduvalli VK, et al. Toward better early-phase brain tumor clinical trials: a reappraisal of current methods and proposals for future strategies. Neuro Oncol. 2002,4(4).274, with permission. [*B–E*] *From* Lang FF, Conrad C, Gomez-Manzano C, et al. Phase I study of DNX-2401 (Delta-24-RGD) oncolytic adenovirus: replication and immunotherapeutic effects in recurrent malignant glioma. J Clin Oncol. 2018;36(14):1419–27; with permission.)

removed at surgery, assessments of radiographic response may be difficult in this design. Therefore, like phase I trial, these phase II trials with biologic end points may include a "standard treatment" arm in which no surgical intervention is undertaken so that the traditional end points of radiographic response, PFS, and OS can be assessed independent of any surgical intervention.[30] In this arm, a pretreatment biopsy may be undertaken to determine the extent to which the molecular target is present in the tumor at baseline. This information can then be used to define whether the presence of the target correlates with higher rates of

radiographic response, longer PFS and longer OS compared with tumors that do not have the target.

In addition to this ideal phase II design, a more cost-effective approach for a window of opportunity phase II study is to randomize patients with surgically accessible lesions to either receive the experimental agent or to receive placebo/no drug, and then to perform a craniotomy and en bloc resection, thereby providing specimens for molecular analyses. In this scenario the placebo/untreated specimens serve as the control for the treated specimens. Biologic efficacy is based on observing a statistically significant higher number of patients in which the target is hit in the treatment group compared with the control group. After the craniotomy for resection, all the patients are treated with the experimental agent and followed for tumor recurrence to define PFS and OS.

When done well, these window of opportunity phase II designs add meaningful biologic data to the standard clinical outcome data, and enhance decision-making around whether the agent should be further studied. In this context, agents that clearly hit their molecular target in most patients in the window arm of the trial and show clinical response and extension of PFS/OS in the standard arm are likely to be efficacious and should be moved to phase III trials. In contrast, agents that do not hit their target and do not show responses should likely be abandoned, although the window of opportunity arm of the trial may provide insight at the molecular or cellular level into the cause of the failure. For example, the biologic studies may reveal that the drug levels were below those needed to kill tumor cells, or the drug may have inhibited the target only partially. These insights may lead to continued pursuit of the target through the development of more effective agents rather than completely abandoning the target. Potentially more interesting are agents that may hit their target in biologic studies, but do not induce clinical responses. Although such a result may suggest that the target is not an independent driver of tumor growth, it may also suggest that the experimental agent may be effective when combined with other agents that hit alternative tumor supportive pathways, thus spurring the rational development of the agent in combination trials.

SUMMARY

The clinical development of new therapeutic agents for GBM could be advanced through improvements in the design of standard phase I and II clinical trials. Window of opportunity trials are such an improvement and should routinely be incorporated into standard early phase clinical trials for GBM (and all brain tumors) because they provide a unique opportunity to capture the complex cellular and molecular changes induced by molecularly targeted agents, thereby providing information about the biologic activity of the agent at its MTD, arguably the most important outcome of any early stage trial. Window of opportunity trials are based on several fundamental principles: acquisition of post-treatment tumor specimens, a clinically applicable assay to detect alterations in molecular targets post-treatment, pretreatment or untreated control specimens that provide a

baseline level of activity against which post-treatment changes can be compared, and therapeutic dosing schedules. Incorporation of molecular end points (pretreatment and post-treatment), and advanced histologic techniques that maintain the integrity of molecular end points during window of opportunity phase I/II clinical trials provide avenues for assessing the distribution of these agents within tumors and directly determining the extent to which these agents actually modify the target for which they were designed to interact, especially in the BBB-protected central nervous system. As more studies incorporate molecular end point concepts in window of opportunity trials, we anticipate uncovering more rationale combinations of therapies that work synergistically against a heterogenous and resilient disease, such as GBM.

CLINICS CARE POINTS

- Window of opportunity clinical trials provide tissue for assessment of the biological effects of therapies on their intended target.
- Window of opportunity clinical trials for brain tumors evaluate whether systemically administered drugs cross the blood brain barrier at biologically effective levels.
- Window of opportunity clinical trials for brain tumors could delineate responders from non-responders based on biological biomarkers within tumors.
- Future clinical trials for brain tumors should incorporate a Windows of Opportunity arm to assess biological efficacy of new agents.

DISCLOSURE

Drs. VM Srinivasan, C Ene, BP Kerrigan has nothing to disclose. Dr. Frederick Lang is a patent holder on DNX-2401.

REFERENCES

1. Louis DN, Perry A, Reifenberger G, et al. The 2016 World Health Organization Classification of Tumors of the Central Nervous System: a summary. Acta Neuropathol 2016;131(6):803–20.
2. Stupp R, Mason WP, van den Bent MJ, et al. Radiotherapy plus concomitant and adjuvant temozolomide for glioblastoma. N Engl J Med 2005;352(10):987–96.
3. Chamberlain MC. Treatment options for glioblastoma. Neurosurg Focus 2006;20(4):E19.
4. American Cancer Society. Clinical trials. 2020. Available at: https://www.cancer.org/treatment/treatments-and-side-effects/clinical-trials.html. Accessed July 20, 2020.

5. Shergalis A, Bankhead A 3rd, Luesakul U, et al. Current challenges and opportunities in treating glioblastoma. Pharmacol Rev 2018;70(3):412–45.
6. Gilbert MR, Dignam JJ, Armstrong TS, et al. A randomized trial of bevacizumab for newly diagnosed glioblastoma. N Engl J Med 2014;370(8): 699–708.
7. Stupp R, Hegi ME, Gorlia T, et al. Cilengitide combined with standard treatment for patients with newly diagnosed glioblastoma with methylated MGMT promoter (CENTRIC EORTC 26071-22072 study): a multicentre, randomised, open-label, phase 3 trial. Lancet Oncol 2014;15(10): 1100–8.
8. Kunwar S, Prados MD, Chang SM, et al. Direct intracerebral delivery of cintredekin besudotox (IL13-PE38QQR) in recurrent malignant glioma: a report by the Cintredekin Besudotox Intraparenchymal Study Group. J Clin Oncol 2007;25(7):837–44.
9. Wen PY, Chang SM, Lamborn KR, et al. Phase I/II study of erlotinib and temsirolimus for patients with recurrent malignant gliomas: North American Brain Tumor Consortium trial 04-02. Neuro Oncol 2014; 16(4):567–78.
10. Bastien JI, McNeill KA, Fine HA. Molecular characterizations of glioblastoma, targeted therapy, and clinical results to date. Cancer 2015;121(4):502–16.
11. Qazi MA, Vora P, Venugopal C, et al. Intratumoral heterogeneity: pathways to treatment resistance and relapse in human glioblastoma. Ann Oncol 2017;28(7):1448–56.
12. Azad TD, Pan J, Connolly ID, et al. Therapeutic strategies to improve drug delivery across the blood-brain barrier. Neurosurg Focus 2015;38(3):E9.
13. Robertson FL, Marques-Torrejon MA, Morrison GM, et al. Experimental models and tools to tackle glioblastoma. Dis Model Mech 2019;12(9).
14. Aldape K, Brindle KM, Chesler L, et al. Challenges to curing primary brain tumours. Nat Rev Clin Oncol 2019;16(8):509–20.
15. Ivy SP, Siu LL, Garrett-Mayer E, et al. Approaches to phase 1 clinical trial design focused on safety, efficiency, and selected patient populations: a report from the Clinical Trial Design Task Force of the National Cancer Institute Investigational Drug Steering Committee. Clin Cancer Res 2010;16(6): 1726–36.
16. Seymour L, Ivy SP, Sargent D, et al. The design of phase II clinical trials testing cancer therapeutics: consensus recommendations from the Clinical Trial Design Task Force of the National Cancer Institute Investigational Drug Steering Committee. Clin Cancer Res 2010;16(6):1764–9.
17. Vivanco I, Robins HI, Rohle D, et al. Differential sensitivity of glioma- versus lung cancer-specific EGFR mutations to EGFR kinase inhibitors. Cancer Discov 2012;2(5):458–71.
18. Chinot OL, Wick W, Mason W, et al. Bevacizumab plus radiotherapy-temozolomide for newly diagnosed glioblastoma. N Engl J Med 2014;370(8): 709–22.
19. Arnedos M, Roulleaux Dugage M, Perez-Garcia J, et al. Window of opportunity trials for biomarker discovery in breast cancer. Curr Opin Oncol 2019; 31(6):486–92.
20. Lang FF, Gilbert MR, Puduvalli VK, et al. Toward better early-phase brain tumor clinical trials: a reappraisal of current methods and proposals for future strategies. Neuro Oncol 2002;4(4): 268–77.
21. Cloughesy TF, Yoshimoto K, Nghiemphu P, et al. Antitumor activity of rapamycin in a phase I trial for patients with recurrent PTEN-deficient glioblastoma. PLoS Med 2008;5(1):e8.
22. Vogelbaum MA, Krivosheya D, Borghei-Razavi H, et al. Phase 0 and window of opportunity clinical trial design in neuro-oncology: a RANO review. Neuro Oncol 2020. [Epub ahead of print].
23. Cloughesy TF, Mochizuki AY, Orpilla JR, et al. Neo-adjuvant anti-PD-1 immunotherapy promotes a survival benefit with intratumoral and systemic immune responses in recurrent glioblastoma. Nat Med 2019;25(3):477–86.
24. Lang FF, Bruner JM, Fuller GN, et al. Phase I trial of adenovirus-mediated p53 gene therapy for recurrent glioma: biological and clinical results. J Clin Oncol 2003;21(13):2508–18.
25. Schmitz S, Duhoux F, Machiels JP. Window of opportunity studies: do they fulfil our expectations? Cancer Treat Rev 2016;43:50–7.
26. Saenz-Antonanzas A, Auzmendi-Iriarte J, Carrasco-Garcia E, et al. Liquid biopsy in glioblastoma: opportunities, applications and challenges. Cancers (Basel) 2019;11(7).
27. Snuderl M, Fazlollahi L, Le LP, et al. Mosaic amplification of multiple receptor tyrosine kinase genes in glioblastoma. Cancer Cell 2011;20(6):810–7.
28. Hentschel SJ, Lang FF. Surgical resection of intrinsic insular tumors. Neurosurgery 2005;57(1 Suppl): 176–83 [discussion: 176–3].
29. Mahase S, Rattenni RN, Wesseling P, et al. Hypoxia-mediated mechanisms associated with antiangiogenic treatment resistance in glioblastomas. Am J Pathol 2017;187(5):940–53.
30. Lang FF, Conrad C, Gomez-Manzano C, et al. Phase I study of DNX-2401 (Delta-24-RGD) oncolytic adenovirus: replication and immunotherapeutic effects in recurrent malignant glioma. J Clin Oncol 2018;36(14):1419–27.
31. Lang FF. US. National Library of Medicine. Oncolytic adenovirus DNX-2401 in treating patients with recurrent high-grade glioma. 2020. Available at: https://clinicaltrials.gov/ct2/show/NCT03896568. Accessed: August 30, 2020.

32. O'Brown NM, Pfau SJ, Gu C. Bridging barriers: a comparative look at the blood-brain barrier across organisms. Genes Dev 2018;32(7–8):466–78.

33. Fu W, Wang W, Li H, et al. Single-cell atlas reveals complexity of the immunosuppressive microenvironment of initial and recurrent glioblastoma. Front Immunol 2020;11:835.

34. Patel AP, Tirosh I, Trombetta JJ, et al. Single-cell RNA-seq highlights intratumoral heterogeneity in primary glioblastoma. Science 2014;344(6190):1396–401.

35. Jun HJ, Appleman VA, Wu HJ, et al. A PDGFRalpha-driven mouse model of glioblastoma reveals a stathmin1-mediated mechanism of sensitivity to vinblastine. Nat Commun 2018;9(1):3116.

36. Fueyo J, Alemany R, Gomez-Manzano C, et al. Preclinical characterization of the antiglioma activity of a tropism-enhanced adenovirus targeted to the retinoblastoma pathway. J Natl Cancer Inst 2003;95(9):652–60.

37. Kawakami M, Kawakami K, Puri RK. Intratumor administration of interleukin 13 receptor-targeted cytotoxin induces apoptotic cell death in human malignant glioma tumor xenografts. Mol Cancer Ther 2002;1(12):999–1007.

38. Gupta UC, Bhatia S, Garg A, et al. Phase 0 clinical trials in oncology new drug development. Perspect Clin Res 2011;2(1):13–22.

39. Sanai N. Phase 0 clinical trial strategies for the neurosurgical oncologist. Neurosurgery 2019;85(6):E967–74.

40. Kummar S, Kinders R, Rubinstein L, et al. Compressing drug development timelines in oncology using phase '0' trials. Nat Rev Cancer 2007;7(2):131–9.

41. Tien AC, Li J, Bao X, et al. A Phase 0 trial of ribociclib in recurrent glioblastoma patients incorporating a tumor pharmacodynamic- and pharmacokinetic-guided expansion cohort. Clin Cancer Res 2019;25(19):5777–86.

42. de Groot J, Penas-Prado M, Alfaro-Munoz K, et al. Window-of-opportunity clinical trial of pembrolizumab in patients with recurrent glioblastoma reveals predominance of immune-suppressive macrophages. Neuro Oncol 2020;22(4):539–49.

43. Jiang H, Gomez-Manzano C, Aoki H, et al. Examination of the therapeutic potential of Delta-24-RGD in brain tumor stem cells: role of autophagic cell death. J Natl Cancer Inst 2007;99(18):1410–4.

Stereotactic Laser Ablation of Glioblastoma

Matthew M. Grabowski, MD[a], Balint Otvos, MD, PhD[a], Alireza M. Mohammadi, MD[b],*

KEYWORDS

- Laser interstitial thermal therapy • LITT • Stereotactic laser ablation • SLA • Glioblastoma • GBM

KEY POINTS

- Over the past decade, laser interstitial thermal therapy (LITT) has emerged as a valuable surgical tool that allows for glioblastoma (GBM) cytoreduction in deep-seated and/or eloquent lesions that are otherwise inoperable.
- When compared with frequently used treatments for GBM, current literature suggests that LITT compares favorably in terms of outcomes, complication rates, preservation of quality of life, and cost-effectiveness when adequate extent of ablation is achieved.
- Given its minimally invasive nature, current research is focused on LITT's potential to disrupt the blood-brain barrier and induce immunomodulatory effects. Clinical trials are currently being conducted using LITT in combination with other therapies, such as immunotherapy, to investigate these phenomena.
- Because no randomized controlled trials have been performed, well-designed, prospective trials are needed to further define the utility and outcomes of LITT for GBM.

INTRODUCTION

Laser interstitial thermal therapy (LITT) is a minimally invasive surgical procedure that uses a laser probe inserted through a burr hole to deliver optical radiation and thermal damage to intracranial lesions.[1] Although the modern concept of using a stereotactically introduced, intracranial laser probe to deliver thermal damage was first formalized in the 1980s and used experimentally in clinical practice shortly thereafter, limitations inherent to the technology of the time prevented its widespread adoption.[2–4] In recent decades although, improvements in equipment such as laser probe design and cooling, stereotactic targeting hardware, and real-time thermography have allowed neurosurgeons to effectively and safely deliver targeted treatments.[5] These key advancements have increased the clinical deployment of LITT as a management option for a variety of neurosurgical pathologies, including gliomas, brain metastases, and radiation necrosis, as well as some indications outside the neuro-oncology sphere, such as epilepsy.[6,7] This review aims to describe the current state of the technology, operative technique, and periprocedural practices, as well as summarize the data regarding outcomes and future directions in the use of LITT for treating glioblastoma (GBM).

SURGICAL METHODOLOGY
Laser Interstitial Thermal Therapy Systems

There have been 2 widely used and Food and Drug Administration (FDA)-approved systems for LITT: the Medtronic Visualase (Medtronic; Minneapolis, Minnesota) and the Monteris NeuroBlate (Monteris; Plymouth, Minnesota) systems (**Fig. 1**). Both systems rely on the principle of selective transmission of laser energy with resultant interstitial

[a] Department of Neurosurgery, Rose Ella Burkhardt Brain Tumor & Neuro-Oncology Center, Cleveland Clinic, Cleveland, OH, USA; [b] Department of Neurological Surgery, Cleveland Clinic Lerner College of Medicine at CWRU, Rose Ella Burkhardt Brain Tumor & Neuro-Oncology Center, Cleveland Clinic, CA-51, 9500 Euclid Avenue, Cleveland, OH 44195, USA
* Corresponding author.
E-mail address: MOHAMMA3@ccf.org

Neurosurg Clin N Am 32 (2021) 105–115
https://doi.org/10.1016/j.nec.2020.08.006
1042-3680/21/© 2020 Elsevier Inc. All rights reserved.

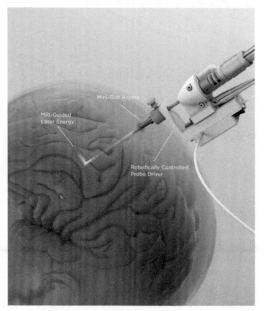

Fig. 1. The NeuroBlate system for stereotactically targeted treatment of intracranial lesions, including GBM. (Used with permission. © 2020 Monteris Medical.)

hyperthermia and tissue ablation based on the Arrhenius equation.[8] The Visualase system uses a liquid saline–cooled, 15W 980 nm diode laser with a 1 cm omnidirectional tip. Emission at 980 nm allows for a higher water absorption coefficient and therefore faster heating of affected tissue and less tissue penetration, allowing for sharper delineation between zones of thermal injury.[9,10] The Visualase system allows operators to set temperature limit points at zones within the affected tissue, usually set at 90°C at the tip of the probe and 50°C at the periphery of the lesion, to prevent carbonization and vaporization of the treated tissue. On initiation of the laser, fast-spoiled gradient-recalled echo (GRE) images are obtained, and test 3 to 4 W pulses are administered to determine the exact location of the 1-cm laser-emitting distal tip of the probe.[6,11,12] The Monteris system uses a 12 W neodymium-doped, yttrium aluminum garnet (Nd:YAG) diode laser with an emission of 1064 nm, which is cooled by gaseous carbon dioxide and has both omnidirectional and directed, side-firing tips.[6,13,14] Emission at 1064 nm allows for greater tissue penetration and therefore greater ablation volumes in regions of high blood perfusion. Use of the side-firing directional tips, although decreasing rate of tissue heating, allows for greater sculpting of thermal injury zones and conformation to tumor margins.[9,10] Monteris systems also have both 3.2 and 2.1 mm probes, allowing for tailoring of treatment plans.[15]

Laser Interstitial Thermal Therapy Procedure

Before the initiation of the procedure, patients undergo contrast-enhanced, T1-weighted volumetric MRI scans for planning and stereotactic navigation, with further imaging depending on tumor location (eg, diffusion tensor imaging [DTI] and functional MRI for characterization of white matter tracts and eloquent cortex).[16–18] Trajectories for biopsy/treatment are planned on neuronavigation software, with an ideal trajectory traveling down the long axis of the targeted lesion while avoiding sulci, vascular structures, and eloquent white matter tracts.[17,19]

The patient is induced under general anesthesia and fixed to the table using an MRI-compatible, 3-point cranial fixation device. Scalp fiducials are registered, a frameless stereotactic guidance system is aligned to the predefined trajectory, and biopsy specimens are obtained for histopathologic diagnosis.[20] Using the same trajectory, the hollow bolt is screwed into the skull for precise passage of the laser. In Monteris systems, the 142-mm lower profile Monteris MiniBolt can be used for single passes, whereas the 197 mm Monteris Axiis frame is required for multiple trajectories instead of using several MiniBolts.[17] The laser probe is then attached to the frame and introduced into the tumor along the planned trajectory. The patient is then further draped, the MRI bore is brought into the operating theater (or the patient is taken to an MRI suite if intraoperative MRI is not available), and a scan is performed confirming the location of the probe.[14] The final position of the probe tip is optimized using the probe driver, and in Visualase setups, 3 to 4 W test pulses administered under continuous image acquisition confirm distal tip location.[18–20] The laser probe output is increased to treatment dosages, and the therapy commences. Throughout the lasing portion of the procedure, GRE MRI sequences are continually obtained at roughly 8-second intervals for acquisition of thermometry data.[21] The images are deconvoluted, displayed at the Visualase or NeuroBlate workstation, and allow for near real-time monitoring and manipulation of laser output, ablation depth, or in the case of NeuroBlate side-firing tips, directionality of thermal damage (**Fig. 2**).

The extent of thermal damage and ablation (EOA) is calculated by an algorithm incorporating temperature and time and is displayed as thermal damage threshold (TDT) lines. Yellow TDT lines indicate regions of tissue exposed to 43°C for 2 minutes, blue TDT lines indicate regions exposed to 43°C for 10 minutes (or higher temperatures for shorter durations), and white TDT lines indicate regions exposed to 43°C for 60 minutes (see

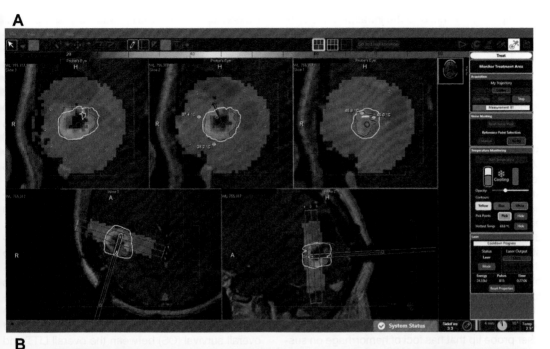

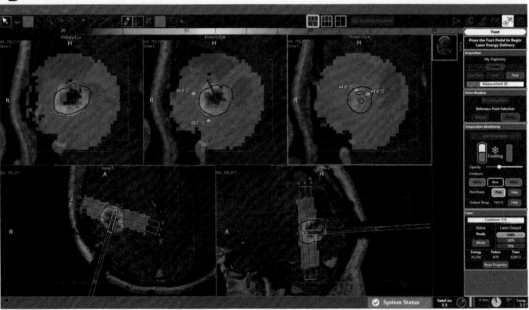

Fig. 2. Intraoperative view from LITT workstation during treatment of a right-sided tumor. The operator is able to manipulate the laser's depth and directionality to conform energy delivery to tumor boundaries (*pink line*). (*A*) Example of a yellow TDT line (defined as the tissue exposed to 43°C for 2 minutes) and (*B*) a blue TDT line (43°C for 10 minutes). (Used with permission. © 2020 Monteris Medical.)

Fig. 2).[14,22] In preclinical studies, tissue within white TDT lines suffered 100% death within 48 hours, whereas tissue outside of the yellow TDT line boundaries demonstrated no irreversible damage.[19] Tumor volumes within the blue TDT lines have been associated with necrosis, whereas volumes inside the yellow line have been associated with apoptosis.[23] Recent histopathologic analysis demonstrated 3 concentric zones of cellular architecture radiating outward from the thermal source. The innermost zone 1 harbors necrotic cells, the middle zone 2 has a rim of granulation tissue, and the outermost zone 3 contains viable tumor cells, although these zones have not been specifically linked to the intraoperative visualized TDT lines.[24] Treatment zones typically stop enlarging about 15 seconds after ceasing of laser activity.[19]

Although most of the tumors in several series (more than 80%) have been successfully treated using one trajectory, larger or more irregular lesions may require multiple trajectories in a single procedure (up to 3 trajectories in a single setting).[17,25] On completion of treatment, the MRI, laser probe, and stereotactic frame are removed, and closure is performed similar to a standard stereotactic biopsy. Postoperatively, patients are placed on dexamethasone to mitigate edema and monitored in a neurosurgical step-down or intensive care unit overnight. In many institutions, a postprocedure MRI is performed on the day after surgery to assess the EOA, extent of edema, and serve as the new baseline for monitoring progression.[17] Postoperative MRIs demonstrate 5 zones of tissue damage post-LITT: the probe track itself, a central zone centered at the laser probe tip that has foci of hemorrhage on susceptibility weighted imaging, a peripheral zone corresponding to the treated tissue, a thin rim surrounding the peripheral zone, and the peritumoral edema.[26] With larger tumors that have undergone LITT, some centers have attempted to mitigate postoperative swelling with minimal-access craniotomies and debulking of thermally treated tumors, although this not routinely performed.[27–29] Patients are typically discharged from the hospital within 1 to 2 days on a rapid steroid taper, with monitoring MRIs typically performed 1 to 2 months postprocedure and every 2 to 4 months subsequently (**Fig. 3**).[30]

DISCUSSION
Current Evidence

The first use of the Nd:YAG laser system to treat brain tumors in humans came in 1990 when Sugiyama and colleagues[3] reported on the outcomes of 5 patients. However, formal FDA approval for the modern LITT systems (ie, Neuro-Blate and Visualase) would not come until decades later. Since then, publications reporting outcomes data in GBM have steadily increased, which will be summarized hereafter.

Outcomes in newly diagnosed glioblastoma
Although there are numerous case series reporting on the outcomes of patients with GBM treated with LITT, most of the early literature did not stratify the outcomes by upfront versus recurrence or glioma World Health Organization (WHO) grade. Because of this, higher-quality outcomes data on nGBM

treated upfront with LITT was very sparse until 2019, when Mohammadi and colleagues[31] published the first and largest multiinstitutional retrospective cohort study. In it, 24 patients with nGBM were treated initially with LITT followed by concurrent chemoradiation therapy (CRT) and were compared with a matched control group who underwent biopsy-only followed by CRT, with median follow-up times of 9.3 months (2–43) and 14.7 months (2–41), respectively. Most of the patients receiving LITT had deep-seated GBMs or were not good candidates for standard microsurgical resection. The 2 groups had similar characteristics, including age, sex, and location (including the thalamus in ~30% of each group). Contrast-enhancing tumor volume (CETV) and Ki-67 was similar between the 2 groups (LITT group with mean CETV of 9.3 cc); however, the biopsy-only group had more favorable molecular markers with respect to IDH1 and MGMT methylation status. There was no statistically significant difference in the median progression-free survival (PFS) and overall survival (OS) between the overall LITT and biopsy groups: PFS: 4.3 versus 5.9 months ($P = .94$), OS: 14.4 versus 15.8 months ($P = .78$).[31] Of note, the landmark trial by Stupp and colleagues in nGBM reported a median OS of 15.8 months with a complete/partial resection followed by CRT and a 9.4-month OS in those with biopsy plus CRT. Therefore, Mohammadi and colleagues's[32] biopsy-only group seems to have above-average outcomes, and this may be partially explained by the favorable molecular markers in that group. However, when LITT patients were stratified by EOA, those with favorable EOA had improved (lower) disease-specific PFS and OS cumulative incidence at 12 months compared with those with biopsy only (disease specific progression free survival, confidence interval [CI]: 25% vs 63%, $P = .05$; DSOS CI: 25% vs 31%, $P = .03$).[33–35] The effect of EOA will be discussed in further detail in a later section.

Other smaller studies have published on LITT as a primary treatment of nGBM. Shah and colleagues[36] reported in 2019 on 11 patients with nGBM who underwent LITT as a primary treatment of deep-seated tumors (median depth 60.4 mm [range 46.2–68.2]). Mean CETV for their cohort was 6.8 cc (1.2–127.0), and mean EOA was 98%. They report a median PFS of 31.9 months and a median OS of 32.3 months. Other studies from 2012 to 2016 with between 2 and 16 patients with nGBM each reported on patients treated with upfront LITT for newly diagnosed high-grade gliomas (nHGGs), showing much shorter average PFS of between 2.0 and 5.1 months (range 2.0–23) and a median OS of

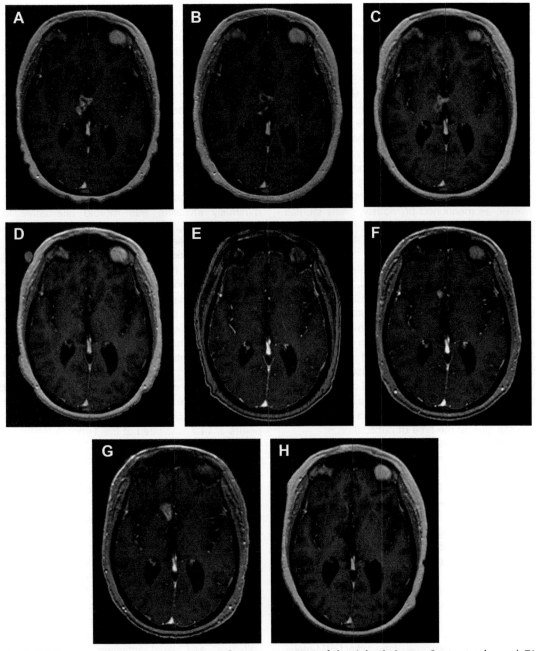

Fig. 3. A 54-year-old patient treated with LITT for recurrent GBM of the right thalamus. Contrast-enhanced, T1-weighted MR images at (*A*) preoperative, (*B*) immediate postoperative, (*C*) 2-, (*D*) 5-, (*E*) 7-, (*F*) 10-, (*G*) 12-, and (*H*) 14-month time points, showing the radiographic evolution of the LITT-treated lesion. The lesion recurred at an adjacent site within the corpus callosum, which was then treated with stereotactic radiosurgery (*F–H*). The patient survived 18.7 months from the time of LITT treatment.

14.2 months (range 0.1–23) in a small meta-analysis of these data.[14,27,30,37–41] The limited sample sizes, lack of consistent availability of EOA, retrospective nature, and outcomes variability limit the interpretability of these data. Therefore, given the evidence to date, LITT has not been established as a first-line therapy for nGBM in most of the cases. Well-designed, prospective trials should be undertaken to assess LITT's impact as an upfront treatment of nGBM, specifically in those for whom surgical resection is infeasible.

Outcomes in recurrent glioblastoma

Compared with LITT for nGBM, a greater number of studies have reported on their outcomes in patients with rGBM.[25,42] One of the earliest publications (first in human study) using a modern LITT system for rGBM was performed by Sloan and colleagues[19] in 2013 from a phase I, thermal dose-escalation trial. Ten patients were included in their initial study, with a mean CETV of 6.8 cc ± 5 and mean EOA of 78% +/− 12%. The median OS was 10.4 months (range 2.0–25.2), with 3 patients improving neurologically, 6 remaining stable, and 1 worsening.[19] Given these promising results, multiple case series were subsequently published; however, as mentioned previously, many studies did not stratify their outcomes by nGBM versus rGBM, or WHO grades 3 versus 4, limiting the interpretability of the data.[43]

More recent studies have stratified their outcomes data by recurrence status, such as the one by Thomas and colleagues[30] in 2016. This paper describes their experience with 13 patients with rGBM undergoing LITT. The mean age was 49 years, with a mean time from diagnosis of 16 months. Sixty-two percent of lesions were located in eloquent areas, and 69% were multifocal, with an average CETV of 14.6 cc. This group had a median PFS of 5 months and a median OS of greater than 7 months from LITT, as 7/13 patients were still alive at the time of publication.[30]

In 2019, Shah and colleagues[36] analyzed outcomes in 14 patients treated with LITT for rGBM. Their patients had a mean age of 54 years and median preoperative CETV of 3.8 cc (range 0.5–15.8). All lesions were considered deep seated and were treated to a median EOA of 87.5% (range 77.0%–99.5%). The investigators report a median PFS of 5.6 months and OS of 7.3 months. Similarly in 2019, Kamath and colleagues[44] reported on their center's outcomes in 41 patients with rGBM treated with LITT, with 35 of them on their first recurrence. Median PFS was 7.3 months (95% CI 5.1–8.9, range 0–32) and median OS was 11.8 months (95% CI 8.6–13.8, range 0–34.2). When calculated from time of the initial GBM diagnosis, their OS was 22.3 months (95% CI 16.2–26.8).

No study has directly compared LITT versus other treatment modalities for rGBM in a prospective format, requiring other literature to derive outcomes from comparator cohorts. A recent study with 299 patients with rGBM reported median OS of 3.1 months for best supportive care, 7.3 months for systemic therapy, and 11 months for reresection followed by adjuvant treatment, with no statistically significant difference found between systemic therapy and reresection groups when controlling for multiple confounders.[45] For the patients receiving systemic therapy and reresection, median PFS was 4.3 months and 9.0 months, respectively. Given the deep-seated nature of many of these rGBM lesions treated with LITT, the current LITT outcomes compare favorably with frequently used treatments for rGBM such as systemic therapy and reresection. Head-to-head trials are needed to further clarify the utility and outcomes with LITT for rGBM.

Preservation of quality of life and functional status

Although LITT has often been presented as a more minimally invasive, less morbid alternative to craniotomy, high-quality prospective data supporting that belief has been lacking until recently. The Laser Ablation of Abnormal Neurologic Tissue Using Robotic NeuroBlate System (LAANTERN) Study is an ongoing, prospective, multicenter registry enrolling patients undergoing treatment with the NeuroBlate system. Its outcome data include cognitive, functional, and quality of life (QoL) metrics, among others, with the first report of these data only recently published for 223 patients with brain tumors.[42] Of these 223 patients, 90 had HGGs, with an estimated survival rate of 59% at 12 months (95% CI 55%–79%). A mean Karnofsky Performance Score (KPS) change of −5.4 points ± 11.7 was seen at the 1-month follow-up compared with baseline KPS (86.2 ± 11.8), which stabilized from the 1-month score until the 12-month time point, where a median decrease of −13.2 points compared with baseline was seen ($P < .0001$). Fifty-one percent of patients had no change or an improvement in their KPS at 6 months. Within the Functional Assessment of Cancer Therapy-Brain data looking at social, emotional, and functional well-being, there was no clinically meaningful changes (>10% of instrument range) seen at the 1-, 3-, 6-, or 12-month time points when compared with baseline. In the EuroQol 5-dimensional questionnaire, improvements were seen in the subscores for mobility, self-care, and usual activities, and scores for pain/discomfort, anxiety/depression, and visual analogue scale were stable.[42] These data suggest that on average, QoL remains stable both in the immediate and long-term post-LITT period and that improvements can be seen in patient mobility, self-care, and ability to participate in usual activities.

Other quantitative measures of the minimally invasive nature of the procedure were also reported in the 2020 LAANTERN data.[42] Mean blood loss for primary tumor cases was minimal at 7.0 ± 18.3 cc and total procedure time averaged

198.8 ± 91.1 minutes. Most of the patients were discharged to home after the procedure (83.2%, with 10.7% discharged to rehab and 1.5% to a nursing facility) following a median 33.8-hour hospital length of stay (LOS, range 20–695). Of note, it has been reported in multiple studies that the procedure length and LOS tend to decline as providers become more familiar with the procedure and the patients' clinical course post-LITT.[25,28]

Complication rates

The complication rate from open surgery and stereotactic biopsy for GBM has historically ranged from 4.5% to 13% and 5% to 7% in large cohorts of patients, respectively.[42,46] Recent publications have shown that the LITT complication profile is comparable with these results, especially when considering the difficult-to-access/deep-seated nature of many of the LITT-treated tumors. Barnett and colleagues[47] performed a meta-analysis comparing proportions of major complications between LITT (n = 79) and craniotomy-treated (n = 1036) patients with HGGs in or near areas of eloquence. The results showed a reduction in major complication rates for LITT compared with craniotomy (5.7% [95% CI: 1.8–11.6] vs 13.8% [95% CI: 10.3–17.9], respectively).[47] In 100 consecutive procedures from 2013 to 2018, Shah and colleagues[36] reported a complication rate of 4%, which included superficial wound infections, seizures, and a transient facial palsy. In the 223 patients reported in the 2020 LAANTERN results, 1.8% of patients experienced an LITT/surgery-related serious adverse event, with the same percentage having readmission within 30 days.[42] In Kamath and colleagues,[25] they report a complication rate of 15.5% overall, with morbidities such as cerebral edema, seizures, hydrocephalus, hyponatremia, and infection seen. Their study also included 2 mortalities—one related to hemorrhage after treatment, whereas the second was due to equipment contamination leading to fulminant Enterobacter meningitis. In the 136 patients who received LITT more recently from 2015 to 2018, Shao and colleagues[28] reported a permanent neurologic deficit rate of 4.4%, no hemorrhages necessitating evacuation, no infections, and a 1.5% 30-day mortality rate. Each of these complication rates were reduced when compared with those in an earlier cohort of 96 patients receiving the procedure in 2011 to 2014 at the same center, which may reflect refined patient selection and/or improvements in operator technical proficiency over time. Taken as a whole, these recent data suggest that LITT has a comparable or favorable safety profile to that of craniotomy and stereotactic biopsy in appropriate-use scenarios for GBM.

Cost-effectiveness of laser interstitial thermal therapy

Research has also focused on the cost-effectiveness of LITT. Leuthardt and colleagues[48] compared acute care costs (inpatient care + aftercare) of LITT versus craniotomy for primary tumors at an academic medical center in year 2015 costs. They found that patients receiving LITT had a significantly shorter hospital LOS and were more likely to be discharged home compared with craniotomy. When looking at primary tumors alone and difficult-to-access primary tumors, there was a trend toward reduced costs with LITT compared with craniotomy, although this did not reach statistical significance.[48] Adding to this literature, Voigt and Barnett performed a cost-effectiveness analysis from a societal perspective in patients with HGG treated with LITT.[46] When compared with other treatments, they found an incremental cost/life year gained (LYG) of $29,340 when using LITT, significantly less than the international threshold value of $32,575/LYG and the US threshold value of $50,000/LYG.

Technical Considerations to Improve Outcomes

Complete lesion coverage

The benefits of resection over biopsy in GBM have been well documented in the neurosurgical literature, as well as the improvements in PFS and OS seen with a higher extent of resection/lower postoperative residual CETV.[33,35,49] Analogous to this, multiple studies have now reported on the importance of maximizing LITT EOA to the blue/yellow TDT lines, with smaller lesions being associated with higher EOA, and higher EOA being predictive of lower disease-specific PFS and OS (see **Fig. 3**).[14,20,31,36] These findings have been replicated across LITT systems, and EOA calculations can be performed with both of the major systems available currently.[31,36]

Shah and colleagues[36] identified an EOA cutoff of 85% to be a significant predictor of longer disease-specific PFS for both nGBM and rGBM (P = .006) using the Visualase system. In patients with nGBM treated with the NeuroBlate system, Mohammadi and colleagues[31] were able to identify 3 prognostic groups that correlated with PFS: favorable—≤0.025 cc of CETV within the yellow-blue TDT transition zone; intermediate—greater than 0.025 cc of CETV in the transition zone and greater than 90% tumor coverage by the blue TDT line; and unfavorable—greater than 0.025 cc and less than 90% tumor coverage by the blue TDT line.[31] These groups were then associated with lower incidence of disease-specific PFS and OS on multivariate analysis. Additionally of note, a systematic review found that LITT is associated with a higher EOA than the extent of resection able to be obtained by craniotomy in GBM lesions located in eloquent or difficult-to-access locations.[47] These findings highlight the importance of maximizing EOA and the utility of LITT in attaining a high EOA with lesions in challenging locations.

Fiber tracking
In an attempt to improve outcomes and minimize neurologic deficit complications, fiber tracking (DTI sequences) has been used successfully in LITT planning. In a group of patients operated on between 2011 and 2015, volume of overlap between the corticospinal tracts (CSTs) and TDT lines were identified that were associated with postoperative motor deficits (PMDs), and cutoff points were determined that provided optimal sensitivity (92%–100%) and specificity (80%–90%).[50] These overlap volumes for the yellow, blue, and white TDT lines equated to 0.103, 0.068, and 0.046 cc, respectively, indicating that PMDs can result from even a minimal overlap of the CSTs and TDT lines.[50] Recently published outcomes comparing the early (2011–2014) versus recent (2015–2018) LITT-treated cohorts revealed a statistically significant reduction in PMDs in the recent cohort (4.4% vs 15.5%, *P* = .005) after routine utilization of fiber tracking in planning.[28]

Future Directions

Laser interstitial thermal therapy, the blood-brain barrier (BBB), and chemoradiation
The BBB is a known impediment to delivering systemically administered chemotherapies in high concentrations to the tumor microenvironment. As LITT induces changes to the perilesional vasculature, Leuthardt and colleagues[16] investigated the disruption of the BBB after LITT through dynamic contrast-enhancement brain MRI and measurements of neuron-specific enolase.[43] They report that disruption of the BBB occurs immediately and peak permeability occurs ~1 to 3 weeks after LITT, returning to normal by 4 to 6 weeks.[16] These pilot data were analyzed in conjunction with a clinical trial investigating the delivery effects and efficacy of early versus late administration of post-LITT doxorubicin in patients with rGBM, as the minimally invasive nature of LITT allows early administration of chemotherapy with minimal impact on wound healing (NCT01851733).

In addition to the effects on the BBB and chemotherapies, there are implications with LITT and radiotherapy. As hyperthermia is known to radiosensitize cells, Man and colleagues[51] investigated the effects of preradiotherapy hyperthermia on glioma stem cells (GSCs) and the PI3K/AKT pathway, which is aberrantly regulated in more than 40% of GBM and is associated with poor patient prognosis. GSCs treated with radiation alone exhibited increased AKT activation, but the addition of hyperthermia before radiotherapy reduced AKT activation and impaired GSC proliferation, an effect that was further enhanced by treatment with a PI3K inhibitor.[51] These preclinical data show the potential combined effects of LITT and other conventional treatment strategies.

Laser interstitial thermal therapy and immunotherapy
Hyperthermia has been found to improve both the innate and adaptive antitumor immune response via several mechanisms, including the release of tumor antigen-dense exosomes with increased tumor antigen presentation; induction of immune-stimulating heat-shock proteins expression; increased cytokine and chemokine production resulting in attraction of and enhanced activity of antigen-presenting cells, cytotoxic T cells, and natural killer cells; and vessel dilation with BBB disruption and increased perfusion permitting greater immune surveillance.[43,52,53] And this effect is not limited to the treated lesion, as multiple animal models in various types of cancers have demonstrated that lesions near or distant to the treatment area shrank or were stable after LITT was performed (abscopal effect).[54–59] These tumors were found to have a significant increase in CD3+ T cells at the tumor-host interface of both ablated and distant tumors, among other immunomodulatory effects. Although more comprehensive data with regard to immunophenotypic changes in the tumor microenvironment exists in other types of ablation techniques and cancer models, several studies have reported favorable preclinical results using hyperthermia via LITT in conjunction with immunotherapies to improve the body's immune response to gliomas.[52] For example, nanoparticle-enhanced thermal ablation paired with anti-PD-L1 immunotherapy improved survival and enabled rejection of tumor rechallenge in a murine model of GBM.[60] At least 2 clinical trials are currently underway investigating the outcomes of combinatorial LITT + immunotherapy for rGBM (NCT03341806: LITT + avelumab; NCT03277638: LITT + pembrolizumab). The field awaits the results of these trials expectantly, both from a clinical outcomes standpoint and any experimental aims examining the systemic immune alterations

in patients, as well as those within the tumor microenvironment.

Nanoparticles

Given the importance of maximizing EOA, researchers have investigated the uses of nanoparticles to act at "lightning rods" to increase the diameter of ablation and specificity for the tumor. Chongsathidkiet and colleagues[61] showed that plasmon-activated gold nanostars have selective tumor uptake and expanded the tumor-conforming zone of cytotoxic edema in a murine model of GBM.[60] In phantoms containing the gold nanostars, blue TDT line coverage expanded to 3.8 cm in diameter from 2.0 cm, with faster heating, higher temperatures, and more homogenous temperature zones attained.[60,61] Development of additional novel techniques to increase LITT coverage area and tumor specificity could confer significant improvements in LITT-related outcomes in GBM.

SUMMARY

The previous decade has seen an expansion in the use of LITT for a variety of pathologies. Although LITT has been used for both nGBM and rGBM, these systems have developed a niche in treating deep-seated, difficult-to-access lesions, where open resection is otherwise infeasible. Improvements in patient outcomes and reductions in complications have stemmed from advances in operative technique to maximize EOA and minimize damage to nearby critical fiber tracts. In appropriately selected patients, LITT outcomes for GBM seem comparable or favorable to that of craniotomy and/or stereotactic biopsy in recent literature. And given its immunomodulatory effects, ability to alter BBB permeability, and potential synergism with chemotherapies and immunotherapies, multiple trials using LITT are currently underway to advance the treatment options and improve outcomes for patients with this near-uniformly fatal disease.

DISCLOSURE

A.M. Mohammadi is a consultant for Monteris Medical, Inc. The other authors have nothing to declare.

REFERENCES

1. Silva D, Sharma M, Juthani R, et al. Magnetic Resonance Thermometry and Laser Interstitial Thermal Therapy for Brain Tumors. Neurosurg Clin N Am 2017;28(4):525–33.

2. Bown SG. Phototherapy of tumors. World J Surg 1983;7(6):700–9.

3. Sugiyama K, Sakai T, Fujishima I, et al. Stereotactic interstitial laser-hyperthermia using Nd-YAG laser. Stereotact Funct Neurosurg 1990;54-55:501–5. Available at: http://ovidsp.ovid.com/ovidweb.cgi?T=JS&PAGE=reference&D=med3&NEWS=N&AN=2080375.

4. Yokote H, Komai N, Nakai E, et al. Stereotactic hyperthermia for brain tumors. Stereotact Funct Neurosurg 1990;54(1–8):506–13.

5. Ashraf O, Patel NV, Hanft S, et al. Laser-Induced Thermal Therapy in Neuro-Oncology: A Review. World Neurosurg 2018;112:166–77.

6. Lee I, Kalkanis S, Hadjipanayis CG. Stereotactic Laser Interstitial Thermal Therapy for Recurrent High-Grade Gliomas. Neurosurgery 2016;79(Suppl 1):S24–34. Available at: http://ovidsp.ovid.com/ovidweb.cgi?T=JS&PAGE=reference&D=medc&NEWS=N&AN=27861323.

7. Wicks RT, Jermakowicz WJ, Jagid JR, et al. Laser Interstitial Thermal Therapy for Mesial Temporal Lobe Epilepsy. Neurosurgery 2016;79(Suppl 1):S83–91. Available at: http://ovidsp.ovid.com/ovidweb.cgi?T=JS&PAGE=reference&D=medc&NEWS=N&AN=27861328.

8. Rahmathulla G, Recinos PF, Valerio JE, et al. Laser interstitial thermal therapy for focal cerebral radiation necrosis: a case report and literature review. Stereotact Funct Neurosurg 2012;90(3):192–200.

9. Kangasniemi M, McNichols RJ, Bankson JA, et al. Thermal therapy of canine cerebral tumors using a 980 nm diode laser with MR temperature-sensitive imaging feedback. Lasers Surg Med 2004;35(1):41–50. Available at: http://ovidsp.ovid.com/ovidweb.cgi?T=JS&PAGE=reference&D=med5&NEWS=N&AN=15278927.

10. Norred SE, Johnson JA. Magnetic resonance-guided laser induced thermal therapy for glioblastoma multiforme: a review. Biomed Res Int 2014;2014:761312.

11. Medvid R, Ruiz A, Komotar RJ, et al. Current applications of MRI-guided laser interstitial thermal therapy in the treatment of brain neoplasms and epilepsy: A radiologic and neurosurgical overview. Am J Neuroradiol 2015;36(11):1998–2006.

12. Jethwa PR, Barrese JC, Gowda A, et al. Magnetic resonance thermometry-guided laser-induced thermal therapy for intracranial neoplasms: initial experience. Neurosurgery 2012;71(1 Suppl Operative):133–5.

13. Borghei-Razavi H, Koech H, Sharma M, et al. Laser Interstitial Thermal Therapy for Posterior Fossa Lesions: An Initial Experience. World Neurosurg 2018;117:e146–53.

14. Mohammadi AM, Hawasli AH, Rodriguez A, et al. The role of laser interstitial thermal therapy in

enhancing progression-free survival of difficult-to-access high-grade gliomas: a multicenter study. Cancer Med 2014;3(4):971–9.

15. Missios S, Bekelis K, Barnett GH. Renaissance of laser interstitial thermal ablation. Neurosurg Focus 2015;38(3):E13.

16. Leuthardt EC, Duan C, Kim MJ, et al. Hyperthermic laser ablation of recurrent glioblastoma leads to temporary disruption of theperitumoral blood brain barrier. PLoS One 2016;11(2). https://doi.org/10.1371/journal.pone.0148613.

17. Kamath AA, Friedman DD, Hacker CD, et al. MRI-Guided Interstitial Laser Ablation for Intracranial Lesions: A Large Single-Institution Experience of 133 Cases. Stereotact Funct Neurosurg 2017;95(6):417–28.

18. Shah AH, Richardson AM, Burks JD, et al. Contemporaneous biopsy and laser interstitial thermal therapy for two treatment-refractory brain metastases. Neurosurg Focus 2018;44(VideoSuppl2):V5.

19. Sloan AE, Ahluwalia MS, Valerio-Pascua J, et al. Results of the NeuroBlate System first-in-humans Phase I clinical trial for recurrent glioblastoma: clinical article. J Neurosurg 2013;118(6):1202–19.

20. Shah AH, Burks JD, Buttrick SS, et al. Laser Interstitial Thermal Therapy as a Primary Treatment for Deep Inaccessible Gliomas. Neurosurgery 2019; 84(3):768–77.

21. Carpentier A, McNichols RJ, Stafford RJ, et al. Laser thermal therapy: real-time MRI-guided and computer-controlled procedures for metastatic brain tumors. Lasers Surg Med 2011;43(10):943–50.

22. Sapareto SA, Dewey WC. Thermal dose determination in cancer therapy. Int J Radiat Oncol Biol Phys 1984;10(6):787–800.

23. Hawasli AH, Ray WZ, Murphy RKJ, et al. Magnetic resonance imaging-guided focused laser interstitial thermal therapy for subinsular metastatic adenocarcinoma: technical case report. Neurosurgery 2012; 70(2 Suppl Operative):332–8.

24. Elder JB, Huntoon K, Otero J, et al. Histologic findings associated with laser interstitial thermotherapy for glioblastoma multiforme. Diagn Pathol 2019; 14(1):19.

25. Kamath AA, Friedman DD, Akbari SHA, et al. Glioblastoma Treated With Magnetic Resonance Imaging-Guided Laser Interstitial Thermal Therapy: Safety, Efficacy, and Outcomes. Neurosurgery 2019;84(4):836–43.

26. Beaumont TL, Mohammadi AM, Kim AH, et al. Magnetic Resonance Imaging-Guided Laser Interstitial Thermal Therapy for Glioblastoma of the Corpus Callosum. Neurosurgery 2018;83(3):556–65.

27. Wright J, Chugh J, Wright CH, et al. Laser interstitial thermal therapy followed by minimal-access trans-sulcal resection for the treatment of large and difficult to access brain tumors. Neurosurg Focus 2016;41(4):E14. Available at: http://ovidsp.ovid.com/ovidweb.cgi?T=JS&PAGE=reference&D=med12&NEWS=N&AN=27690658.

28. Shao J, Radakovich NR, Grabowski M, et al. Lessons Learned in Using Laser Interstitial Thermal Therapy (LITT) for Treatment of Brain Tumors: A Case Series of 238 Patients from A Single Institution. World Neurosurg 2020. https://doi.org/10.1016/j.wneu.2020.03.213.

29. Habboub G, Sharma M, Barnett GH, et al. A novel combination of two minimally invasive surgical techniques in the management of refractory radiation necrosis: Technical note. J Clin Neurosci 2017;35:117–21.

30. Thomas JG, Rao G, Kew Y, et al. Laser interstitial thermal therapy for newly diagnosed and recurrent glioblastoma. Neurosurg Focus 2016;41(4):E12. Available at: http://ovidsp.ovid.com/ovidweb.cgi?T=JS&PAGE=reference&D=med12&NEWS=N&AN=27690657.

31. Mohammadi AM, Sharma M, Beaumont TL, et al. Upfront Magnetic Resonance Imaging-Guided Stereotactic Laser-Ablation in Newly Diagnosed Glioblastoma: A Multicenter Review of Survival Outcomes Compared to a Matched Cohort of Biopsy-Only Patients. Clin Neurosurg 2019;85(6):762–72.

32. Stupp R, Hegi ME, Mason WP, et al. Effects of radiotherapy with concomitant and adjuvant temozolomide versus radiotherapy alone on survival in glioblastoma in a randomised phase III study: 5-year analysis of the EORTC-NCIC trial. Lancet Oncol 2009;10(5):459–66.

33. Lacroix M, Abi-Said D, Fourney DR, et al. A multivariate analysis of 416 patients with glioblastoma multiforme: prognosis, extent of resection, and survival. J Neurosurg 2001;95(2):190–8.

34. Sanai N, Polley M-Y, McDermott MW, et al. An extent of resection threshold for newly diagnosed glioblastomas. J Neurosurg 2011;115(1):3–8.

35. Grabowski MM, Recinos PF, Nowacki AS, et al. Residual tumor volume versus extent of resection: predictors of survival after surgery for glioblastoma. J Neurosurg 2014;121(5):1115–23.

36. Shah AH, Semonche A, Eichberg DG, et al. The Role of Laser Interstitial Thermal Therapy in Surgical Neuro-Oncology: Series of 100 Consecutive Patients. Neurosurgery 2019;3(2):54–67.

37. Schroeder JL, Missios S, Barnett GH, et al. Laser interstitial thermal therapy as a novel treatment modality for brain tumors in the thalamus and basal ganglia. Photon Lasers Med 2014;3(2):151–8.

38. Hawasli AH, Bagade S, Shimony JS, et al. Magnetic resonance imaging-guided focused laser interstitial thermal therapy for intracranial lesions: single-institution series. Neurosurgery 2013;73(6):1007–17.

39. Jethwa P, Barrese J, Gowda A, et al. Magnetic resonance thermometry-guided laser-induced thermal therapy for intracranial neoplasms: initial experience. Neurosurgery 2012;71(1 Supplement): 133–45.

40. Pisipati S, Smith KA, Shah K, et al. Intracerebral laser interstitial thermal therapy followed by tumor resection to minimize cerebral edema. Neurosurg Focus 2016;41(4). https://doi.org/10.3171/2016.7. FOCUS16224.

41. Ivan ME, Mohammadi AM, De Deugd N, et al. Laser Ablation of Newly Diagnosed Malignant Gliomas: a Meta-Analysis. Neurosurgery 2016;79(Suppl 1): S17–23. Available at: http://ovidsp.ovid.com/ ovidweb.cgi?T=JS&PAGE=reference&D=medc& NEWS=N&AN=27861322.

42. Kim AH, Tatter S, Rao G, et al. Laser Ablation of Abnormal Neurological Tissue Using Robotic Neuro-Blate System (LAANTERN): 12-Month Outcomes and Quality of Life After Brain Tumor Ablation. Neurosurgery 2020. https://doi.org/10.1093/neuros/ nyaa071.

43. Lee I, Kalkanis S, Hadjipanayis CG. Stereotactic laser interstitial thermal therapy for recurrent high-Grade gliomas. Clin Neurosurg 2016;79:S24–34.

44. Kamath AA, Friedman DD, Akbari SHA, et al. Glioblastoma Treated With Magnetic Resonance Imaging-Guided Laser Interstitial Thermal Therapy: Safety, Efficacy, and Outcomes. Neurosurgery 2019;84(4):836–43.

45. van Linde ME, Brahm CG, de Witt Hamer PC, et al. Treatment outcome of patients with recurrent glioblastoma multiforme: a retrospective multicenter analysis. J Neurooncol 2017;135(1):183–92.

46. Voigt JD, Barnett G. The value of using a brain laser interstitial thermal therapy (LITT) system in patients presenting with high grade gliomas where maximal safe resection may not be feasible. Cost Eff Resour Alloc 2016;14:6.

47. Barnett GH, Voigt JD, Alhuwalia MS. A Systematic Review and Meta-Analysis of Studies Examining the Use of Brain Laser Interstitial Thermal Therapy versus Craniotomy for the Treatment of High-Grade Tumors in or near Areas of Eloquence: An Examination of the Extent of Resection and Major Comp. Stereotact Funct Neurosurg 2016;94(3):164–73.

48. Leuthardt EC, Voigt J, Kim AH, et al. A Single-Center Cost Analysis of Treating Primary and Metastatic Brain Cancers with Either Brain Laser Interstitial Thermal Therapy (LITT) or Craniotomy. Pharmacoecon Open 2017;1(1):53–63.

49. McGirt MJ, Chaichana KL, Gathinji M, et al. Independent association of extent of resection with survival in patients with malignant brain astrocytoma. J Neurosurg 2009;110(1):156–62.

50. Sharma M, Habboub G, Behbahani M, et al. Thermal injury to corticospinal tracts and postoperative motor deficits after laser interstitial thermal therapy. Neurosurg Focus 2016;41(4):E6. Available at: http:// ovidsp.ovid.com/ovidweb.cgi?T=JS&PAGE= reference&D=med12&NEWS=N&AN=27690653.

51. Man J, Shoemake JD, Ma T, et al. Hyperthermia sensitizes Glioma stem-like cells to radiation by inhibiting AKT signaling. Cancer Res 2015;75(8):1760–9.

52. Srinivasan ES, Sankey EW, Grabowski MM, et al. The intersection between immunotherapy and laser interstitial thermal therapy (LITT): A multi-pronged future of neuro-oncology. Int J Hyperthermia 2020; 37(2):27–34.

53. Skitzki JJ, Repasky EA, Evans SS. Hyperthermia as an immunotherapy strategy for cancer. Curr Opin Investig Drugs 2009;10(6):550–8.

54. Qian L, Shen Y, Xie J, et al. Immunomodulatory effects of ablation therapy on tumors: Potentials for combination with immunotherapy. Biochim Biophys Acta Rev Cancer 2020;1874(1):188385.

55. Takaki H, Cornelis F, Kako Y, et al. Thermal ablation and immunomodulation: From preclinical experiments to clinical trials. Diagn Interv Imaging 2017; 98(9):651–9.

56. Slovak R, Ludwig JM, Gettinger SN, et al. Immunothermal ablations - boosting the anticancer immune response. J Immunother Cancer 2017;5(1):78.

57. Lin WX, Fifis T, Malcontenti-Wilson C, et al. Induction of Th1Immune responses following laser ablation in a murine model of colorectal liver metastases. J Transl Med 2011;9:83.

58. Isbert C, Ritz JP, Roggan A, et al. Enhancement of the immune response to residual intrahepatic tumor tissue by Laser-Induced Thermotherapy (LITT) compared to hepatic resection. Lasers Surg Med 2004;35(4):284–92.

59. Haen SP, Pereira PL, Salih HR, et al. More than just tumor destruction: Immunomodulation by thermal ablation of cancer. Clin Dev Immunol 2011;2011. https://doi.org/10.1155/2011/160250.

60. Liu Y, Chongsathidkiet P, Crawford BM, et al. Plasmonic gold nanostar-mediated photothermal immunotherapy for brain tumor ablation and immunologic memory. Immunotherapy 2019;11(15): 1293–302.

61. Chongsathidkiet P, Liu Y, Kemeny H, et al. EXTH-23. A novel nanotechnology-based platform improves laser interstitial thermal therapy for intracranial tumors. Neuro Oncol 2018;20(suppl_6):vi89–90.

Radiosurgery for Glioblastoma

Adomas Bunevicius, MD, PhD, Jason P. Sheehan, MD, PhD*

KEYWORDS

- Glioblastoma • Stereotactic radiosurgery • Gamma knife radiosurgery • Prognosis • Survival

KEY POINTS

- Glioblastoma (GBM) is the most common primary malignant brain tumor with annual incidence rate of 3.21 per 100,000 population.
- First-line treatment of patients with GBM usually includes gross total surgical resection followed by adjuvant chemotherapy with temozolomide and concurrent fractionated radiotherapy and maintenance temozolomide chemotherapy.
- Stereotactic radiosurgery allows spatially precise targeted delivery of high-dose radiation with submillimeter accuracy.

INTRODUCTION

Glioblastoma (GBM) is the most common primary malignant brain tumor with annual incidence rate of 3.21 per 100,000 population.[1] Prognosis remains poor with median survival of approximately 15 months, and survival rarely exceeds 2 years after the diagnosis.[2] First-line treatment of patients with GBM usually includes gross total surgical resection followed by adjuvant chemotherapy with temozolomide and concurrent fractionated radiotherapy (FRT) and maintenance temozolomide chemotherapy.[2,3] Patients harboring GBM tumors in surgically inaccessible brain locations receive only biopsy. FRT for GBM is typically achieved by delivering 60 Gy over 30 fractions.[4] Target volume of FRT usually includes tumor resection cavity, contrast-enhancing areas on T1-weighted MRI (which suggests residual tumor), and T2/FLAIR hyperintense region (which suggests tumor infiltration/edema).[4] Other external beam radiation dose-fractionation schedules can be considered depending on a patients' age, functional status, and prior radiation therapies. Unfortunately, GBM progression after multimodal first-line therapies is almost inevitable, and effective second-line treatment options are limited.

Stereotactic radiosurgery (SRS) allows spatially precise targeted delivery of high-dose radiation with submillimeter accuracy. It is commonly used for treatment of small-to-moderate volume discrete brain lesions residing in deeper and/or functionally eloquent brain regions. On one hand, it might seem counterintuitive to use SRS for treatment of highly invasive GBM in which tumor cells can typically be found well outside of T1-weighted (T1w) contrast-enhancing areas and in every lobe of the brain at the time of diagnosis and local treatment.[5,6] Therefore, volume constraints and highly conformal treatment fields of radiosurgery are often considered as important limiting factors of SRS for treatment of infiltrative disorders that necessitate large treatment fields, such as the GBM. On the other hand, it is well established that GBM responds to radiation treatment at least as well, if not better, as it responds to every other treatment, and 60 Gy fractionated radiation therapy is insufficient for prolonged and adequate local control of the tumor from progression even when used together with multimodal adjuvant therapies.[7,8] Furthermore, sublethal doses of irradiation can even promote migration and invasiveness of human glioma cells.[9] Conformal irradiation of well-delineated targets may confer therapeutic benefits because (1) gross

Department of Neurosurgery, University of Virginia Health System, Charlottesville, VA 22908, USA
* Corresponding author.
E-mail address: jps2f@hscmail.mcc.virginia.edu

Neurosurg Clin N Am 32 (2021) 117–128
https://doi.org/10.1016/j.nec.2020.08.007

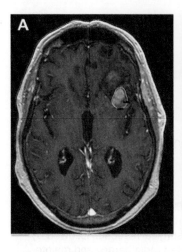 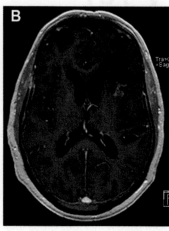

Fig. 1. An 85-year-old man with a 3-year history of IDH1-mutated, MGMT hypermethylated left insular GBM s/p tumor biopsy, and fractionated radiation therapy (60 Gy in 30 fractions) with concurrent temozolomide presented with tumor progression. He was on bevacizumab and was treated with radiosurgery delivering 14 Gy to 50% isodose line (A). A 2-month follow-up brain MRI demonstrated less avid contrast enhancement in the nodular enhancing component of the tumor (B). IDH1, isocitrate dehydrogenase 1.

total resection of all T1w contrast-enhancing GBM tumor tissue is not always possible, and subtotal resection is associated with inferior overall and progression-free survival and (2) most of the GBM recurrences occur within 2 cm of the enhancing portion of the original tumor.[10] Another potential advantage of SRS for treatment of previously irradiated recurrent GBM is that conformal targeting of residual or recurrent GBM tissue could mitigate risks of toxicity and radionecrosis associated with repeated wide-field FRT.

STEREOTACTIC RADIOSURGERY TECHNIQUE

SRS can be accomplished using various methods that include (1) Gamma Knife radiosurgery (GKRS) (Elekta Instruments AB, Stockholm, Sweden) using multiple cobalt-60 gamma radiation emitting radiation beams; (2) Cyberknife Robotic Radiosurgical System (Accuray, Sunnyvale, CA, USA); (3) charged particle; and (4) linear accelerator–based photon radiosurgery. SRS is usually delivered in a single-fraction targeting gadolinium-enhancing tumor areas on thin-sliced T1w brain MRI. T2w/FLAIR MRI sequences can be used to define areas of increased cellularity when T1w images are not sufficient (**Fig. 1**).[11,12] There have been attempts to increase SRS treatment volume of GBM by including FLAIR hyperintense areas outside of contrast-enhancing tumor nidus[13] or by adding 5 mm margins to gross tumor volume.[14]

Radiation dose is selected based on several considerations that include patient's performance status, tumor volume, prior radiation dose to the area, interval from prior cranial irradiation, and proximity to radiation sensitive neural structures. In general, lower radiation doses are used for larger tumors or tumors residing in close proximity to critical structures. Hypofractionated SRS (usually in 5 fractions) can be used for treatment of larger tumors and tumors residing in close proximity to or encasing critical neural structures. Multiple isocenters are frequently used for conformal dose planning for optimized precision and maximized dose gradient.

STEREOTACTIC RADIOSURGERY FOR RECURRENT GLIOBLASTOMA

SRS, is most commonly used for locally recurrent GBMs, was shown to be associated with longer survival of patients with GBM when compared with historic controls (**Table 1**).[15,16] Independent predictors of survival of patients with GBM treated with SRS were younger age, smaller tumor volume, use of multiple chemotherapy agents before SRS, SRS prescription dose, less homogeneous treatment plans, time from surgery to SRS, and MGMT methylation status.[11,16–21] Median-reported SRS-treated GBM volumes ranged from 3.75 cm^3 to 14 cm.[3,16,22] The most commonly used median prescription dose was 16 Gy.[11,15,17,23] Adverse event rate of SRS for GBM was less than 26% and radiation necrosis developed in less than 24% of patients.[11,15–18,20,23,24] However, these results should be interpreted cautiously in the context of institutional variations in patient follow-up protocols and definition of adverse events and radiation necrosis.

A series of 297 consecutive patients treated with SRS for residual or recurrent GBM reported median survival after diagnosis and after SRS of 18 months and 9 months, respectively, which was superior when compared with historical data.[16] Smaller tumor volume, younger age, and use of chemotherapy were associated with longer survival. Twenty-three percent of patients

Table 1
Major series of stereotactic radiosurgery for recurrent glioblastoma

Author, y	SRS Modality	Period	Number of Patients	Follow-up after SRS Median (Range)	Median Age (Range)	Median Time from Diagnosis to SRS (Range)	Median Tumor Volume in cm³ (Range)	Median Marginal Dose in Gy (Range)	Median Survival Time after Diagnosis (mo)	Median Survival Time after SRS (mo)	1-y Survival	2-y Survival	Median PFS after SRS (mo)	Adverse Event Rate	Multivariate Predictors of Overall Survival
Niranjan e al,[16] 2018	GKRS	-	297	8.6 (1.1–173)	58 (23–89)	-	14 (0.26–84.2)	15 (9–25)	18	9	72.5%	29.5%	4.3	Any: 23%	Age at diagnosis (<60 y), smaller tumor volume (<14 cm3), use of chemotherapy during primary treatment, radiosurgical treatment of tumor recurrence
Imber et al,[11] 2017	GKRS	1991–2013	174	8.7 (0–120.1)	54.1 (21.8–85.3)	8.7 (0.4–195.8)	7.0 (0.3–39.0)	16 (10–22)	21.1	10.6	-	-	-	Radiation necrosis: 29/46 (63%)	Time from initial surgery to SRS, age at SRS and SRS prescription dose
Guseynova et al,[22] 2018	GKRS	1992–2014	126	n/r	56 (17–80)	12 (1–96)	3.75 (0.04–37.1)	12 (10–25)	20	7	27%	8%	8.5	None detected	-
Kong et al,[15] 2007	LINAC and GKRS	2000–2006	65	11.2 (1.5–99.5)	49 (5–75)	4.3 (1.5–27.0)	10.6 (0.09–79.6)	16 (12–50)	23	13	20.5%	-	4.6	Radiation necrosis: 24.4% [a]	-
Kim et al,[17] 2017	GKRS	2004–2015	61	7.5 (0.1–36.0)	58 (27–79)	9.8 (1.7–101.5)	7.0 (0.033–35.1)	16 (9–25)	22.1	11	43.7%	13.7%	5	Radiation necrosis: 8.2% Hemorrhage: 1 patient	MGMT methylation status

(continued on next page)

Table 1
(continued)

Author, y	SRS Modality	Period	Number of Patients	Follow-up after SRS Median (Range)	Median Age (Range)	Median Time from Diagnosis to SRS (Range)	Median Tumor Volume in cm³ (Range)	Median Marginal Dose in Gy (Range)	Median Survival Time after Diagnosis (mo)	Median Survival Time after SRS (mo)	1-y Survival	2-y Survival	Median PFS after SRS (mo)	Adverse Event Rate	Multivariate Predictors of Overall Survival
Sharma et al,[19] 2018	GKRS	1997–2016	53	10.1 (0.8–51.4)	58 (19–82)	9.0 (0.07–71.5)	3.80 (0.01–29.7)	18 (12–24)	-	11	-	-	4.4	n/r	KPS score ≥80, small tumor volume (<15 cm³) and less homogeneous treatment plans (homogeneity index >1.75)
Skeie et al,[20] 2012	GKRS	1996–2007	51	55.3 (27–73)[e]	55.3 (27–73)[e]	10.3[e]	12.4	12.2 (8–20)	19	12	43.1%	17.6%	6	Any: 9.8%	SRS (vs resection) at progression
Cuneo et al,[18] 2012	LINAC + Bev	2002–2010	49	31	47[b]	20[b]	4.8	15 (12.5–25)[b]	47/25[c]	11.2/3.9[c]	50%/22%[c]	-	5.2/2.1[c]	Radiation necrosis: 10% Grade 3–4 toxicity: 13%	KPS score > 70 and age ≤50 y
Mahajan et al,[48] 2005	LINAC	<2003	48	21 (3–61)[d]	54 (17–69)	11 (3–49)	4.7 (0.15–16.3)	-	26	11	39%	-	-	n/r	-
Morris et al,[21] 2019	GKRS + Bev	2009–2015	45	-	57 20–78	-	2.2 (0.1–25.2)	17 (13–24)	31	13.2	-	-	5.2	-	Multiple chemotherapy agents before SRS
Frischer et al,[24] 2016	GKRS	-	42	n/r	55.6 (14.1–81.1)	17 (3.9–57.9)	5.1 (0.6–15.0)	10 (6–16)	25.6	9.6	-	-	4.4	Any: 26%	-
Dodoo et al,[49] 2014	GKRS	2001–2007	35	17.2 (2.5–114.2)	51.1 (17.0–81.1)	-	4.80 (0.03–38.10)	20 (14–22)	24.5	11.3	-	51.4%	-	-	-

| Park et al,[23] 2012 | GKRS + Bev | 1987–2010 | 11 | 13.7 (4.6–28.3) | 62 (46–72) | 17 (5–34.5) | 13.6 (1.2–45.1) | 16 (13–18) | 33.2 | 18 | 73% | n/r | 15 | Radiation necrosis: 9% | - |

Abbreviations: bev, bevacizumab; LINAC, linear accelerator.

[a] Out of a total sample of 114 patients with glioma treated with SRS.
[b] Total sample: World Health Organization grade IV (n = 49) and grade III (n = 14) glioma.
[c] Bevacizumab/no bevacizumab.
[d] From diagnosis.
[e] In the total sample (SRS or surgery).

experienced new neurologic symptoms that were successfully managed with corticosteroids. Another series of 174 patients treated with SRS for recurrent GBM reported median overall survival time after SRS of 10.6 months.[11] Shorter time from surgery to SRS, younger age at SRS, and greater prescription dose were associated with longer survival. Forty-six (26%) patients required craniotomy, and radionecrosis with or without GBM recurrence was diagnosed in 29 patients. Guseynova and colleagues treated 126 patients with SRS for locally recurrent GBM and reported median survival after diagnosis and after SRS of 20 months and 7 months, respectively.[22] Kong with colleagues used salvage SRS for 65 patients with recurrent GBM[15] and found that median survival after GBM diagnosis and after SRS was 23 months and 13 months, respectively. Survival was longer in patients with GBM treated with SRS than in a historic cohort of patients with GBM (23 vs 12 months). Kim and colleagues treated 61 recurrent patients with GBM with SRS[17] and reported median survival after SRS of 11 months. Radiation necrosis was diagnosed in 8% of patients. Only MGMT methylation status was associated with overall survival in multivariate analysis. Skeie and colleagues compared SRS (n = 51) versus reoperation (n = 26) for management of recurrent GBM.[20] They found that SRS, when compared with reoperation, was associated with longer progression-free survival (6 vs 2 months, respectively), longer survival time after recurrence (12 vs 6 months, respectively), greater 1-year (43.1% vs 15.4%, respectively) and 2-year (17.6% vs 0%) survival rates, and lower complication rate (9.8% vs 25.2%, respectively). SRS was an independent predictor of longer overall survival after diagnosis and after disease recurrence.

SRS is a reasonable treatment approach for salvage therapy for recurrent GBM that can improve survival with limited toxicity of this challenging and devastating disease. However, the quality of available evidence of SRS for recurrent GBM is limited to nonrandomized retrospective institutional series. Prospective studies exploring safety and efficacy of SRS and comparing it with other salvage therapies for recurrent GBM are encouraged.

UPFRONT AND BOOST STEREOTACTIC RADIOSURGERY

Escalation of radiation dose for treatment of GBM can have therapeutic advantage, given dose-response relationship between fractionated radiation dose and control rate of malignant gliomas.[25,26] Initial retrospective institutional series have documented that radiation dose escalation can improve prognosis of patients with malignant glioma (**Table 2**).[27,28]

A multiinstitutional prospective randomized phase III Radiation Therapy Oncology Group (RTOG) trial (RTOG 93–05) evaluated potential clinical value of SRS boost delivered upfront of FRT for GBM.[29] Two-hundred three patients with GBM with a tumor diameter of less than 4 cm and KPS of greater than or equal to 60 were randomly assigned either to (1) postoperative SRS followed by FRT (60 Gy) plus bis-chloroethylnitrosourea (BCNU) (80 mg/m^2 days 1–3 every 8 weeks for 6 cycles) or to (2) FRT with BCNU alone. SRS was delivered 1 week before FRT (60 Gy in 2 Gy daily fractions) using GKRS- or linear accelerator–based techniques. SRS boost dose was selected based on the tumor size and ranged from 15 Gy to 24 Gy. The median survival time was similar in the SRS + FRT and external beam radiation therapy (EBRT)-only groups (13.5 vs 13.6 months, respectively). There were 4 cases of grade 3 toxicities in the SRS group, and 7 out of 28 operated patients in the SRS arm were diagnosed with radiation necrosis. Quality of life and cognitive status trajectories were also not different between the 2 treatment arms. However, the design of the RTOG 93–05 trial has raised some concerns, including the decision to study upfront rather than boost SRS, which is the more commonly used approach in GBM setting,[30] patterns and criteria of GBM recurrence, and the use of BCNU rather that temozolomide for adjuvant chemotherapy.[31] In a small retrospective series (n = 10) SRS was delivered the same day after biopsy (ie, before FRT) for unresectable GBMs of less than 3 cm in diameter.[32] Median survival in the SRS group was 52 weeks when compared with 8 weeks in the control group that received FRT alone for biopsy-proven GBM. Progression-free survival at 3 months was 75% in the GKRS group and 45% in the control group.

Retrospective series have shown largely beneficial results of boost SRS (ie, delivered after FRT) for patients with GBM. For example, Shrieve and colleagues used boost SRS (after FRT and within 14.2 weeks after diagnosis) to treat 78 patients with GBM.[33] The median actuarial survival time from the diagnosis was 19.9 months with 2-year overall survival of 35.9%. There were no serious acute complications associated with SRS; however, 39 (50%) patients required reoperation, and radiation necrosis was diagnosed in 19 (48.7%) of reoperated patients. Nwokedi and colleagues compared FRT plus boost SRS (n = 31) with FRT-only (n = 33) for recurrent GBM. SRS was administered within 4 weeks of EBRT

Table 2
Major series of upfront or boost stereotactic radiosurgery for glioblastoma

Author, y	SRS Modality	Period	Number of Patients	Median Follow-Up (mo) (Range)	Timing of SRS	Median Time from Diagnosis to SRS	Median Age (Range)	Median KPS	Pre-SRS Therapy	Median Tumor Volume in cm³	Median Marginal Dose (Gy)	Median Survival Time after Diagnosis (mo)	Median Survival Time after SRS (mo)	Median PFS after SRS (mo)	Adverse Event Rate
Duma et al,[13] 2016	GKRS	2000–2016	174	-	Before or during FRT	18 d	59 (22–87)	-	Surgery ± FRT	48.5 (2.5–220)	8 (6–14)	23	-	-	Permanent complications: 6%
Souhami et al,[29] 2004[a]	GKRS or LINAC	1994–2000	89	61	Before FRT (1 wk)	-	Mean: 56.4 (18–79)	≥60	Surgery	3 (0.7–6)	15–24 Gy	13.5	-	-	Grade 3 toxicities: 5% Radiation necrosis: 7/28
Shrieve et al,[33] 1999	LINAC	1988–1995	78	40.8 (25.5–79.4)	After FRT	14.2 wk	51 (12–84)	90	FRT + TMZ, surgery	9.4 (0.86–72)	12 (6–24)	19.9	-	-	Radiation necrosis: 39/20
Nwokedi et al,[34] 2002	GKRS	1993–1998	31	17.5	After FRT (within 4 wk)	6 wk	50.4	80	Surgery, FRT	25	17.1 (10–28)	25	-	-	No acute events
Azoulay et al,[14] 2020	CyberKnife	2010–2015	30	13.8 (1.7–64.4)	After surgery (no FRT)	4.1 wk	66 (51–86)	80	Resection	PTV: 60 (14.7–137.3) GTV: 27 (4–81)	25–40	14.8	-	8.2	N = 8
Hsieh et al,[35] 2005	GKRS	1998–2003	25	21	After FRT	-	60.3	70	Surgery, FRT	23.6	12	10	8	-	No acute, 16 cases of radionecrosis
Pouratian et al,[12] 2009	GKRS	1991–2007	22	9.5 (2.7–51.1)	After (n = 19) or before (n = 2)FRT	-	60.1 (12.9–76.9)	80	Chemotherapy (n = 22), FRT (n = 44)	13.4	17	15.1	10	8.3	None
Kong et al,[50] 2006	GKRS	2002	10	53	Before FRT	Before EBRT	Mean: 7.2	90	Surgery, EBRT (60 Gy)	8.1 (1–31)	12 (9–16)	52 wk	-	-	none

(continued on next page)

Table 2
(continued)

Author, y	SRS Modality	Period	Number of Patients	Median Follow-Up (mo) (Range)	Timing of SRS	Median Time from Diagnosis to SRS	Median Age (Range)	Median KPS	Pre-SRS Therapy	Median Tumor Volume in cm³	Median Marginal Dose (Gy)	Median Survival Time after Diagnosis (mo)	Median Survival Time after SRS (mo)	Median PFS after SRS (mo)	Adverse Event Rate
Bir at al,[51] 2015	GKRS	2000–2013	7	7.2 (0.2–32.1)	Before FRT	-	53	-	Resection (100%), ERBT (86%), chemotherapy (58%)	Mean: 11.1	14 (10–20)	18.2	7.25	-	39%

Abbreviations: EBRT, external beam radiation therapy; LINAC, linear accelerator; TMZ, temozolomide.
[a] Randomized clinical trial.

completion.[34] Overall survival was significantly longer in the FRT plus SRS group than FRT-only group (25 vs 13 months, respectively). No patients experienced acute grade 3 to 4 toxicities, and 2 (7%) patients in FRT plus SRS group developed radiation necrosis that was managed with medical therapy. Another retrospective institutional series by Hsieh and colleagues compared SRS given as initial boost (25 patients) with SRS given at GBM progression (26 patients) in consecutive series of patients with GBM referred for GKRS.[35] SRS was delivered after surgery and FRT. They found a trend ($P = .09$) for longer overall survival in patients who received SRS at recurrence than upfront SRS (16.7 vs 10 months, respectively), but the study was limited by small sample size. There were no acute toxicities; however, radiation necrosis was noted in 16 patients using serial imaging or histologic examination.[35] A series from the University of Virginia compared outcomes of patients with GBM treated with SRS as part of initial treatment paradigm after FRT (n = 22) versus at GBM progression (n = 26).[12] Patients treated at the time of disease progression had longer overall survival than patients treated at initial presentation (17.4 vs 15.1 months, respectively). RTOG class and extent of resection were independent predictors of overall survival.

Finally, in a recent phase I/II trial of 5-fraction SRS with 5-mm margins for newly diagnosed GBM, 30 patients were treated with escalating radiation dose levels from 25 Gy to 40 Gy that was delivered to a median target volume of 60 cm^3.[14] SRS was delivered at median of 4.1 weeks after surgery. The median progression-free survival was 8.2 months, and median overall survival was 14.8 months. Late grade 1 to 2 adverse radiation events that occurred in 8 patients were associated with longer overall survival (27.2 vs 11.7 months, respectively).

RTOG 93–05 study indicates that SRS should not be used before FRT for all patients with GBM. However, post-FRT SRS can have therapeutic advantage for carefully selected patients with GBM, and this remains to be validated in prospective studies. The potential roles of upfront SRS should be defined in patients with GBM treated with contemporary chemotherapeutic regimens that includes temozolomide that has been shown to have radiosensitizing effects.[36]

LEADING EDGE STEREOTACTIC RADIOSURGERY

Glioma cells migrate along the brain structures with white matter tracts being significant conduits of glioma cell spread.[37] Targeting of areas that enhance on T1w MRI aims to improve local tumor control, but cells migrating along white matter tracts remain untreated.[13] Treatment of white matter tracts adjacent to glioma could slow glioma spread.[13] Indeed, GBM resection beyond contrast-enhancing areas (supratotal or supramarginal resection) is associated with greater survival benefit than gross total resection.[38]

Duma and colleagues introduced the concept of "leading-edge" SRS.[13] They targeted FLAIR signal abnormality surrounding the resection cavity of GBM with irradiation doses ranging from 10 Gy for 0 to 20 cm^3 lesions to 7 Gy for 61 to 80 cm^3 lesions. In their experience with 174 patients, median survival from diagnosis was 23 months, with 2- and 5-year survival rates of 39% and 16%, respectively. Although these results were superior to traditionally used estimates of GBM prognosis, retrospective single-institutional design and single-user determination of the SRS target were the main limitation of the study. Direct targeting of adjacent white matter conduits of glioma cell migration could be achieved by using diffusion tensor imaging for delineation of white matter tracts.

STEREOTACTIC RADIOSURGERY AND BEVACIZUMAB

GBM is a hypoxic tumor, and its progression depends on angiogenesis, and elevated vascular endothelial growth factor (VEGF) expression correlates with worse prognosis.[39] Bevacizumab is a humanized monoclonal antibody to VEGF-A, resulting in blockade of endothelial cell proliferation. Bevacizumab is used as second-line agent for GBM progression and has been shown to control peritumoral edema and prolong time to progression, but its effectiveness for prolonging patient survival is less evident.[40] Blockage of VEGF with bevacizumab can increase radiosensitivity and act synergistically with ionizing radiation.[41,42]

A handful of institutional series have demonstrated that concurrent use of bevacizumab with SRS is associated with prolonged survival of patients with GBM.[16,18,23,43] For example, a study in 49 patients with recurrent GBM found that SRS + bevacizumab (n = 33) when compared with SRS alone (n = 16) was associated with better 1-year survival rate (50% and 22%, respectively) and longer progression-free survival (5.2 and 2.1 months, respectively).[18] Bevacizumab therapy was an independent predictor of longer overall and progression-free survival in multivariate analyses. The incidence rate of treatment-related grade 3/4 toxicities was similar in SRS + bevacizumab and

SRS-only cohorts (10% and 14%, respectively). Park and colleagues reported that bevacizumab administered 4 to 10 weeks after SRS for GBM (n = 11) at a dose of 10 mg/kg every 2 weeks on a 28-day cycle was associated with longer progression-free and overall survival rate when compared with 44 case-matched controls treated with SRS alone (15 vs 7 months and 18 vs 12 months, respectively).[23] The incidence rate of radiation necrosis requiring resection was significantly lower in the SRS plus bevacizumab when compared with SRS-only cohorts (9% vs 46%, respectively). Bevacizumab also allows for safe dose escalation of SRS up to 22 Gy in recurrent GBM.[44] Concurrent administration of bevacizumab should be considered for patients with GBM selected for SRS therapy, and prospective studies exploring safety and efficacy of such combination therapy are encouraged.

MOLECULAR PROFILES AND STEREOTACTIC RADIOTHERAPY

Molecular profiles of GBM, including MGMT promotor methylation, carry important prognostic value in patients with GBM.[45,46] Larger radiation doses can overcome radioresistance and negative prognostic impact of molecular phenotypes.[14,47]

A handful of studies explored prognostic value of MGMT methylation in patients with GBM treated with SRS and found that MGMT unmethylated status was associated with worse prognosis.[18,21,28] For example, a study on 61 patients with GBM (41% MGMT methylated and 59% MGMT unmethylated) treated with SRS found that MGMT promoter methylation when compared with MGMT unmethylated status was associated with longer median progression-free (8.9 vs 4.6 months) and overall (14 vs 9 months) survival.[17] MGMT methylation status predicted survival independently from other clinical indexes. Others also reported that patients with GBM treated with SRS harboring MGMT methylated or hypermethylated tumors lived longer than patients with MGMT unmethylated GBMs.[14,24]

SUMMARY

SRS for recurrent GBM is associated with improved survival and acceptable safety profile. SRS is also used after FRT; however, a randomized trial did not find survival benefits of SRS administered before FRT. Administration of bevacizumab with SRS was shown to improve patient survival and decrease the incidence of radiation necrosis. Prospective studies exploring optimal SRS treatment approaches for GBM are encouraged.

CLINICS CARE POINTS

- Based on retrospective institutional series, SRS is associated with improved survival and a reasonable safety profile for recurrent patients with GBM.
- SRS delivered after FRT has therapeutic benefits based on institutional series; however, randomized RTOG 93–05 study did not find survival benefits of upfront SRS administered before fractionated radiation.
- Bevacizumab administered during SRS is associated with improved survival, decreased incidence of radiation necrosis, and can allow safe dose escalation of SRS, and therefore, this approach should be considered.
- Prospective studies exploring the possible impact of SRS timing relative to fractionated radiation therapy, fractionation schedule, treatment dose, and target volume delineation are encouraged so as to provide clinicians with higher quality evidence that could be used for treatment guidance of patients with GBM.

DISCLOSURE

The authors have nothing to disclose.

REFERENCES

1. Ostrom Quinn T, Gittleman H, Gabrielle T, et al. CBTRUS Statistical Report: Primary Brain and Other Central Nervous System Tumors Diagnosed in the United States in 2011-2015. Neuro Oncol 2018; 20(suppl_4):iv1–86.
2. Roger S, Mason Warren P, van den Bent Martin J, et al. Radiotherapy plus Concomitant and Adjuvant Temozolomide for Glioblastoma. N Engl J Med 2005;352(10):987–96.
3. Sulman Erik P, Ismaila Nofisat, Armstrong Terri S, et al. Radiation therapy for glioblastoma: American Society of Clinical Oncology Clinical Practice Guideline Endorsement of the American Society for Radiation Oncology Guideline. J Clin Oncol 2017;35(3): 361–9.
4. Cabrera Alvin R, Kirkpatrick John P, Fiveash John B, et al. Radiation therapy for glioblastoma: Executive summary of an American Society for Radiation Oncology evidence-based clinical practice guideline. Pract Radiat Oncol 2016;6(4):217–25.
5. Kelly PJ, Daumas-Duport C, Kispert DB, et al. Imaging-based stereotaxic serial biopsies in untreated intracranial glial neoplasms. J Neurosurg 1987; 66(6):865–74.

6. Yamahara T, Numa Y, Oishi T, et al. Morphological and flow cytometric analysis of cell infiltration in glioblastoma: a comparison of autopsy brain and neuroimaging. Brain Tumor Pathol 2010;27(2):81–7.

7. Roger S, Taillibert S, Kanner A, et al. Effect of tumor-treating fields plus maintenance temozolomide vs maintenance temozolomide alone on survival in patients with glioblastoma: a randomized clinical trial. JAMA 2017;318(23):2306–16.

8. Roger S, Hegi Monika E, Mason Warren P, et al. Effects of radiotherapy with concomitant and adjuvant temozolomide versus radiotherapy alone on survival in glioblastoma in a randomised phase III study: 5-year analysis of the EORTC-NCIC trial. Lancet Oncol 2009;10(5):459–66.

9. Wild-Bode C, Weller M, Rimner A, et al. Sublethal Irradiation Promotes Migration and Invasiveness of Glioma Cells: Implications for Radiotherapy of Human Glioblastoma. Cancer Res 2001;61(6): 2744–50.

0. Sherriff J, Tamangani J, Senthil L, et al. Patterns of relapse in glioblastoma multiforme following concomitant chemoradiotherapy with temozolomide. Br J Radiol 2013;86(1022):20120414.

1. Imber Brandon S, Kanungo I, Steve B, et al. Indications and efficacy of gamma knife stereotactic radiosurgery for recurrent glioblastoma: 2 decades of institutional experience. Neurosurgery 2017;80(1): 129–39.

2. Nader P, Webster CR, Sherman Jonathan H, et al. Gamma Knife radiosurgery after radiation therapy as an adjunctive treatment for glioblastoma. J Neurooncol 2009;94(3):409–18.

3. Duma CM, Kim Brian S, Chen Peter V, et al. Upfront boost Gamma Knife "leading-edge" radiosurgery to FLAIR MRI-defined tumor migration pathways in 174 patients with glioblastoma multiforme: a 15-year assessment of a novel therapy. J Neurosurg 2016; 125(Suppl 1):40–9.

4. Azoulay M, Chang Steven D, Gibbs Iris C, et al. A phase i/ii trial of 5-fraction stereotactic radiosurgery with 5-mm margins with concurrent temozolomide in newly diagnosed glioblastoma: primary outcomes. Neuro Oncol 2020. https://doi.org/10.1093/neuonc/noaa019.

5. Kong DS, Lee J-Il, Park K, et al. Efficacy of stereotactic radiosurgery as a salvage treatment for recurrent malignant gliomas. Cancer 2008;112(9): 2046–51.

6. Niranjan A, Monaco EA, Kano H, et al. Stereotactic radiosurgery in the multimodality management of residual or recurrent glioblastoma multiforme. Prog Neurol Surg 2018;31:48–61.

7. Kim BS, Kong D-S, Seol Ho J, et al. MGMT promoter methylation status as a prognostic factor for the outcome of gamma knife radiosurgery for recurrent glioblastoma. J Neurooncol 2017;133(3):615–22.

18. Cuneo Kyle C, Vredenburgh James J, Sampson John H, et al. Safety and efficacy of stereotactic radiosurgery and adjuvant bevacizumab in patients with recurrent malignant gliomas. Int J Radiat Oncol Biol Phys 2012;82(5):2018–24.

19. Sharma M, Schroeder Jason L, Paul E, et al. Outcomes and prognostic stratification of patients with recurrent glioblastoma treated with salvage stereotactic radiosurgery. J Neurosurg 2018;131(2): 489–99.

20. Skeie Bente Sandvei. Enger Per Øyvind., Brøgger Jan., et al. γ knife surgery versus reoperation for recurrent glioblastoma multiforme. World Neurosurg 2012;78(6):658–69.

21. Morris SL, Zhu P, Rao M, et al. Gamma knife stereotactic radiosurgery in combination with bevacizumab for recurrent glioblastoma. World Neurosurg 2019;127:e523–33.

22. Guseynova K, Roman L, Simonova G, et al. Gamma knife radiosurgery for local recurrence of glioblastoma. Neuro Endocrinol Lett 2018;39(4):281–7.

23. Park K-J, Kano H, Iyer A, et al. Salvage gamma knife stereotactic radiosurgery followed by bevacizumab for recurrent glioblastoma multiforme: a case-control study. J Neurooncol 2012;107(2):323–33.

24. Frischer JM, Christine M, Woehrer A, et al. Gamma knife radiosurgery in recurrent glioblastoma. Stereotact Funct Neurosurg 2016;94(4):265–72.

25. Bleehen NM, Stenning SP. A Medical Research Council trial of two radiotherapy doses in the treatment of grades 3 and 4 astrocytoma. The Medical Research Council Brain Tumour Working Party. Br J Cancer 1991;64(4):769–74.

26. Walker MD, Strike TA, Sheline GE. An analysis of dose-effect relationship in the radiotherapy of malignant gliomas. Int J Radiat Oncol Biol Phys 1979; 5(10):1725–31.

27. Loeffler JS, Alexander E, Shea WM, et al. Radiosurgery as part of the initial management of patients with malignant gliomas. J Clin Oncol 1992;10(9): 1379–85.

28. Sarkaria JN, Mehta MP, Loeffler JS, et al. Radiosurgery in the initial management of malignant gliomas: survival comparison with the RTOG recursive partitioning analysis. Radiation Therapy Oncology Group. Int J Radiat Oncol Biol Phys 1995;32(4): 931–41.

29. Souhami L, Seiferheld W, Brachman D, et al. Randomized comparison of stereotactic radiosurgery followed by conventional radiotherapy with carmustine to conventional radiotherapy with carmustine for patients with glioblastoma multiforme: report of Radiation Therapy Oncology Group 93-05 protocol. Int J Radiat Oncol Biol Phys 2004; 60(3):853–60.

30. Douglas K, Dade LL, Flickinger John C. In regard to Dr. Souhami et al. (Int J Radiat Oncol Biol Phys 2004;

60:853–860). Int J Radiat Oncol Biol Phys 2005; 62(2):614–5.

31. Vordermark D, Oliver K. Lack of survival benefit after stereotactic radiosurgery boost for glioblastoma multiforme: Randomized comparison of stereotactic radiosurgery followed by conventional radiotherapy with carmustine to conventional radiotherapy with carmustine for patients with glioblastoma multi-forme: Report of Radiation Therapy Oncology Group 93-05 protocol: In regard to Souhami et al. (Int J Radiat Oncol Biol Phys 2004;60:853–860). Int J Radiat Oncol Biol Phys 2005;62(1):296–7.

32. Kong D-S, Kim Y-H, Kim YH, et al. Long-term effi-cacy and tolerability of gamma knife radiosurgery for growth hormone-secreting adenoma: a retro-spective multicenter study (MERGE-001). World Neurosurg 2019;122:e1291–9.

33. Shrieve DC, Alexander E, Black PM, et al. Treatment of patients with primary glioblastoma multiforme with standard postoperative radiotherapy and radiosur-gical boost: prognostic factors and long-term outcome. J Neurosurg 1999;90(1):72–7.

34. Nwokedi Emmanuel C, DiBiase Steven J, Jabbour Salma, et al. Gamma knife stereotactic ra-diosurgery for patients with glioblastoma multiforme. Neurosurgery 2002;50(1):41–6 [discussion: 46–7].

35. Hsieh Patrick C, Chandler James P, Sandeep B, et al. Adjuvant gamma knife stereotactic radiosur-gery at the time of tumor progression potentially im-proves survival for patients with glioblastoma multiforme. Neurosurgery 2005;57(4):684–92 [dis-cussion: 684–92].

36. van Nifterik Krista A, van den Berg Jaap, Stalpers Lukas JA, et al. Differential radiosensitizing potential of temozolomide in MGMT promoter methylated glioblastoma multiforme cell lines. Int J Radiat Oncol Biol Phys 2007;69(4):1246–53.

37. Vishnu Anand C, Robel S, Watkins S, et al. A neurocentric perspective on glioma invasion. Nat Rev Neurosci 2014;15(7):455–65.

38. Fatih I, Koene S, Vincent Arnaud JPE, et al. Associ-ation between supratotal glioblastoma resection and patient survival: a systematic review and meta-anal-ysis. World Neurosurg 2019;127:617–24.e2.

39. Cheng W-Y, Shen C-C, Ming-Tsang C, et al. High expression of a novel splicing variant of VEGF, L-VEGF144 in glioblastoma multiforme is associated with a poorer prognosis in bevacizumab treatment. J Neurooncol 2018;140(1):37–47.

40. Gilbert MR, Dignam James J, Armstrong Terri S, et al. A randomized trial of bevacizumab for newly diagnosed glioblastoma. N Engl J Med 2014; 370(8):699–708.

41. Gorski DH, Beckett MA, Jaskowiak NT, et al. Blockage of the vascular endothelial growth factor stress response increases the antitumor effects of ionizing radiation. Cancer Res 1999;59(14):3374–8.

42. Nieder C, Nicole W, Andratschke Nicolaus H, et al. Radiation therapy plus angiogenesis inhibition with bevacizumab: rationale and initial experience. Rev Recent Clin Trials 2007;2(3):163–8.

43. Gutin Philip H, Iwamoto Fabio M, Kathryn B, et al. Safety and efficacy of bevacizumab with hypofrac-tionated stereotactic irradiation for recurrent malig-nant gliomas. Int J Radiat Oncol Biol Phys 2009; 75(1):156–63.

44. Mahmoud A, Symeon M, Barnett Gene H, et al. Phase I trial of radiosurgery dose escalation plus bevacizumab in patients with recurrent/progressive glioblastoma. Neurosurgery 2018;83(3):385–92.

45. Hegi Monika E, Annie-Claire D, Gorlia T, et al. MGMT gene silencing and benefit from temozolomide in glioblastoma. N Engl J Med 2005;352(10): 997–1003.

46. Williams PD, Jones S, Zhang X, et al. An integrated genomic analysis of human glioblastoma multiforme. Science 2008;321(5897):1807–12.

47. Omuro A, Kathryn B, Gutin P, et al. Phase II study of bevacizumab, temozolomide, and hypofractionated stereotactic radiotherapy for newly diagnosed glio-blastoma. Clin Cancer Res 2014;20(19):5023–31.

48. Mahajan A, McCutcheon Ian E, Suki D, et al. Case-control study of stereotactic radiosurgery for recur-rent glioblastoma multiforme. J Neurosurg 2005; 103(2):210–7.

49. Dodoo E, Beate H, Peredo I, et al. Increased survival using delayed gamma knife radiosurgery for recur-rent high-grade glioma: a feasibility study. World Neurosurg 2014;82(5):e623–32.

50. Kong D-S, Nam D-H, Lee J-Il, et al. Preservation of quality of life by preradiotherapy stereotactic radio-surgery for unresectable glioblastoma multiforme. J Neurosurg 2006;105(Suppl):139–43.

51. Bir SC, Connor David E, Ambekar S, et al. Factors predictive of improved overall survival following ste-reotactic radiosurgery for recurrent glioblastoma. Neurosurg Rev 2015;38(4):705–13.

Challenges Associated with Reoperation in Patients with Glioma

Rasheed Zakaria, PhD, FRCS, Jeffrey S. Weinberg, MD*

KEYWORDS

- Reoperation • Recurrence • Redo surgery • Progression • Glioblastoma • Glioma

KEY POINTS

- Indications for reoperation in patients with glioma are numerous.
- Inherent risks at each stage of the surgery should be anticipated.
- For glioma resection, consider the approach for a recurrent operation when planning the incision aat the first surgery.

BACKGROUND

Glioma is a disease with an increasing variety of treatment modalities and combinations, but surgical resection, when feasible, remains the first intervention, with a well-established evidence base. Repeat tumor resection, or rather reoperation for glioma, was first reported more than 30 years ago[1] but with increased survival and advances in surgical technology it is arguably more common in clinical practice now than at any other time.[2–4] The critical appraisal of reoperation for glioma in the neurosurgical literature is mixed. Although individual surgeons may recall patients with exceptionally good outcomes from reoperation and individual centers may report favorable results, all these accounts are tainted by selection bias in so far as surgeons tend to select younger, better performance status patients with focal disease where further adjuvant oncologic treatments are known to be available.[5,6] These are, more than likely, the patients who would have better survival regardless of intervention. Furthermore, the variation in treatments for recurrent or progressive glioma (including chemotherapy, cavity chemotherapy, brachytherapy, immunotherapy, vascular endothelial growth factor inhibitors, tumor treating fields, laser ablation, repeat external beam radiation, radiosurgery, and various trial agents) is greater than at first surgery because of lack of a standard of care, leading to more heterogeneous populations and less clear statistical comparisons.[7] This article offers a concise overview of the real world indications for reoperation, aids to patient selection offered by the evidence available, and the practical issues facing the surgeon at reoperation relating to surgical technique and technologies.

INDICATIONS FOR REOPERATION AND SURGICAL GOALS

Of primary import, is to have a clear outline of what the rationale for offering reoperation is, rather than simply determining whether it is surgically feasible.

Cytoreduction remains the principle reason for reoperation and national guidelines, albeit several years old, reflect this in recommending "repeat cytoreductive surgery... in symptomatic patients with locally recurrent or progressive malignant glioma."[8] Attempts to quantify the degree of cytoreduction needed for survival benefit have suggested 80% of the contrast-enhancing mass is the optimum threshold,[9] but a more recent meta-analysis identified radiographic gross total resection is most strongly associated with overall

Department of Neurosurgery, The University of Texas M.D. Anderson Cancer Center, 1515 Holcombe Boulevard, Unit 442, Houston, TX 77030, USA
* Corresponding author.
E-mail address: jweinberg@mdanderson.org

Neurosurg Clin N Am 32 (2021) 129–135
https://doi.org/10.1016/j.nec.2020.09.004
1042-3680/21/© 2020 Elsevier Inc. All rights reserved.

survival advantage.[10] Biopsy and/or cytoreduction may be indicated for multiple reasons: inadequate initial surgery, regrowth at the operated site, regrowth at a separate site, or new radiographic change in an old lesion necessitating pathologic confirmation.

Excising residual disease after a first inadequate surgery is justified because increased extent of resection correlates with extended overall survival in the newly diagnosed population[11] including lower grades,[12] and conversely residual disease after first surgery is associated with worse cognitive function and poorer patient-reported outcomes.[13] Larger series in the literature support this idea that reoperation salvages the effect of incomplete first resection, with overall survival and time to progression from the date of first surgery being extended in reoperated cases but not interval time from reoperation to death.[14,15]

There are additional benefits to obtaining more tissue, however, because diagnosis may also be improved or reclassified because of additional tissue acquired during reoperation. In patients where the diagnosis has been established at the first surgery by biopsy, it has been shown that the diagnosis is changed in 38% of cases because of availability of a greater volume of tissue for the neuropathologist to analyze.[16] Limited tissue volume for analysis, such as after biopsy or subtotal resection, leads to a higher chance of a sampling error. It has been shown for glioblastoma, for example, that the diagnosis is two-fold greater for individual surgical specimens greater than 10 mL than those of lower volume.[17] Furthermore, so-called "adaptive brain tumor studies," such as GBM-AGILE[18] in North American and BRAIN-MATRIX[19] in the United Kingdom, are heavily leveraged on tissue and so ongoing changes in tumor biomarkers and genetics obtained at reoperation are likely to be increasingly important if not essential for pivoting the patient into new and different clinical trial arms.

Beyond just upgrading or augmenting the original diagnosis, reoperation may help resolve diagnostic uncertainty in progressive tumor versus radionecrosis or pseudoprogression. Despite studies evaluating the utility of sophisticated imaging techniques, tissue remains the gold standard for diagnosis. This diagnostic uncertainty preoperatively should not prevent intervention in the symptomatic patient, because resection of radionecrosis as a treatment goal in and of itself seems to reduce edema and improves symptoms.[20]

Improving symptoms is a key feature of reoperation in general and caution should be exercised with the asymptomatic patient[21] who has only radiologic progression because the evidence of

morbidity from reoperation is not insignificant (18% neurologically worse compared with 8% after first craniotomy).[22] Exceptions may include patients requiring high doses of steroids where reoperation may reduce their steroid dependence[23] or the need for bevacizumab.[6] Finally, seizures are a major symptom contributing to morbidity and reduced quality of life in patients with glioma and reoperation may have a role in reducing seizure frequency in this population.[24]

With regards to patient selection, systemic reviews suggest younger age and better performance status as patient factors predicting a better prognosis[25] but tumor factors, such as location adjacent to eloquent areas and volume, should also be considered.[8] An important tumor factor in the modern World Health Organization classification era is genetic markers and molecular classification. It has been shown that IDH1 mutant malignant astrocytomas may do better with aggressive resection and performing additional surgery after incomplete resection may be beneficial compared with patients with wild-type tumors.[26] Also, older patients with O-6-Methylguanine-DNA Methyltransferase (MGMT)-unmethylated tumors may actually have more to gain by reoperation despite the additional morbidity risk because there are limited second-line chemotherapy options for them.[27,28] Scoring systems have been devised for determining the benefit of reoperation[29] and in one pediatric study blinded external review of imaging helped provide an objective opinion on "resectability" for reoperation without the bias of the original surgeon.[30]

Lastly, from a practical perspective, reoperation allows unparalleled access to the brain-tumor interface and remaining infiltrated brain. Until drug delivery to this brain improves either via improved pharmacology (allowing the drug to reach the tumor cells in adequate concentration), via blood-brain barrier opening,[31] convection-enhanced delivery mechanisms,[32] or future unrealized methods, surgery offers the only possibility to place chemotherapy (as biodegradable polymers or wafers[33]) or brachytherapy[34] agents that treat the infiltrative region around the resection margin.

PRACTICAL CHALLENGES DURING REOPERATION

Repeat resection is complicated because of several factors, which are discussed in the order they are encountered from skin to tumor cavity.

Regarding the skin incision, there is undoubtedly a modern trend for smaller, straight incisions at first surgery, dividing skin, galea, muscle, and periosteum in the same cut. This may have immediate benefits for the patient in terms of minimal hair shave, a faster opening, less blood loss, faster closure in as few as two layers, reduced postoperative pain and swelling compared with raising a larger scalp flap, and potentially faster wound healing and suture removal. Although these gains are palpable for diseases where a single surgery over the life of the patient is expected (eg, small vertex meningioma), these benefits may be less beneficial for patients with glioma who may need repeat surgeries and for recurrent disease, which may be under, nearby, or at a considerable distance from the first craniotomy. In addition, radiation therapy is invariably required after tumor resection, and as illustrated in **Fig. 1**, may directly traverse the scar when the incision is fashioned directly over the tumor. Furthermore, nearly all patients with glioma are treated with dexamethasone, which is known to increase the incidence of wound breakdown and infection frequently resulting in reoperation.[35] Scars invariably contract and once radiation therapy and steroids have been administered, tissue tension is likely to be significantly increased by the time of reoperation. When positioning for reoperation, an assistant can be asked to advance the scalp on either side of the scar toward the incision before pinning to ensure there is not further tension placed during

clamp application. Some creativity with the scar, such as curving or bending previous incisions and/or undermining the galea from the pericranium, also helps to relieve direct tension on the wound and aid healing. In extremis, plastic surgery colleagues should be consulted for assistance with wound closure. Several studies suggest it may be possible to predict where glioblastoma recurrence will occur[36] from the preoperative scans even before the first surgery. This information should be strongly considered when planning the first incision, taking into account how it can accommodate surgery for a future recurrence in the predicted location. Consideration of how recurrent tumor may be approached at a future surgery and planning of the incision and opening for reoperation at first surgery is the recommended practice. Scalp closure is typically performed using suture. If the galea is incompetent, one can consider using nylon suture using full-thickness, interrupted, vertical mattress technique. Lastly, sutures should be removed cautiously, and wounds reviewed early, especially if any patient-reported concerns.

Moving deeper, it is advisable to try and separate and retain periosteum as a vascularized flap to "underlie" the skin and galeal closure. When placing bioplates and burrhole covers in particular, consideration should be given to where

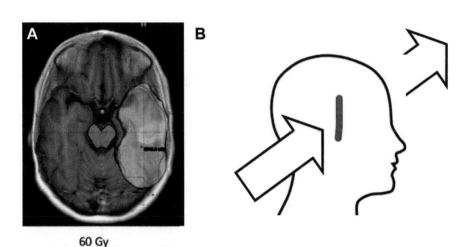

60 Gy

Fig. 1. A "simple" temporal high-grade glioma that lies superficially may be amenable to a small, straight pre-auricular incision (*B*) that is quick to open and close, heals nicely, and is covered by hair. Consider, however, the typical radiation field (*A*) that is needed to treat such a tumor and how this interacts with the incision. At a potential reoperation this small, straight incision is wholly inadequate and may need to be curved forward or backward to obtain enough exposure to access recurrent/progressive tumor and any adjacent cortical areas that may need to be mapped. In regards to the skin, the irradiated scar is devascularized, contracted orthogonal to the cut, thinned because of steroids, and exacerbated further by bioplates or burrhole covers directly underlying the incision. It is better to take the time to raise a larger flap initially that serves for future operations and keeps the scalp and bone over the tumor well covered and vascularized. (*Adapted from* Gzell C, Back M, Wheeler H, et al. Radiotherapy in glioblastoma: the past, the present and the future. Clin Oncol (R Coll Radiol). 2017;29(1):18; with permission.)

these will lie in relation to the skin incision. Without periosteum or muscle (eg, temporalis) atop a plate, the risk of hardware exposure and biofilm adherence to it by bacteria is more likely in the event of a superficial wound breakdown (**Fig. 2**). It is advised that these prostheses be placed away from the suture line under the scalp or at least covered with vascularized periosteum (**Fig. 3**). At reoperation, one can always relocate the plates away from the incision line, discarding the existing covers or plates. One might consider removing the fibrous plug in a prior burrhole because it represents an avascular nidus for future infection.

The bony opening should be considered at the first surgery with the temptation to perform a limited craniotomy to access the tumor balanced against the thought of where recurrence might occur and what further exposure might be needed in future. Frequently, the flap is anticipated to be adherent to the dura. One should tailor the craniotomy flap as need for the recurrence, to be the same, outside and encompassing the prior flap, or even inside a previous larger flap to help minimize interaction with scar at the prior defect between flap and surrounding skull or to give better exposure with which to dissect and preserve dura rather than injuring during flap elevation. One should be prepared and anticipate that the dura may be missing or dehisced creating a

potential interaction between the pia and inner craniotomy surface.

Beneath the bone the dura is often adherent and scarred because of radiation, peritumoral inflammation, tumor growth, scar from prior surgery, and necrosis. It is advisable to circumferentially free the cortex from the underlying dura around the dural opening and classic sharp dissection with attention to microsurgical technique should be applied especially when the pia and cortical vessels are adherent. Preserving the pia is of critical importance to preserving the integrity and function of the underlying brain. Adherence of the pia to the dura at the margins, in addition to scar adhering veins to the dura, may prevent passing subdural electrodes for monitoring. During closure, a lip of free dura needs to be dissected to accept suture. If the dura seems inadequate for coverage of the defect then duroplasty may be considered; because cerebrospinal fluid leak is problematic for these patients (and a particular problem with intracavity chemotherapy[37]),

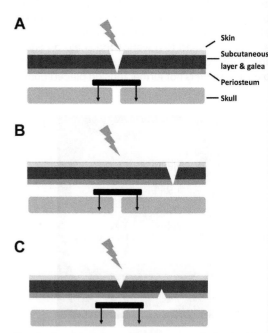

A

Skin
Subcutaneous layer & galea
Periosteum
Skull

B

C

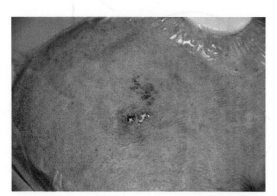

Fig. 2. The result of operation, adjuvant chemoradiotherapy, reoperation, and wound failure in a patient with glioblastoma. Multiple incisions, hardware (eg, bioplates and burrhole covers directly under the incision), the scalp in the direct line of radiation beam, and prolonged steroid therapy may lead to wound failure with exposure of hardware and ultimately delays in therapy and reduced quality of life. Careful planning of the incision at the first surgery may prevent wound-related issues, but judicious closure, reduced skin tension, thoughtful siting of plates, and plastic surgery involvement should be used.

Fig. 3. Consideration of placement of the incision, plates, and craniotomy should prevent the situation in *A* where the radiotherapy beam directly crosses the scar and the burrhole cover or dog boneplate is beneath the incision. Ideally the scar should be offset from the line of radiation therapy as in *B* with the burrhole cover or plate protected by full thickness scalp. As a compromise, the situation in *C* is preferable to *A*. The scar overlies the edge of the craniotomy but an underlay of periosteum provides some coverage and reduces the possibility of hardware exposure should the superficial wound fail.

watertight closure and reinforcement with an onlay graft and synthetic "glue" as needed may be used.

Many of the conventional tools for identifying tumor boundaries preoperatively and intraoperatively[38] are rendered less useful at reoperation. With respect to neuronavigation, the T2 and FLAIR signal are altered following irradiation and the volume of FLAIR hyperintensity, for example, no longer seems to be prognostic[39] making it more challenging to plan the limits of resection preoperatively. Fluid or cyst cavities are often drained early but conversely this may lead to brain shift inaccuracy with image guidance. Functional MRI activation areas have also been shown to alter with radiotherapy[40] and plasticity may have led to reorganization of cortical functions. Therefore, previously noneloquent areas should not be assumed to be safe for resection. Intraoperative ultrasound is a tremendously useful tool in intrinsic brain tumor resection but in a systematic review, performance has been shown to be worsened during reoperation.[41] Borders are less well defined and the radiation-induced hyperintensity seen on FLAIR and T2 MRI sequences blurs the acoustic interface, typically well-defined during a first surgery. 5-Aminolevulinic acid (5-ALA) is an increasingly available adjunct in glioma surgery in North America and has been proposed to be standard of care for reoperation.[42] This is despite reports from Europe, which suggest caution when trying to use fluorescence to discriminate tumor from treatment change.[43] As with primary surgeries, use of 5-ALA must be accompanied by thoughtful preoperative planning and judicious intraoperative monitoring to prevent increased resection at the expense of function. Overall, more careful preoperative planning for the intracranial phase of the surgery is needed for reoperation with a clear plan for the intended margin, perhaps giving greater credibility to more immutable landmarks, such as sulci, ventricles, or dural boundaries and en bloc or circumferential resection rather than internal debulking.

SUMMARY

Reoperation carries many potential benefits in terms of cytoreduction, diagnostic yield, symptom relief, reduction of steroids, increased effectiveness of adjuvant therapies, delivery of adjuvant therapies, and ultimately survival. One should select patients logically and with a clear surgical goal, taking account of the previous operations, diagnosis (including prior pathology, grade, and genetics), age, tumor location and volume, performance status, and adjuvant options. Once the decision to reoperate has been made, functional and advanced imaging should be updated as necessary with a clear plan for surgery created with regards planned extent of resection and approach. Careful attention to detail in the operating room includes wound preparation; extending or reopening the incision to allow the necessary bony exposure; and maneuvers to reduce tension, such as advancing the scalp during pinning. Insight and humility are required if wounds look likely to fail because of atrophic scalp necessitating assistant from a plastic surgeon. Careful intraoperative progress should address adhesions of dura to cortex and fluid in the previous cavity. Surgical neuronavigation, ultrasound, and 5-ALA may all be used but with the knowledge that the utility of all these modalities are altered by previous surgery, chemotherapy, and radiotherapy. Closure must be meticulous and the dura watertight. Careful consideration of these principles results in fewer complications and improved patient outcome.

CLINICS CARE POINTS

- Consider the indications for reoperation: cytoreduction because of inadequate first surgery or tumor regrowth, obtain further diagnostic tissue to confirm diagnosis, for trials or to guide adjuvant therapy, symptom control (including seizures), steroid reduction, possible radionecrosis with diagnostic uncertainty, place chemotherapy or radiotherapy delivering implant in cavity.

- Consider patient factors: age, performance status, symptoms, ability to tolerate future therapy.

- Consider the tumor factors: location, volume, isocitrate dehydrogenase (IDH), and MGMT status.

- Wound issues: plot target with image guidance and consider incision location and scalp integrity.

- Be prepared for pia adherence to the dura using sharp dissection to preserve pia. Be wary of ultrasound and MRI as sole guide to distinguishing tumor from invaded brain. Consider adjuncts, such as 5-ALA.

- Ensure watertight dural closure, use fresh bioplates, attempt underlay skin with vascularized periosteum, wean steroids as soon as possible, and review wound early especially if any patient-reported concerns.

DISCLOSURE

The authors have nothing to disclose.

REFERENCES

1. Harsh GRt, Levin VA, Gutin PH, et al. Reoperation for recurrent glioblastoma and anaplastic astrocytoma. Neurosurgery 1987;21(5):615–21.
2. Chen YR, Sole J, Ugiliweneza B, et al. National trends for reoperation in older patients with glioblastoma. World Neurosurg 2018;113:e179–89.
3. Chaul-Barbosa C, Marques DF. How we treat recurrent glioblastoma today and current evidence. Curr Oncol Rep 2019;21(10):94.
4. Lu VM, Jue TR, McDonald KL, et al. The survival effect of repeat surgery at glioblastoma recurrence and its trend: a systematic review and meta-analysis. World Neurosurg 2018;115:453–9.e3.
5. Ortega A, Sarmiento JM, Ly D, et al. Multiple resections and survival of recurrent glioblastoma patients in the temozolomide era. J Clin Neurosci 2016;24:105–11.
6. Sastry RA, Shankar GM, Gerstner ER, et al. The impact of surgery on survival after progression of glioblastoma: a retrospective cohort analysis of a contemporary patient population. J Clin Neurosci 2018;53:41–7.
7. Franceschi E, Bartolotti M, Tosoni A, et al. The effect of re-operation on survival in patients with recurrent glioblastoma. Anticancer Res 2015;35(3):1743–8.
8. Ryken TC, Kalkanis SN, Buatti JM, et al. The role of cytoreductive surgery in the management of progressive glioblastoma: a systematic review and evidence-based clinical practice guideline. J Neurooncol 2014;118(3):479–88.
9. Oppenlander ME, Wolf AB, Snyder LA, et al. An extent of resection threshold for recurrent glioblastoma and its risk for neurological morbidity. J Neurosurg 2014;120(4):846–53.
10. Lu VM, Goyal A, Graffeo CS, et al. Survival benefit of maximal resection for glioblastoma reoperation in the temozolomide era: a meta-analysis. World Neurosurg 2019;127:31–7.
11. Lacroix M, Abi-Said D, Fourney DR, et al. A multivariate analysis of 416 patients with glioblastoma multiforme: prognosis, extent of resection, and survival. J Neurosurg 2001;95(2):190–8.
12. Brown TJ, Bota DA, van Den Bent MJ, et al. Management of low-grade glioma: a systematic review and meta-analysis. Neurooncol Pract 2019;6(4):249–58.
13. Hall WA, Pugh SL, Wefel JS, et al. Influence of residual disease following surgical resection in newly diagnosed glioblastoma on clinical, neurocognitive, and patient reported outcomes. Neurosurgery 2019;84(1):66–76.
14. Ringel F, Pape H, Sabel M, et al. Clinical benefit from resection of recurrent glioblastomas: results of a multicenter study including 503 patients with recurrent glioblastomas undergoing surgical resection. Neuro Oncol 2016;18(1):96–104.
15. Suchorska B, Weller M, Tabatabai G, et al. Complete resection of contrast-enhancing tumor volume is associated with improved survival in recurrent glioblastoma-results from the DIRECTOR trial. Neuro Oncol 2016;18(4):549–56.
16. Jackson RJ, Fuller GN, Abi-Said D, et al. Limitations of stereotactic biopsy in the initial management of gliomas. Neuro Oncol 2001;3(3):193–200.
17. Kim BYS, Jiang W, Beiko J, et al. Diagnostic discrepancies in malignant astrocytoma due to limited small pathological tumor sample can be overcome by IDH1 testing. J Neurooncol 2014;118(2):405–12.
18. Alexander BM, Ba S, Berger MS, et al. Adaptive Global Innovative Learning Environment for Glioblastoma: GBM AGILE. Clin Cancer Res 2018;24(4):737–43.
19. Watts C, Apps J, Ansorg O, et al. RBTT-06. Tessa Jowell BRAIN MATRIX Study: a British feasibility study of molecular stratification and targeted therapy to optimise the clinical management of patients with glioma. Neuro Oncol 2019;21(Supplement_6):vi219–20.
20. Grossman R, Shimony N, Hadelsberg U, et al. Impact of resecting radiation necrosis and pseudoprogression on survival of patients with glioblastoma. World Neurosurg 2016;89:37–41.
21. Barker FG 2nd, Chang SM, Gutin PH, et al. Survival and functional status after resection of recurrent glioblastoma multiforme. Neurosurgery 1998;42(4):709–20 [discussion: 720–3].
22. Chang SM, Parney IF, McDermott M, et al. Perioperative complications and neurological outcomes of first and second craniotomies among patients enrolled in the Glioma Outcome Project. J Neurosurg 2003;98(6):1175–81.
23. Vecil GG, Suki D, Maldaun MV, et al. Resection of brain metastases previously treated with stereotactic radiosurgery. J Neurosurg 2005;102(2):209–15.
24. Wang DD, Deng H, Hervey-Jumper SL, et al. Seizure outcome after surgical resection of insular glioma. Neurosurgery 2018;83(4):709–18.
25. Barbagallo GM, Jenkinson MD, Brodbelt AR. 'Recurrent' glioblastoma multiforme, when should we reoperate? Br J Neurosurg 2008;22(3):452–5.
26. Beiko J, Suki D, Hess KR, et al. IDH1 mutant malignant astrocytomas are more amenable to surgical resection and have a survival benefit associated with maximal surgical resection. Neuro Oncol 2014;16(1):81–91.
27. Chun SJ, Park SH, Park CK, et al. Survival gain with re-Op/RT for recurred high-grade gliomas depends upon risk groups. Radiother Oncol 2018;128(2):254–9.
28. Pala A, Schmitz AL, Knoll A, et al. Is MGMT promoter methylation to be considered in the decision making for recurrent surgery in glioblastoma patients? Clin Neurol Neurosurg 2018;167:6–10.

29. Park JK, Hodges T, Arko L, et al. Scale to predict survival after surgery for recurrent glioblastoma multiforme. J Clin Oncol 2010;28(24):3838–43.

30. Millward CP, Mallucci C, Jaspan T, et al. Assessing 'second-look' tumour resectability in childhood posterior fossa ependymoma-a centralised review panel and staging tool for future studies. Childs Nerv Syst 2016;32(11):2189–96.

31. Dréan A, Lemaire N, Bouchoux G, et al. Temporary blood-brain barrier disruption by low intensity pulsed ultrasound increases carboplatin delivery and efficacy in preclinical models of glioblastoma. J Neurooncol 2019;144(1):33–41.

32. Barua NU, Hopkins K, Woolley M, et al. A novel implantable catheter system with transcutaneous port for intermittent convection-enhanced delivery of carboplatin for recurrent glioblastoma. Drug Deliv 2016;23(1):167–73.

33. Brem H, Piantadosi S, Burger PC, et al. Placebo-controlled trial of safety and efficacy of intraoperative controlled delivery by biodegradable polymers of chemotherapy for recurrent gliomas. The Polymer-brain Tumor Treatment Group. Lancet 1995;345(8956):1008–12.

34. Brachman DG, Youssef E, Dardis CJ, et al. Resection and permanent intracranial brachytherapy using modular, biocompatible cesium-131 implants: results in 20 recurrent, previously irradiated meningiomas. J Neurosurg 2018; 131(6):1819–28.

35. Patel S, Thompson D, Innocent S, et al. Risk factors for surgical site infections in neurosurgery. Ann R Coll Surg Engl 2019;101(3):220–5.

36. Yan JL, Li C, Hoorn AV, et al. A neural network approach to identify the peritumoral invasive areas in glioblastoma patients by using MR radiomics. Sci Rep 2020;10(1):9748.

37. Subach BR, Witham TF, Kondziolka D, et al. Morbidity and survival after 1,3-bis(2-chloroethyl)-1-nitrosourea wafer implantation for recurrent glioblastoma: a retrospective case-matched cohort series. Neurosurgery 1999;45(1):17–22 [discussion: 22–3].

38. Krivosheya D, Prabhu SS, Weinberg JS, et al. Technical principles in glioma surgery and preoperative considerations. J Neurooncol 2016;130(2):243–52.

39. Woodroffe RW, Zanaty M, Soni N, et al. Survival after reoperation for recurrent glioblastoma. J Clin Neurosci 2020;73:118–24.

40. Kovács Á, Emri M, Opposits G, et al. Changes in functional MRI signals after 3D based radiotherapy of glioblastoma multiforme. J Neurooncol 2015; 125(1):157–66.

41. Trevisi G, Barbone P, Treglia G, et al. Reliability of intraoperative ultrasound in detecting tumor residual after brain diffuse glioma surgery: a systematic review and meta-analysis. Neurosurgical Review 2019;43(5):1221–33.

42. Chohan MO, Berger MS. 5-Aminolevulinic acid fluorescence guided surgery for recurrent high-grade gliomas. J Neurooncol 2019;141(3): 517–22.

43. Kamp MA, Felsberg J, Sadat H, et al. 5-ALA-induced fluorescence behavior of reactive tissue changes following glioblastoma treatment with radiation and chemotherapy. Acta Neurochir 2015; 157(2):207–13 [discussion: 213–4].

Surgery for Glioblastoma in Elderly Patients

Marco Conti Nibali, MD[a,b,*], Lorenzo G. Gay, MD[a,b], Tommaso Sciortino, MD[a,b], Marco Rossi, MD[a,b], Manuela Caroli, MD[c], Lorenzo Bello, MD[a,b], Marco Riva, MD[b,d]

KEYWORDS

- GBM • Elderly • Resection • Adjuvant treatment • Elderly patients • Radiotherapy • Chemotherapy • Survival

KEY POINTS

- The incidence of glioblastoma increases with age, with highest rate in the population between 75 and 84 years old. Given the increased life expectancy, elderly patients represent up to 25% of patients with glioblastoma.
- Age alone is not a predictor of survival in glioblastoma. General condition and performance status strongly influence and guide therapy.
- In this age group, biological age is more relevant than chronologic age.
- Surgery aimed at the maximal safe resection, when feasible, followed by adjuvant therapy according to O^6-methylguanine-DNA methyl-transferase methylation might be the first therapeutic option.
- Future clinical trials focusing on glioblastomas in the elderly subjects could provide more specific data for patient's selection.

INTRODUCTION AND BACKGROUND

Glioblastoma (GBM) is the most common primary malignant tumor of the central nervous system, accounting for 48.3% of primary malignant brain tumors and 57.3% of all gliomas. The incidence of GBMs increases with age. The highest rate is recorded in the population between 75 and 84 years old; the disease is 2 times more frequent in this age range than in the population aged between 55 and 64 years.[1]

Despite advances in surgery and adjuvant treatments, the prognosis remains poor, with a median overall survival (OS) of fewer than 18 months in the adult population. An analysis conducted on more than 88,000 patients with GBM treated between 2004 and 2013 reports a mild increase in the number of patients surviving 3 years after the initial diagnosis.[2]

The definition of "elderly" is controversial. The elderly age starts at 65 year old, according to the World Health Organization; as for patients with GBM, the National Comprehensive Cancer Network sets the age to consider a patient into the "elderly category" at 70 years.[3,4] The real-life evidence shows that subjects up to 70 years may still have an active social and intellectual life. Especially in high-income countries, a longer life expectancy is recorded than in the past and or in comparison with low- and middle-income countries. In this age range, the physiologic age is becoming more relevant than the date of birth to shape the indication and intention to treat. Age is a negative prognostic factor, and every year of increase in age is associated with a statistically significant decrease in survival in patients with GBM.[4–6]

[a] Department of Oncology and Hemato-Oncology, Via Festa del Perdono 7, Milan 20122, Italy; [b] IRCCS Istituto Ortopedico Galeazzi, Neurochirurgia Oncologica, Milan, Italy; [c] Unit of Neurosurgery, Fondazione IRCCS Ca' Grande Ospedale Maggiore Policlinico, Milan, Italy; [d] Department of Medical Biotechnology and Translational Medicine, Universita' degli Studi di Milano, Via Festa del Perdono 7, Milan 20122, Italy
* Corresponding author. Department of Oncology and Hemato-Oncology, Via Festa del Perdono 7, Milan 20122, Italy.
E-mail address: marco.continibali@gmail.com

Neurosurg Clin N Am 32 (2021) 137–148
https://doi.org/10.1016/j.nec.2020.08.008
1042-3680/21/© 2020 Elsevier Inc. All rights reserved.

Having this being premised, it is thus mandatory to review the best (current) management of GBMs in the elderly population, because life expectancy (ie, adding years to life) is growing throughout the world (in Italy life expectancy in 2017 was 83.2 years according to the World Health Organization) and elderly patients represent up to 25% of patients with GBM. In addition, numbers are expected to double in the next 2 decades.[7,8]

The management of GBMs is currently multidisciplinary. A balance among available options, such as surgery, chemotherapy, radiation therapy (RT), and experimental approaches, is essential to grant the best feasible outcome and preserve the quality of life (ie, adding life to years).[9] The scope of this review is to report and discuss the state of the art of surgical and adjuvant treatment in elderly patients affected by GBMs.

CURRENT EVIDENCE
Histomolecular Features

Phenotypic differences across age ranges are only partially explained by differences in known molecular features, such as IDH mutational status, O^6-methylguanine-DNA methyl-transferase (MGMT) methylation, and TP53 mutation. IDH mutation, the most important positive prognostic factor in gliomas, is differently expressed in GBM between adult and elderly: IDH1/2 mutations are rarely present in adult GBM and virtually missing in the elderly.[10–12] Although the physiologic methylation of cells of the central nervous system decreases with age, the results of the NOA-08 trial revealed that age does not affect the MGMT promoter methylation frequency.[13] The expression of vascular endothelial growth factor increases in patients older than 55 years with recurrent GBM.[14] Moreover, TP53 mutation and CDKN1A/p16 alteration are negative markers in patients older than 70 years, conversely than younger subjects.[11,13]

Prognostic Factors

The first study about prognostic factors using the recursive partitioning analysis was conducted on data collected in the 1970s and 1980s, therefore in the pre-temozolomide (TMZ) era.[15] With a plethora of variables, the authors identified 6 different classes of risk based on preoperative (age, race, gender, Karnofsky performance status [KPS], neurologic examination, comorbidity, tumor location and size) and postoperative (histology, Extent Of Resection (EOR), adjuvant therapies) variables, correlating risk classes with oncologic outcome. Further updates were released in the following years, with fewer prognostic classes.[16] In the latest edition, the extent of resection and

the MGTM promoter methylation were reported as the most relevant prognostic factors for survival in the elderly subjects.[13,16–20]

Along with the previous factors, in elderly patients a special emphasis should be given to performance status and to general condition as variables strongly influencing and guiding therapies. In this context, the process of selection of those patients who could benefit from treatments, especially surgery, remains a crucial issue. Physiologic assessment taking in to account organ function and associated comorbidities may better predict patient health status than chronologic age itself.[21] Elderly patients are not identical and age per se is not a synonymous of frail, that, instead, concerns much more with the physical status of the individual patient. Frailty is generally defined as an unintentional weight loss, self-reported exhaustion, weakness, slow walking speed, and low physical activity.[22] In the elderly patient assessment, surgeons and neuro-oncologists along with the individual patient and family interview, are helped in the decision-making process by the use of scales or questionnaires of evaluation aimed at a more personalized approach.[11,23–26] In addition to the well-known KPS, various scales of frailty have been proposed, such as the Instrumental Activities of Daily Living (IDAL) questionnaire, that assess the ability and motivation to use the phone, to go shopping, or food preparation, to do household work, to take medication, or to use transportation or to handle finances; other are the Oncodage G8 questionnaire, the Mini Mental State Examination or the Charlson Comorbidity Index.[11,27,28]

Surgery

Maximum safe resection is an important prognostic factor in all patients with GBM.[29,30] Surgery aims at impacting on the progression-free survival (PFS) and on the OS, as well as to fulfill other relevant goals such as histologic and molecular diagnosis, the relief of the mass effect, the improvement of the neurologic status, and the reduction of the use of steroids.

The extent of resection is also a prognostic factor for survival in elderly patients. A recent prospective study conducted on 1452 elderly patients showed that craniotomy for tumor resection was a feasible and safe procedure.[31] A pioneering randomized trial analyzed the differential outcome of a group of elderly patients undergoing either surgical resection or biopsy: data showed an improvement in survival of 3 months for the group undergoing resection.[32] Although the difference in survival was small, the randomized design made this study a milestone in the field. A later retrospective case-control study demonstrated a gain of 40% in survival in the resection group (OS 5.7 months vs 4.0 months) compared with the biopsy group.[33] Further retrospective studies confirmed these initial findings in primary GBMs.[19,34–39] A wide meta-analysis included a large group of more than 12,000 patients older than 60 years from 34 studies.[35] Patients who underwent gross total resection experienced a gain in OS of 7.05 months on the average, a better functional recovery, a longer PFS, and comparable mortality and morbidity compared with those submitted to biopsy only. A further single-institution retrospective study evaluated the outcome and its associated prognostic factors in 178 elderly subjects, treated from 2004 to 2015. The results confirmed that the elderly population submitted to resection have a statistically significant increase in survival when the complete resection of the contrast enhancement tumor was achieved, with a 2-year OS that is 3 times longer than that recorded in patients submitted to biopsy alone.[40]

Further studies introduced the concept of EOR thresholds stratification, and assessed the association between the achieved threshold and the outcome: Oszvald[41] showed that a significant increase in survival was observed when the residual volume was less than 5%; Pessina and colleagues[40] reported less than 2 cm³, as an absolute value. Multiples tools are described to increase EOR: intraoperative fluorescence surgery has been recently approved by the US Food and Drug Administration, and it is widely available in neuro-oncologic centers. Efficacy on OS of 5-aminolevulinic acid in GBM surgery was first proved with a randomized prospective phase III trial.[42] Despite its widespread use, there are no studies in literature focused only on elderly patients.[43,44]

When resection is pushed toward a maximal level, the issue of preserving patient integrity is becoming crucial. The use of mapping and monitoring techniques is helpful. There is no dedicated report on the feasibility and safety of awake surgery in elderly patients; generally, age is not considered an absolute contraindication for an awake anesthesia, although strict and careful patient selection is strongly advised.

Regarding patient selection, a low preoperative KPS, a tumor bigger than 4 cm, and the existence of preoperative deficits (motor, language) have been found to factors negatively influence surgical outcome[40,45]; in particular regarding elderly patients, the evaluation of the functional status is the most important prognostic factor; it thus represents an essential selection criteria[18,19,40,46] to establish the indication for surgery. **Table 1**

describes the principal studies that investigated oncologic outcome of elderly patients after the introduction of TMZ in to the clinical routine; works that compared outcome of biopsy and resection were included.

In patients where stereotaxic biopsy is not feasible owing to a high risk of complications, advanced MRI (perfusion and/or spectroscopy study) or metabolic imaging (11-C-methionine PET, O-(2-[18F]fluoroethyl-)-L-tyrosine PET) are recommended.[47]

In the preoperative stage, it is also important to exclude potential differential diagnoses. To perform a total body computed tomography scan with an iodine contrast agent is advisable to rule out a possible metastatic origin of the brain lesion, or to carefully look at diffusion-weighted images to exclude infection.

Last, surgery (resection or biopsy) has also the goal of providing adequate tissue for complete histomolecular characterization, considering that the assessment of the MGMT methylation status is incorporated in the clinical routine[17,18,48] owing to its relevant prognostic predictivity, in first-line treatments and potential newer therapeutic regimes.[49]

Adjuvant Treatments

Several studies support the role of adjuvant treatments in elderly patients. If evidence about surgery has been available since the early 1990s, data about the safety and efficacy of postsurgical RT in the elderly were published in 2007. The French database (ANOCEF) showed that RT (50 Gy in 1.8 Gy fractions) is superior to the best supportive care in elderly patients with a KPS of 70 or greater, because it led to an OS of 29.1 weeks versus 16.9 weeks and a PFS of 14.9 versus 5.4 weeks.[50] Initially, the use of a hypofractionated protocol was reserved for patients with unfavorable prognostic factors defined by age or performance status[51] to minimize the radiation time exposure. The Canadian Phase II trial and NORDIC phase III randomized trial demonstrated that a hypofractionated regimen is preferable in most cases, both for oncologic and functional reasons. The hypofractionated schedule is nowadays the standard therapy in patients with unmethylated MGMT promoter. The NORDIC trial showed in patients older than 70 years a survival of 7.0 months when the hypofractionated protocol was applied and in of 5.2 months when the standard (60 gy in 2 Gy fractions over 6 weeks) RT was used.[17]

The NOA-08 trial confirmed these findings, comparing 2 arms of treatment: RT (60 Gy in 30 fractions) versus continuative TMZ (1 week on/

Table 1
Studies comparing oncologic outcome of elderly patients that underwent either resection or biopsy after the introduction of TMZ

First Author (Year of Publication)	No. of Patients	Elderly Definition	KPS	Type of Surgery	Postoperative Deficits	Morbidity or Mortality	Adjuvant Treatment	PFS	OS
Kleinschmidt,[71] 2005	18	≥75	n.a.	6 Biopsy 12 Resection	n.a.	n.a.	6 RT 1 CT 2 RT + CT	n.a	3.08 Biopsy 5.42 Resection
Combs,[72] 2008	43	≥65	26 ≥ 70	14 Biopsy 17 STR 12 GTR	n.a.	n.a.	43 RT + CT	n.a.	6.0 Biopsy 16.0 STR 18.0 GTR
Sijben,[73] 2008	39	≥65	≥60	11 Biopsy 28 Resection	n.a	n.a.	20 RT 19 RT + CT	4.5 Biopsy 5.2 Resection	5.0 Biopsy 8.5 Resection
Gerstein,[74] 2010	51	≥65	44 ≥ 70	23 Biopsy 15 STR 13 GTR	n.a.	n.a.	51 RT + CT	4.73 Biopsy 4.17 STR 9.5 GTR	7.89 Biopsy 15.5 STR 27.4 GTR
Kimple,[75] 2010	30	≥70	Mean ≥63.3	14 Biopsy 7 STR 9 GTR	n.a.	n.a.	9 RT 9 RT + CT	n.a.	7.0 Biopsy 4.6 STR 8.3 GTR
Lai,[76] 2010	1355	≥65	n.a.	296 Biopsy 485 STR 574 GTR	n.a.	n.a.	1005 RT 350 RT + CT	n.a.	5.6 Biopsy 8 STR 9.3 GTR
Laigle-Donadey,[77] 2010	39	≥70	Mean ≥73.6	21 Biopsy 14 STR 3 GTR	n.a.	n.a.	39 CT	n.a.	8.4 Biopsy 9.07 STR 9.07 16.0 GTR
Chaicana,[32] 2011	80	≥65	Mean ≥80	40 Biopsy 25 STR 15 GTR	4 Biopsy 7 Resection	1 Biopsy 0 Resection	64 RT 8 CT	n.a.	4.0 Biopsy 5.4 STR 5.8 GTR
Ewelt,[33] 2011	103	≥65	66 ≥ 70	43 Biopsy 37 STR 23 GTR	n.a.	n.a.	37 RT 35 RT + CT	2.1 Biopsy 3.4 STR 6.4 GTR	2.2 Biopsy 7.0 STR 13.9 GTR
Kushnir,[78] 2011	74	≥65	68 ≥ 65	26 Biopsy 42 Resection	n.a.	n.a.	8 RT 27 RT + CHT 34 CT	n.a.	5.56 Biopsy 11.83 Resection
Hashem,[79] 2012	20	≥65	13 ≥ 70	10 Biopsy 8 STR 2 GTR	n.a.	n.a.	20 RT + CHT	n.a.	8.26 Biopsy 15.41 STR 21.25 GTR

Study	N	Age	Median/Mean						
Oszvald,[40] 2012	146	≥65	Median = 70	66 Biopsy / 61 STR / 19 GTR	n.a.	n.a.	63 RT / 58 RT + CT	n.a.	4.0 Biopsy / 11.4 STR / 17.7 GTR
Scott,[18] 2012	702	≥70	387 ≥ 70	324 Biopsy / 231 STR / 141 GTR	n.a.	n.a.	419 RT / 234 CT	n.a.	3.1 Biopsy / 8.0 Resection
Tanaka,[80] 2013	105	≥65	Mean = 74.9	52 Biopsy / 53 Resection	16 Biopsy / 10 Resection	4 Biopsy / 0 Resection	23 RT / 41 RT + CT / 1 CT	n.a.	6.5 Biopsy 6.5 / 11.0 Resection
Fariselli,[81] 2013	33	≥70	≥70	4 Biopsy / 13 STR / 16 GTR	n.a.	n.a.	26 RT / 7 RT + CT	n.a.	7 Biopsy / 8 STR / 11 GTR
Lee,[82] 2013	20	≥70	n.a.	4 Biopsy / 13 STR / 16 GTR	n.a.	n.a.	16 RT + CT	n.a.	11.8 Biopsy / 5.0 STR / 28.9 GTR
Uzuka (2014)	79	≥75	Median = 60	32 Biopsy / 21 STR / 26 GTR	n.a.	n.a.	33 RT / 19 RT + CT / 27 CT	n.a.	9.1 Biopsy / 13 GTR
Almenawer,[34] 2014	211	≥65	Mean = 74.2	73 Biopsy / 71 STR / 67 GTR	20 Biopsy / 9 STR / 4 GTR	4 Biopsy / 2 STR / 1 GTR	101 RT / 72 CT	2 Biopsy / 3.9 STR / 5.6 GTR	5.4 Biopsy / 8.6 STR / 10.6 GTR
Hoffermann,[83] 2014	124	≥65	Mean = 70	17 Biopsy / 62 STR / 35 GTR	n.a.	0 Biopsy / 5 STR / 0 GTR	7 RT / 60 RT + CT / 6 CT	n.a.	4 Biopsy / 9 STR / 15 GTR
Abdullah,[35] 2015	58	≥80	≥60	40 STR / 12 GTR	12	2	10 RT / 10 RT + CT	n.a.	4.2 Resection
Lombardi,[84] 2015	237	≥65	≥60	40 STR / 12 GTR	n.a.	n.a.	237 RT + CT	n.a.	16.1 STR / 17.7 GTR
Welzel,[85] 2015	146	≥65	79 ≥ 70	113 Resection / 33 Biopsy	n.a.	n.a.	n.a.	4.8 Resection / 3.5 Biopsy	4.4 Biopsy / 8.1 Resection
Babu,[36] 2016	120	≥65	Median = 80	63 STR / 174 GTR	n.a.	n.a.	110 RT + CHT	n.a.	9.6 STR / 14.1 GTR
Di Cristofori,[26] 2017	117	≥65	Median = 70	38 STR / 79 GTR	6 Resection	Resection 13	84 RT + CT / 16 CT	n.a.	7 STR / 11 GTR
Karsy,[86] 2018	82	≥75	Median = 80	18 Biopsy / 33 STR / 19 GTR	2 Biopsy / 5 STR / 2 GTR	6 Biopsy / 10 STR / 6 GTR	32 RT / 22 CT	n.a.	3.7 Biopsy / 5 STR / 12.1 GTR

(continued on next page)

Table 1
(continued)

First Author (Year of Publication)	No. of Patients	Elderly Definition	KPS	Type of Surgery	Postoperative Deficits	Morbidity or Mortality	Adjuvant Treatment	PFS	OS
Hager,[57] 2018	59	≥65	Median = 90	17 Biopsy 17 STR 25 GTR	n.a.	n.a.	11 RT 41 RT + CT 25 CT	9.7 Resection 5.6 Biopsy	20.7 Resection 7.4 Biopsy
Pessina,[39] 2018	178	≥65	142 ≥ 70	45 Biopsy 62 STR 63 GTR 8 CR	4 Biopsy 4 STR 3 GTR 0 CR	1 Biopsy 0 STR 2 GTR 0 CR	46 RT 132 RT + CT	n.a.	8.1 Biopsy 11.9 STR 15.1 GTR 24.5 CR

Studies without a report of the OS were excluded. Number are reported as absolute value. We report the sample size included, age threshold, KPS (median, mean, or majority patients' value), type of surgery, postoperative deficits, postoperative morbidity and mortality, type of adjuvant treatment, months of PFS and OS. Not available (n.a.) is indicated when the study did not explicitly report the information requested. References are quoted in the main text.

Abbreviations: CCR, complete resection; CT, chemotherapy; CHT, chemotherapy; GTR, gross total resection; STR, subtotal resection.

week off). RT improved survival in patients with an unmethylated MGMT (PFS of 4.6 months in the RT group vs 3.3 months in the TMZ group), although TMZ yielded to better PFS in patients with a methylated MGMT promoter (PFS of 8.4 months in the TMZ group vs 4.6 in the RT group).[18] Both the NORDIC and NOA-08 trials confirmed the prognostic relevance of MGMT methylation status and the consequent use of TMZ in patients who underwent biopsy or partial resection. However, data on the combination of RT and on the best therapeutic strategy for elderly patients with an unmethylated MGMT promoter are still lacking.[18]

Because the association with short course RT proved to be safe and useful in elderly patients, TMZ became the subject of a further trial (CCTG CE.6/EORTC 26062) that enrolled 281 patients with resectable tumors, in 2 arms: short-course RT (15 fractions of 2.67 Gy each) with TMZ and up to 12 cycles of maintenance versus exclusive RT.[52,53] The results favored the chemoradiation arm with an impact on PFS (5.3 months vs 3.9 months) and on OS (9.3 months vs 7.6 months). The trial confirmed the importance of MGMT promoter methylation as a favorable prognostic factor; methylated patients had almost a 2 times greater OS than the comparison study arm. The results showed also an advantage in the use of TMZ in the patients with an unmethylated MGMT promoter: OS was 10.0 months versus 7.9 months.

Globally, RT is associated with an improvement in OS (with controversial evidence of decreases in cognitive function and quality of life); for this reason, a short course of RT delivered by targeted radiation technique is usually recommended.

Conversely, TMZ therapy is largely effective and well-tolerated in the elderly, with a rate of severe side effects (<15%). TMZ is recommended in patients with methylation of the MGMT promoter after RT. Exclusive TMZ is also an option for patients with a very unfavorable prognosis.[54] Although chemoradiation is used in selected patients with MGMT promoter methylation, the stand-alone hypo-RT treatment or TMZ chemotherapy is delivered according to MGMT promoter methylation status. Based on the most recent evidence, first-line treatments are reported in **Fig. 1**.

Management of Recurrences

Despite the best optimal multidisciplinary treatments, GBMs inevitably recur and progress. The is no consensus or evidence on the choice of the best strategy to apply on recurrence. However, 2 recent studies[55,56] proved that any treatment (ie, chemotherapy, RT, surgery) is superior (in terms of PFS and OS) to supportive or palliative care alone. The most important limitation of those studies was that they did not considered the quality of life of enrolled patients as a goal.

To the best of our knowledge, only 2 retrospective studies have addressed the issue of surgery for recurrent GBM in the elderly. Considering the limitations of the studies, such as the selection bias of the population selected for surgery and the small size of the cohort, an improvement in survival of at least 7 months[57] was reported in the group who underwent a second surgery for recurrent GBM. Previous work,[58] conversely, did not show any advantage in survival (4 months) in the group of patients that underwent a second

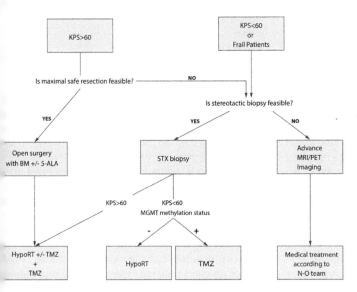

Fig. 1. Flow-chart for the treatment of elderly patients with GBM. 5-ALA, 5-aminolevulinic acid; BM, brain mapping; HypoRT, hypofractionated radiotherapy; MGMT, O[6]-methylguanine-DNA methyltransferase; N-O, neuro-oncologic; STX, stereotactic.

surgery; no data about alternative treatments were reported.

Reirradiation (re-RT) is a well-established option for treatment of recurrent GBM in young adults also after a second surgery. A recent study investigated the feasibility and safety of re-RT in a cohort of elderly patients with good success in term of OS (6.9 months after re-RT) with only minor side effects.[59] The decision about re-RT should not be based on age per se.

As a good clinical practice point, by a meticulous patient's selection, evaluating KPS, previous treatment, tumor volume, location of recurrence, and the time between last treatment and recurrence, a surgical removal of the recurrent tumors could be considered with the consensus of a neuro-oncologic tumor board, while taking patient quality of life into account.

Epilepsy and Corticosteroids

As in the younger population, there is no consensus on the use of anti-epilepsy drug prophylactic therapy in patients with no history of seizures or on the fast tapering of anti-epilepsy drugs when the tumor is stable.[60,61] The onset of seizures can severely compromise the clinical status of an older patient. The choice of the drug to administer should be made carefully, especially considering comorbidity or aggressive behavior side effects, along with the compliance on daily drug intake. The starting dose should be lower than in the younger patients, and monotherapy with a new anti-epilepsy drug is usually the first choice.[48,62] About the use of corticosteroids, a consensus agreement advocates keeping the use at a minimum. Steroids are usually given to control preoperative edema, and a rapid tapering is generally recommended in the postoperative period. A plethora of patients receiving a complete resection can accomplish RT without or with a limited dosage of steroids.

Thromboembolic Event

GBM is one of the more prothrombotic tumors across all age groups.[48] However, the risk is not age related as it is for other diseases. The reported risk is approximately 18% per year despite pharmacologic thromboprophylaxis. The event is related to decreased mobility, presence of a moderate or severe motor deficit, steroid intake, RT, and the disease itself by the release of vasoactive molecules.

For prophylaxis, low-molecular-weight heparin is the first choice for its safety profile. An inferior vena cava filter might be an option for patients who are suitable for pharmacologic anticoagulation.[63–66]

The timing of prophylaxis after surgery should be individualized, especially in this class of patients. A prompt start (24–48 hours after surgery) of administration of low-molecular-weight heparin should be considered. A synergy with hematologists is encouraged to evaluate patients with a high-risk profile in the preoperative stage, such as those with preexisting multiple cardiovascular diseases, with previous thrombotic or thromboembolic events, and those who take anticoagulant or antiplatelet drugs to establish the timing of suspension and the best protocol to restart therapy.

Supportive and Palliative Care

The end after an oncologic disease (ie, an end of the disease) is a delicate issue. A single surgical article cannot cope with such a delicate complexity. However, it is relevant to observe that the end-of-the-disease issue faces end-of-life issues in the elderly population. In this context, physicians are often asked to answer some troublesome questions during the initial consultation for an elderly patients with such a lethal form of cancer right from the clinical and radiologic presentation of the disease. Addressing these ethical questions with patients and their caregivers is also frequent during the clinical course of the disease. These issues touch each individual and his or her own beliefs and behaviors. Such issues also have a different understanding and legal ramifications in different countries and, therefore, result in differential attitudes in approaching and dealing with them. A reasonable albeit simplistic piece of advice is to individualize the medical management with the family or caregivers.

Future Directions

Compared with the younger adult population, elderly patients undergo fewer salvage therapies. Bevacizumab, a monoclonal antibody targeting vascular endothelial growth factor, is approved for recurrent GBM outside Europe, where may be administered as an off-label regimen. The antibody is not proven to be superior to lomustine,[67] but plays an important role in symptom relief and steroid-sparing effects.[68] The AVAglio trial investigated the likely efficacy in the elderly, given the significant vascular endothelial growth factor overexpression in tumors in this age group. The trial reported a significant increase in the PFS in all patients included, but the elderly constituted only 8% of enrolled patients. Their efficacy and safety in the elderly should be addressed in future trials.[69]

Tumor treating fields, instead, represents a novel promising treatment. A randomized phase III trial proved a significantly longer survival in patients receiving tumor treating fields in association with TMZ with a longer median OS of 20 months.[70] Further studies should be performed in the elderly population, assessing compliance in handling the device, cost effectiveness, and effect after hypofractionated RT.

SUMMARY

The management of GBM in the elderly population represents a field of growing interest owing to the epidemiologic relevance, increase in time to live, and life to years in the general population. Although prognosis remains poor, aggressive safe surgical treatment, with brain mapping and monitoring techniques, can be pursued after careful preoperative assessment. In this age group, biological age is more relevant than chronologic age. A multidisciplinary team should to be encouraged and assembled.

Future clinical trials focusing on GBMs in the elderly patients could provide with more specific data for patient's selection and biomarkers for patients and family counseling about the risk–benefit ratio of the therapeutic management.

CLINICS CARE POINTS

- GBMs in elderly patients represents a field of growing interest due a longer life expectancy.
- Age is not per se a contraindication to aggressive treatment as surgery; general clinical condition guides treatment.
- When feasible a Maximum Safe Resection is to address in order to guarantee access to the best treatment options and a longer Overall Survival.
- Adjuvant treatments will be based on MGMT methylation statuts, expecially if complete resection could not be achieved.
- At Recurrence multiple option can be considered as for young adults.
- More space in future clinical trial should be reserve to elderly patients.

DISCLOSURE

The authors have nothing to disclose.

REFERENCES

1. Ostrom QT, Gino C, Gittleman H, et al. CBTRUS statistical report: primary brain and other central nervous system tumors diagnosed in the United States in 2012-2016. Neuro Oncol 2019;21(5). v1–100.
2. Zreik J, Moinuddin FM, Yolcu Yagiz U, et al. Improved 3-year survival rates for glioblastoma multiforme are associated with trends in treatment: analysis of the national cancer database from 2004 to 2013. J Neurooncol 2020. https://doi.org/10.1007/s11060-020-03469-w.
3. NCCN Clinical Practice Guidelines in Oncology. Available at: https://www.nccn.org/professionals/physician_gls/default.aspx. Accessed May 31, 2020.
4. T Lawrie, Um A. Hanna C, et al, Treatment of newly diagnosed glioblastoma in the elderly: a network meta-analysis. 2020. https://doi.org/10.1002/14651858.CD013261.pub2. Available at: www.cochranelibrary.com.
5. Thumma Sudheer R, Fairbanks Robert K, Lamoreaux Wayne T, et al. Effect of pretreatment clinical factors on overall survival in glioblastoma multiforme: a Surveillance Epidemiology and End Results (SEER) population analysis. World J Surg Oncol 2012;10. https://doi.org/10.1186/1477-7819-10-75.
6. Lorimer CF, Hanna C, Saran F, et al. Challenges to treating older glioblastoma patients: the influence of clinical and tumour characteristics on survival outcomes. Clin Oncol 2017;29(11):739–47.
7. Cohen-Inbar O. Geriatric brain tumor management part II: glioblastoma multiforme. J Clin Neurosci 2019;1–4. https://doi.org/10.1016/j.jocn.2019.05.064.
8. Gately L, Collins A, Murphy M, et al. Age alone is not a predictor for survival in glioblastoma. J Neurooncol 2016;129(3):479–85.
9. Glaser Scott M, Dohopolski Michael J, Balasubramani Goundappa K, et al. Glioblastoma multiforme (GBM) in the elderly: initial treatment strategy and overall survival. J Neurooncol 2017;134(1):107–18.
10. Louis David N, Perry A, Guido R, et al. The 2016 World Health Organization classification of tumors of the central nervous system: a summary. Acta Neuropathol 2016;803–20.
11. Wick A, Kessler T, Elia Andrew EH, et al. Glioblastoma in elderly patients: solid conclusions built on shifting sand? Neuro Oncol 2018;20(2):174–83.
12. Benedikt W, Rainer C, Hartlieb Sabine A, et al. Malignant astrocytomas of elderly patients lack favorable molecular markers: an analysis of the NOA-08 study collective. Neuro Oncol 2013;15(8):1017–26.
13. Arvold Nils D, Reardon David A. Treatment options and outcomes for glioblastoma in the elderly patient. Clin Interv Aging 2014;9:357–67.
14. Nghiemphu PL, Liu W, Lee Y, et al. Bevacizumab and chemotherapy for recurrent glioblastoma: a single-institution experience. Neurology 2009;

72(14):1217–22.   https://doi.org/10.1212/01.wnl.0000345668.03039.90.

15. Curran Walter J, Scott Charles B, Horton John, et al. Recursive partitioning analysis of prognostic factors in three radiation therapy oncology group malignant glioma trials. J Natl Cancer Inst 1993; 85(9):704–10.

16. Bell EH, Pugh Stephanie L, McElroy Joseph P, et al. Molecular-based recursive partitioning analysis model for glioblastoma in the temozolomide era a correlative analysis based on NRG oncology RTOG 0525. JAMA Oncol 2017;3(6):784–92.

17. Malmström A, Grønberg BH, Christine M, et al. Temozolomide versus standard 6-week radiotherapy versus hypofractionated radiotherapy in patients older than 60 years with glioblastoma: the Nordic randomised, phase 3 trial. Lancet Oncol 2012; 13(9):916–26.

18. Wick W, Platten M, Meisner C, et al. Temozolomide chemotherapy alone versus radiotherapy alone for malignant astrocytoma in the elderly: the NOA-08 randomised, phase 3 trial. Lancet Oncol 2012; 13(7):707–15.

19. Scott JG, Bauchet L, Fraum Tyler J, et al. Recursive partitioning analysis of prognostic factors for glioblastoma patients aged 70 years or older. Cancer 2012;118(22):5595–600.

20. Wick A, Kessler T, Platten M, et al. Superiority of temozolomide over radiotherapy for elderly patients with RTK II Methylation Class, MGMT promoter-methylated malignant astrocytoma. Neuro Oncol 2020. https://doi.org/10.1093/neuonc/noaa033.

21. Laigle-Donadey F, Greffard S. Management of glioblastomas in the elderly population. Rev Neurol (Paris) 2020;1–9. https://doi.org/10.1016/j.neurol.2020.01.362.

22. Fried Linda P, Tangen Catherine M, Jeremy W, et al. Frailty in older adults: evidence for a phenotype. J Gerontol A Biol Sci Med Sci 2001;56(3): M146–57.

23. Lin HS, Watts JN, Peel NM, et al. Frailty and postoperative outcomes in older surgical patients: a systematic review. BMC Geriatr 2016. https://doi.org/10.1186/s12877-016-0329-8.

24. Rockwood K, Song X, Chris M, et al. A global clinical measure of fitness and frailty in elderly people. CMAJ 2005;173(5):489–95.

25. Pallis AG, Ring A, Fortpied C, et al. EORTC workshop on clinical trial methodology in older individuals with a diagnosis of solid tumors. Ann Oncol 2011;22(8):1922–6.

26. Soubeyran P, Bellera C, Goyard J, et al. Screening for vulnerability in older cancer patients: the ONCODAGE prospective multicenter cohort study. PLoS One 2014;9(12):e115060.

27. Di Cristofori A, Zarino B, Claudia F, et al. Analysis of factors influencing the access to concomitant chemo-radiotherapy in elderly patients with high grade gliomas: role of MMSE, age and tumor volume. J Neurooncol 2017;134(2):377–85.

28. Lawton MP, Brody Elaine M. Assessment of older people: self-maintaining and instrumental activities of daily Living 1. n.d. Gerontologist. Autumn 1969; 9(3):179-86.

29. Nader S, Polley MY, McDermott MW, et al. An extent of resection threshold for newly diagnosed glioblastomas: clinical article. J Neurosurg 2011;115(1): 3–8.

30. Molinaro AM, Hervey-Jumper S, Morshed Ramin A, et al. Association of maximal extent of resection of contrast-enhanced and non-contrast-enhanced tumor with survival within molecular subgroups of patients with newly diagnosed glioblastoma. JAMA Oncol 2020;6(4):495–503.

31. Schär Ralph T, Shpend T, Mattia B, et al. How safe are elective craniotomies in elderly patients in neurosurgery today? A prospective cohort study of 1452 consecutive cases. J Neurosurg 2020; 1(aop):1–9.

32. Vuorinen V, Hinkka S, Färkkilä M, et al. Debulking or biopsy of malignant glioma in elderly people - a randomised study. Acta Neurochir (Wien) 2003; 145(1):5–10.

33. Chaichana KL, Garzon-Muvdi T, Parker S, et al. Supratentorial glioblastoma multiforme: the role of surgical resection versus biopsy among older patients. Ann Surg Oncol 2011;18(1):239–45.

34. Christian E, Mathias G, Marion R, et al. Glioblastoma multiforme of the elderly: the prognostic effect of resection on survival. J Neurooncol 2011;103(3): 611–8.

35. Almenawer SA, Badhiwala JH, Waleed A, et al. Biopsy versus partial versus gross total resection in older patients with high-grade glioma: a systematic review and meta-analysis. Neuro Oncol 2015;17(6): 868–81.

36. Abdullah KG, Ramayya A, Thawani JP, et al. Factors associated with increased survival after surgical resection of glioblastoma in octogenarians. PLoS One 2015;10(5):127202.

37. Ranjith B, Komisarow Jordan M, Agarwal Vijay J, et al. Glioblastoma in the elderly: the effect of aggressive and modern therapies on survival. J Neurosurg 2016;998–1007. https://doi.org/10.3171/2015.4.JNS142200.

38. Arvold Nils D, Matthew C, Wang Y, et al. Comparative effectiveness of radiotherapy with vs. without temozolomide in older patients with glioblastoma. J Neurooncol 2017;131(2):301–11.

39. Abraham N, Tang JA, Marcus Logan P, et al. Gross-total resection outcomes in an elderly population with glioblastoma: a SEER-based analysis. Clinical article. J Neurosurg 2014; 120(1):31–9.

50. Pessina F, Navarria P, Luca C, et al. Is surgical resection useful in elderly newly diagnosed glioblastoma patients? Outcome evaluation and prognostic factors assessment. Acta Neurochir (Wien) 2018; 160(9):1779–87.

51. Oszvald Á, Güresir E, Matthias S, et al. Glioblastoma therapy in the elderly and the importance of the extent of resection regardless of age: clinical article. J Neurosurg 2012;116(2):357–64.

52. Walter S, Pichlmeier U, Meinel T, et al. Fluorescence-guided surgery with 5-aminolevulinic acid for resection of malignant glioma: a randomised controlled multicentre phase III trial. Lancet Oncol 2006;7(5): 392–401.

53. Walter S, Hanns Jürgen R, Meinel T, et al. Extent of resection and survival in glioblastoma multiforme: identification of and adjustment for bias. Neurosurgery 2008;62(3):564–74.

54. Walter S, Christian TJ, Maximilian MH, et al. Counterbalancing risks and gains from extended resections in malignant glioma surgery: a supplemental analysis from the randomized 5-aminolevulinic acid glioma resection study: clinical article. J Neurosurg 2011;114(3):613–23.

55. Laws Edward R, Parney Ian F, Huang Wei, et al. Survival following surgery and prognostic factors for recently diagnosed malignant glioma: data from the glioma outcomes project. J Neurosurg 2003; 99(3):467–73.

56. Bauchet L, Mathieu-Daudé H, Pascale F-P, et al. Oncological patterns of care and outcome for 952 patients with newly diagnosed glioblastoma in 2004. Neuro Oncol 2010;12(7):725–35.

57. Sciortino T, Fernandes B, Marco CN, et al. Frameless stereotactic biopsy for precision neurosurgery: diagnostic value, safety, and accuracy. Acta Neurochir (Wien) 2019;161(5). https://doi.org/10.1007/s00701-019-03873-w.

58. Weller M, van den Bent M, Hopkins K, et al. EANO guideline for the diagnosis and treatment of anaplastic gliomas and glioblastoma. Lancet Oncol 2014;15(9):395–403.

59. Reardon David A, Brandes Alba A, Omuro A, et al. Effect of nivolumab vs bevacizumab in patients with recurrent glioblastoma: the checkmate 143 phase 3 randomized clinical trial. JAMA Oncol 2020. https://doi.org/10.1001/jamaoncol.2020.1024.

60. Keime-Guibert F, Olivier C, Taillandier L, et al. Radiotherapy for Glioblastoma in the Elderly. N Engl J Med 2007;356(15):1527–35.

61. Wilson R, Brasher PMA, Bauman G, et al. Abbreviated course of radiation therapy in older patients with glioblastoma multiforme: a prospective randomized clinical trial. J Clin Oncol 2004;22(9): 1583–8.

62. Perry JR, Laperriere N, O'Callaghan Christopher J, et al. Short-course radiation plus temozolomide in elderly patients with glioblastoma. N Engl J Med 2017;376(11):1027–37.

53. Perry JR, Laperriere N, O'Callaghan Christopher J, et al. A phase III randomized controlled trial of short-course radiotherapy with or without concomitant and adjuvant temozolomide in elderly patients with glioblastoma (CCTG CE.6, EORTC 26062-22061, TROG 08.02, NCT00482677). J Clin Oncol 2016;34(18_suppl):LBA2.

54. Pérez-Larraya JG, François D, Olivier C, et al. Temozolomide in elderly patients with newly diagnosed glioblastoma and poor performance status: an ANOCEF phase II trial. J Clin Oncol 2011; 29(22):3050–5.

55. Socha J, Kepka L, Ghosh S, et al. Outcome of treatment of recurrent glioblastoma multiforme in elderly and/or frail patients. J Neurooncol 2016;126(3): 493–8.

56. Giuseppe L, Bellu L, Pambuku A, et al. Clinical outcome of an alternative fotemustine schedule in elderly patients with recurrent glioblastoma: a mono-institutional retrospective study. J Neurooncol 2016;128(3):481–6.

57. Fariña Nuñez MT, Franco P, Debora C, et al. Resection of recurrent glioblastoma multiforme in elderly patients: a pseudo-randomized analysis revealed clinical benefit. J Neurooncol 2020; 146(2):381–7.

58. Hager J, Herrmann E, Kammerer S, et al. Impact of resection on overall survival of recurrent Glioblastoma in elderly patients. Clin Neurol Neurosurg 2018;174(July):21–5.

59. Christoph S, Antoni S, Gempt J, et al. Re-irradiation in elderly patients with glioblastoma: a single institution experience. J Neurooncol 2019;142(2): 327–35.

60. Simon K, Grant R. Antiepileptic drugs for treating seizures in adults with brain tumours. Cochrane Database Syst Rev 2011;8. https://doi.org/10.1002/14651858.cd008586.pub2.

61. Tremont-Lukats Ivo, Ratilal BO, Armstrong T, et al. Antiepileptic drugs for preventing seizures in people with brain tumors. Cochrane Database Syst Rev 2008. https://doi.org/10.1002/14651858.CD004424.pub2.

62. Anna R, Luciano B, Roberto S, et al. Efficacy and safety of levetiracetam in patients with glioma: a clinical prospective study. Arch Neurol 2010;67(3):343–6.

63. Perry James R. Thromboembolic disease in patients with high-grade glioma. Neuro Oncol 2012;14(Suppl 4):iv73–80.

64. Perry JR, Julian JA, Laperriere NJ, et al. PRODIGE: a randomized placebo-controlled trial of dalteparin low-molecular-weight heparin thromboprophylaxis in patients with newly diagnosed malignant glioma. J Thromb Haemost 2010;8(9): 1959–65.

65. Brandes AA, Scelzi E, Salmistraro G, et al. Incidence and risk of thromboembolism during treatment of high-grade gliomas: a prospective study. Eur J Cancer 1997;33(10):1592–6.

66. Shahzaib N, Pushpinderdeep K, Bozorgnia F, et al. Predictors of venous thromboembolism in patients with glioblastoma multiforme. J Clin Oncol 2015; 33(15_suppl):e13022.

67. Wick W, Gorlia T, Martin B, et al. Lomustine and bevacizumab in progressive glioblastoma. N Engl J Med 2017;377(20):1954–63.

68. Walter T, Oosterkamp Hendrika M, Walenkamp Annemiek ME, et al. Single-agent bevacizumab or lomustine versus a combination of bevacizumab plus lomustine in patients with recurrent glioblastoma (BELOB trial): a randomised controlled phase 2 trial. Lancet Oncol 2014;15(9):943–53.

69. Chinot Olivier L, Wick W, Mason W, et al. Bevacizumab plus Radiotherapy–Temozolomide for Newly Diagnosed Glioblastoma. N Engl J Med 2014; 370(8):709–22.

70. Stupp R, Taillibert S, Kanner A, et al. Effect of tumor-treating fields plus maintenance temozolomide vs maintenance temozolomide alone on survival in patients with glioblastoma a randomized clinical trial. JAMA 2017;318(23):2306–16.

71. Kleinschmidt-DeMasters BK, Lillehei KO, Varella-Garcia M. Glioblastomas in the Older Old. Arch Pathol Lab Med 2005;129(5). https://doi.org/10. 1043/1543-2165(2005)129<0624:GITOO>2.0.CO;2.

72. Combs Stephanie E, Wagner J, Marc B, et al. Post-operative treatment of primary glioblastoma multiforme with radiation and concomitant temozolomide in elderly patients. Int J Radiat Oncol Biol Phys 2008;70(4):987–92.

73. Sijben Angelique E, McIntyre John B, Roldán Gloria B, et al. Toxicity from chemoradiotherapy in older patients with glioblastoma multiforme. J Neurooncol 2008;89(1):97–103.

74. Gerstein J, Franz K, Steinbach Joachim P, et al. Postoperative radiotherapy and concomitant temozolomide for elderly patients with glioblastoma. Radiother Oncol 2010;97(3):382–6.

75. Kimple Randall J, Grabowski S, Papez M, et al. Concurrent temozolomide and radiation, a reasonable option for elderly patients with glioblastoma multiforme? Am J Clin Oncol Cancer Clin Trials 2010; 33(3):265–70.

76. Lai R, Hershman Dawn L, Doan T, et al. The timing of cranial radiation in elderly patients with newly diagnosed glioblastoma multiforme. Neuro Oncol 2010; 12(2):190–8.

77. Laigle-Donadey F, Figarella-Branger D, Olivier C, et al. Up-front temozolomide in elderly patients with glioblastoma. J Neurooncol 2010;99(1):89–94.

78. Kushnir I, Tzuk-Shina T. Efficacy of treatment for glioblastoma multiforme in elderly patients (65+): a retrospective analysis. IMAJ 2011;13(5):290–4.

79. Hashem Sameh A, Ahmed S, Al-Rashdan A, et al. Radiotherapy with concurrent or sequential temozolomide in elderly patients with glioblastoma multiforme. J Med Imaging Radiat Oncol 2012;56(2): 204–10.

80. Tanaka S, Meyer Fredric B, Buckner Jan C, et al. Presentation, management, and outcome of newly diagnosed glioblastoma in elderly patients. J Neurosurg 2013;118(4):786–98.

81. Fariselli L, Pinzi V, Milanesi I, et al. Short-course radiotherapy in elderly patients with glioblastoma: Feasibility and efficacy of results from a single centre. Strahlentherapie Und Onkol 2013;189(6): 456–61.

82. Lee JH, Jung TY, Jung S, et al. Performance status during and after radiotherapy plus concomitant and adjuvant temozolomide in elderly patients with glioblastoma multiforme. J Clin Neurosci 2013; 20(4):503–8.

83. Hoffermann M, Ali Kariem M, et al. Treatment results and outcome in elderly patients with glioblastoma multiforme - A retrospective single institution analysis. Clin Neurol Neurosurg 2015;128:60–9.

84. Lombardi G, Pace A, Francesco P, et al. Predictors of survival and effect of short (40 Gy) or standard-course (60 Gy) irradiation plus concomitant temozolomide in elderly patients with glioblastoma: a multicenter retrospective study of AINO (Italian Association of Neuro-Oncology). J Neurooncol 2015;125(2):359–67.

85. Welzel G, Gehweiler J, Brehmer S, et al. Metronomic chemotherapy with daily low-dose temozolomide and celecoxib in elderly patients with newly diagnosed glioblastoma multiforme: a retrospective analysis. J Neurooncol 2015;124(2):265–73.

86. Karsy M, Yoon N, Boettcher L, et al. Surgical treatment of glioblastoma in the elderly: the impact of complications. J Neurooncol 2018;138(1):123–32.

Moving?

Make sure your subscription moves with you!

To notify us of your new address, find your **Clinics Account Number** (located on your mailing label above your name), and contact customer service at:

Email: journalscustomerservice-usa@elsevier.com

800-654-2452 (subscribers in the U.S. & Canada)
314-447-8871 (subscribers outside of the U.S. & Canada)

Fax number: 314-447-8029

Elsevier Health Sciences Division
Subscription Customer Service
3251 Riverport Lane
Maryland Heights, MO 63043

*To ensure uninterrupted delivery of your subscription, please notify us at least 4 weeks in advance of move.

ELSEVIER

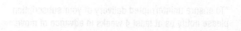